PORTALS OF POWER

PORTALS OF POWER

SHAMANISM IN SOUTH AMERICA

Edited by

E. JEAN MATTESON LANGDON
and GERHARD BAER

UNIVERSITY OF NEW MEXICO PRESS
Albuquerque

A variation of chapter 5 was published in *Anthropos* 82 (1987): 567–580, under the title "Shamanistic Symptoms and Symbols."

Chapter 9, originally titled "Personne n'est là pour écouter," was published in French in *Amerindia,* no. 12 (1987).

A slightly different version of chapter 11 appeared in *Ethnohistory* vol. 33, no. 1 (Winter 1986).

Library of Congress Cataloging-in-Publication Data

Portals of power: Shamanism in South America/edited by E. Jean Matteson Langdon and Gerhard Baer.—1st. ed.
p. cm.
Includes bibliographical references and index.
ISBN 0–8263–1345–0
1. Indians of South America—Religion and mythology.
2. Indians of South America—Rites and ceremonies.
3. Shamanism—South America.
4. Folk medicine—South America.
5. Hallucinogenic drugs and religious experience.
I. Langdon, E. Jean Matteson, 1944-
II. Baer, Gerhard, 1934-
F2320.1.R3P67 1992
299′.8—dc2091–42609
CIP

Design by Stephanie Jurs

First edition.

C O N T E N T S

PORTALS OF POWER

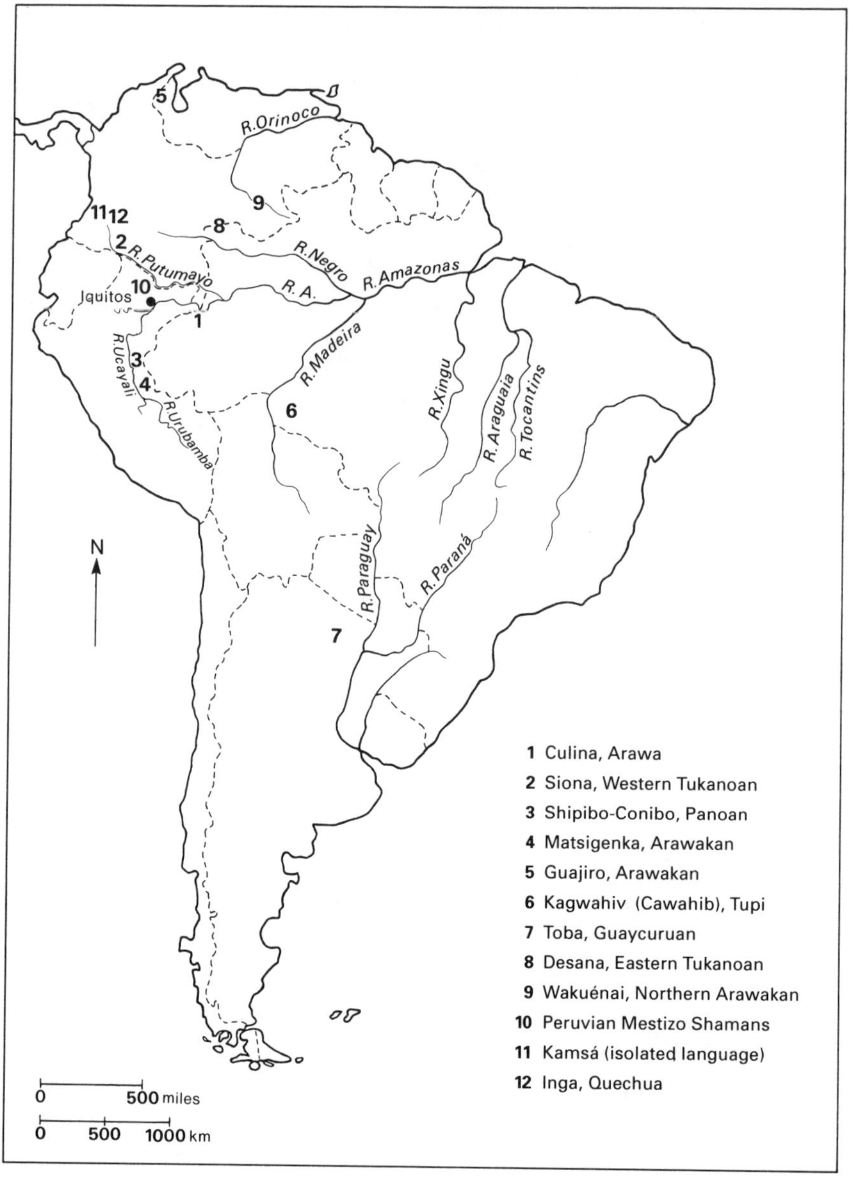

R. Orinoco
R. Negro
R. Amazonas
R. Putumayo
R. A.
Iquitos
R. Ucayali
R. Urubamba
R. Madeira
R. Xingu
R. Araguaia
R. Tocantins
R. Paraguay
R. Paraná
N
0 500 miles
0 500 1000 km
1 Culina, Arawa
2 Siona, Western Tukanoan
3 Shipibo-Conibo, Panoan
4 Matsigenka, Arawakan
5 Guajiro, Arawakan
6 Kagwahiv (Cawahib), Tupi
7 Toba, Guaycuruan
8 Desana, Eastern Tukanoan
9 Wakuénai, Northern Arawakan
10 Peruvian Mestizo Shamans
11 Kamsá (isolated language)
12 Inga, Quechua

FIGURE 1.1. Geographic location of groups presented in this volume.

INTRODUCTION
Shamanism and Anthropology

E. JEAN MATTESON LANGDON

Shamanism has always presented a challenge to anthropology. Since the early ethnographic reports, shamans and their practices have fascinated Western civilization. Characterized by hysteria, ecstasy, magic, and transvestism, shamanism is alien to the rational positivistic worldview of science. Anthropology, dominated by the positivistic sciences, has failed until recently to understand shamanism as an important dynamic force in today's world, or to develop adequate analytical models for comprehending it. However, the events of the last three decades have forced us to recognize its importance and to look for new models and fresh perspectives on the topic.

From the beat generation in the 1950s (Huxley 1954), to the current popularity of oriental religions and parapsychology, shamanism has held a heightened status in both intellectual and popular cultures. The beats were followed by the hippies and the use of hallucinogens, common to shamanic systems, diffused throughout the middle classes in Europe and the United States. Timothy Leary's challenge to "turn on, tune in, and drop out" promised a new vision for those disillusioned with consumerism and a positivist worldview. Carlos Castaneda's books about his journeys with Don Juan began to be published in 1968, rocking the imagination of those looking for a new vision and further challenging assumptions about the nature of reality and perception (Zolla 1983). Interest in right and left brain capacities became popular topics, posing intuitive thinking against the logical as a legitimate way of knowing and experiencing the world (Grof 1985). More recently, popular books and workshops on the shamanic state of consciousness have been in vogue (Doore 1988; Harner 1982). All of this has been aided by native Americans, such as Jamake Highwater (1982), who have chosen to speak directly about their worldview. Finally, in many Third World countries, popular culture has incorporated both shamans and their practices (Henman 1986; Ramírez de Jara and Pinzón 1986; Taussig 1987).

The stimulus of these trends upon new research in psychotropic plant substances, as well as a revival of shamanism as a focus of research, was first noted by Weston La Barre (1969, xi) in the republication of his 1938 doctoral dissertation *The Peyote Cult.* Since then the number of research projects and publications has continued to multiply.[1] Anthropologists, historians, botanists, chemists, and others have joined forces to produce serious studies of the widespread and complex phenomenon known as shamanism (see for example *América Indígena* 1986).

This book aims to provide new insights by presenting the cultural and social context of shamanism in South America. Our focus is on the traditional forms of shamanism, and on the development of these traditions as native South Americans meet with European society. The articles represent trends in research conducted since the 1960s, and they cover diverse issues. It is our belief that this diversity provides new clues for the understanding of shamanism from the "emic" (that is, the native) and sociological points of view. Shamanism has been a central force in native cultures, permeating all aspects of native life. Moreover, the institution of shamanism has been important in the interethnic contacts of the twentieth century and has played a role in the processes of ethnic identity and interethnic contacts (Langdon 1985, 1991; Taussig 1980a, 1987). Thus, the articles in this book represent not only a gathering of new ethnographic data, but also discuss the most recent trends in which shamanism is being studied.

Before highlighting the contributions of this book, it will be helpful to review the history of shamanism within anthropology. One reason for the lack of an adequate theory of shamanism has been the concentration upon the exotic nature of shamans and the problem of "primitive mentality" that has permeated the study of shamanic practices classified as magical rites. These concerns have led to three areas of debate. First, the problem of the definition of a shaman; second, a concern with the psychic experience of the shaman; and third, the problem of the definition of shamanism as religion or magic.

Although these issues have dominated the analysis of shamanism until recently, they have fragmented the understanding of shamanism as a pervasive and encompassing phenomenon which persists, although modified, in the face of the rapid changes occurring throughout this century.

THE DEFINITION OF SHAMAN

The first extended reports of shamanism appeared in the nineteenth century and the first years of the twentieth. These were written primarily by explorers, natural historians, or travelers among the Siberian and Arctic shamans (Bogoraz 1904; Jochelson 1905; Olhmarks 1939; Rasmussen 1929; Shirokogoroff 1923). The term shaman comes from the Tungusic word used to describe the ritual specialists whose activities are marked by ecstasy, ritual flight, death, rebirth, journeys to the underworld and heavens, alliances with animals, curing, and other magical feats (Eliade 1964, 495). Similar characteristics of ecstatic practitioners were reported throughout the world. The term shaman became interchangeable with other terms, such as "medicine man," "sorcerer," and "magician," to designate such practitioners in entirely different cultural complexes in different geographical areas (Eliade 1964, 3; Hoppál 1987, 93; Viertler 1981).

Eliade's classic work (1964), first published in 1951, was the first attempt at unifying the various ethnographic sources to construct a more precise definition that would permit a historical study of shamanism and the exploration of its essential ideological features. Central to his definition is the technique of ecstasy, in which the soul is believed to leave the body and ascend to the sky or descend to the underworld. The shamanic trance involves a relationship between spirits and the shaman who attempts to control them for a specific purpose. This is distinguished from possession trance in which the individual is controlled by the spirit. Other essential elements include training that is both ecstatic (dreams, trance, etc.) and traditional (techniques, identification of spirits, geneology, secret language, etc.). The aim of training is to accumulate mystical power for social and personal use. A shamanic calling is marked by the onset of a psychotic crisis or an illness. Initiation involves mystical death and resurrection, indicating a change of personality. Finally, the shaman is the specialist in the human soul, standing apart from the rest of the community by his possession of mystical powers.

Eliade is preoccupied with locating the origin of shamanism and its purest form in order to examine parallels throughout the world. Strictly speaking, true shamanism is found in Siberia and Central Asia, where the shaman is central to religious practices. It is also found in its nearly pure form in native cultures of the New World. Yet Eliade (1964, 322) discards as true shamanism such examples as the ghost dance of the North American Indians, since it lacks initiation and a secret traditional teaching. Instead, he considers it a parallel phenomenon separate from shamanism while preserving essential ideology and techniques. Other parallels are found in Indonesia, Oceania, Australia, the rest of Asia, and in ancient Indo-European cultures.

Others have also utilized this approach and have focused on the distribution of shamanic systems with a concern to define essential features or to identify the more pure and archaic forms (Baer 1982; Métraux 1944, 1967; Motzki 1977; Vajda 1959). The difference between soul flight and possession has been important in determining whether the practitioners are shamans, thus eliminating most of the cultures of Africa and religions of African influence.

Although Eliade's work must be recognized as the first important attempt to treat shamanism comparatively, his efforts, and those of others, have concentrated too much on the shaman as an individual and on the presence of archaic elements, rather than viewing shamanism as a globalizing and dynamic social and cultural phenomenon (Chaumeil 1983), which is the perspective of this book. We have centered on one geographical area in which the complex presents general features due primarily to the sharing of a general cultural tradition. Our intent is not to define shamanism as limited to specific individuals, nor to argue essential features, but to understand its various forms and expressions as a dynamic cultural-social complex in various societies over time and space.

Since Eliade's work, there have been attempts to understand trance from the purely social perspective (Crapanzano and Garrison 1980; Douglas 1973; Lewis 1971). Lewis's work on ecstatic religions was the first attempt at formulating a theory of ecstatic states not based on psychological explanations. He examines possession states in general, rather than those limited only to shamanism. Based on Eliade, Lewis distinguishes shamanic possession from other states as being primarily controlled voluntary soul flight, as contrasted with nonvoluntary uncontrolled possession. He correlates the sociological determinants of these two forms as they occur in peripheral cults and in central possession religions, such as shamanism. He does not propose to study the cultural forms of possession.

Douglas, on the other hand, follows a tradition closer to Durkheim and attempts to demonstrate how ideological systems emerge from social structure. One important aspect of her work is the elimination of the separation between magical techniques in primitive societies and the sacraments of institutionalized religions in complex societies. However, by categorizing and generalizing ideological systems as derived from social structure, and viewing the function of ritual in primitive societies as being primarily one of social control, the full importance of shamanic systems in native tradition is ignored, as are the creative and expressive aspects. Likewise, we do not agree with Lewis (1971, 13) that cultural distinctions are often of much less consequence than functional similarities. Full appreciation and comprehension of shamanism can only be achieved through examining both aspects. The study of the shamanic tradition as an expressive system and as a social system continues to lack an explanatory paradigm.

THE PSYCHIC EXPERIENCE

Although Eliade clearly rejects the mystical experience as one of a neurotic or psychotic, there has been a long-standing debate in anthropology as to the psychic stability of shamans. Various scholars have argued that shamans have universally psychotic personalities, citing the characteristics of hysteria, trance, and transvestism as symptoms of psychoses (Devereaux 1970; Nadel 1946; Silverman 1967; Wallace 1966, 145–63). They also draw upon the "psychotic episode" that marks the initial calling and training of shamans in various cultures. Others, particularly those influenced by the culture and personality school, have argued the reverse, that shamanic personalities are molded by their cultures and present features distinct from psychotics in that they control their periods of hysteria and trance while psychotics do not (Kennedy 1973; Noll 1983; Schweder 1979). They often conclude that shamans are, in fact, more stable and more imaginative, having a capacity to interpret the events of daily life more adequately than the other members of the culture. Neither side of the debate, however, ignores the importance of culture in defining what is abnormal, nor do they ignore the fact that shamans maintain a positive role that is culturally constructed and without stigma.

We believe that a final answer to the shaman's stability cannot be given for all cultures or shamans in general. Perrin, in this volume, provides the most satisfactory answer. It is necessary to look at collective representations rather than at external behavior to understand normality and marginality. These collective representations, which form a single, logical pattern of general ideas, exist before the individual shamanic calling. As will be seen in the articles here, the shamanic calling through illness occurs in some South American cultures, such as the Guajiro of Venezuela and the Toba of Argentina, however it is not a necessary criterion. The control of trance is the defining characteristic in all cases. Transvestism is also uncommon, although it was present among the Mapuche of the last century. Sexuality, ambivalence between the sexes, and androgenous characteristics of shamanic ideology and ritual is a more fruitful approach for analysis than is the question of transvestism (d'Anglure 1986; see Baer, Landgon, Perrin and Pollock in this volume).

Shamanic Séances as Therapy

Investigations as to the efficacy of shamanic curing séances has had productive results with respect to practical issues regarding therapy and curing (Devereux 1958; Doore 1988; Jilek 1978; Kiev 1962, 1964, 1968; La Barre 1947; Murphy 1964; Pfister 1932; Torrey 1972; Wallace 1958). These investigations have stressed the techniques common in psychotherapy and shamanic curing, such as confession, group therapy, shock therapy, psychodrama, and so forth. Since ethnic and minority groups have concepts regarding sickness, treatment, and patient-practitioner relations that diverge from the dominant medical system, there has also been an interest in integrating shamans and other curers in health services for ethnic groups (Kleinman 1980; Luce 1971).

Ecstasy as Therapy

Concentration on ecstasy as therapy has led to new developments stimulated by research on the psychology of trance and the implications of its effectiveness for altering behavior and erasing past habits (Prince 1982; Sargant 1973; Winkelman 1986). These researchers define the key elements of a shaman as a person who "(1) can access alternate states of consciousness at will; (2) fulfills needs of their community which otherwise are not met; and (3) mediates between the sacred and the profane" (Heinze 1987, 3). Many western therapists identify themselves, as well as others exhibiting these characteristics in therapeutic practices, as shamans (see in particular the Proceedings of the Third and Fourth International Conferences on the Study of Shamanism and Alternate Modes of Healing [Heinze 1987, 1988]). Such works doubtlessly have great practical importance for issues regarding the psychobiological levels of healing, although many anthropologists argue that the utilization of shamanic techniques in cultures without the social and cultural basis of shamanism does not qualify such modern practitioners as true shamans.

THE PROBLEM OF MAGIC AND RELIGION

The problem of the definition of shamanism as religion or as magic has plagued the study of shamanism since the first evolutionary theories in anthropology. Shamanism was fragmented by separating belief systems from ritual. As an ideological system, it was considered to be an example of animism since shamanic ideology includes the belief in souls of inanimate objects, animate beasts, and humans (Tylor 1871). Within the scheme of cultural evolution, animism represents an archaic survival of primitive religion and mentality of the "lower cultures," and thus is destined to be replaced by higher forms. Tylor attributed the origin of the idea of souls to primitive speculations about beings seen in dreams and the problem of explaining death. Marrett (1900, 15) placed the origins of religion in the primitives' awe and fear of nature. Schmidt (1931) viewed primitive religion as a degeneration from a higher form of primeval monotheism. In all cases, these views represented a negative concept of a primitive whose fears blocked the functioning of his mind (Douglas 1966, 12).

Shamanic practices and rituals were treated as analytically separate from ideology and were classified as magic. Frazer in his 1890 publication was the first to deal with magic systematically (see Frazer 1980). He distinguished magic from religion because magic is directed at altering events rather than toward worship. He called magic a pseudoscience in which the primitive not only has a logic but also a faulty perception of reality. This logic, based on the laws of sympathy, leads him to perform technical acts that have the goal of altering the world but, in reality, are inefficacious, since acts based on such laws cannot affect anything. Guided by his logic, he fails to see that magic does not work. Eventually, with the evolution of human mentality, true science would replace magic.

Although the unilineal theory of evolution was rejected for its ethnocentrism and lack of evidence about the general stages of cultural progress, concern with universal definitions of religion and magic have continued to exercise a negative influence on the study of shamanism. Shamanism became linked with the biased concepts of primitive mentality and magic.

Durkheim's classic 1912 work on religion incorporated the importance of ritual for religion, but continued to distinguish it from magic (see Durkheim 1965). Magic belongs to the private realm and therefore is not part of religion, which is collective. Drawing from this, Mauss (1974) constructed his theory of magic with the intention of extending beyond Frazer. Magic, as a private act, does not create an ideal for society and tends to "evil" and to individual goals. Although it is secret, it is a fact of tradition transmitted and believed in by the group. Its efficacy is based on a priori belief and therefore continues to be practiced. Of course, the practice of magic, thus defined, cannot result in cohesion, a function of religious ritual.

Like Frazer, Mauss saw magic as dominating the most primitive levels of culture and as becoming less common and complex in civilized cultures. This is the reverse of religion, which, according to Durkheim, is more simple among primitives and more complex among the civilized. In addition to the magical acts discussed by Frazer, Mauss examined the magician and symbolic representations, including conceptions about the power of magical instruments and beliefs in personal forces in the universe that intervene in events.

His discussion of magical agents summarized a great number of ethnographic resources. For Mauss, the magician represents a social category in that he is usually different from others physically. He experiences ecstasy, which links him to the supernatural world; he owns magical power; he is defined by his relation with animals and spirits; and he must pass through an initiation rite involving mystical death and personality change. These characteristics follow closely those of shamans, but for Mauss (1974, 65), the term magician is more inclusive and the shaman is classified as a kind of magician.

The articles herein clearly demonstrate that the shaman's work is not secret, nor primarily for private ends, and that his leadership of public ritual is essential to religious life. It is Mauss's discussion of representations that is perhaps his most important contribution for a model of shamanism. Mauss focused upon notions of power, indicating that the concept of power as it operates in magic is a collective explanation of existence. As will be seen, power is central to the representational systems of South American shamanism. It is not, however, a "magical" conception of power, but rather concerns general conceptions of power in a worldview that unifies what the early anthropologists wanted to divide—religion and magic.

A slightly different resolution on the relationship between religion and magic was presented by van Gennep (1903). In his article on shamanism he stated that it is not a religion, but that rather the role of shaman is a social position of a magical practitioner in societies where the religion is animism. Later, without reference to shamans but with respect to animistic and dynamistic religions, he identified the rites of such religions as magic and adopted Marrett's term "magico-religious" to speak of such systems (van Gennep 1909, 33). This term has been commonly adopted to refer to primitive religious systems, including shamanism. However, it tends to preserve the problem of the distinction between magic and religion rather than to indicate its solution (van Ball and van Beek 1985, 76).

The early English anthropologists continued to divide religion and magic. Malinowski, although not working directly with shamanism, stated that magic exists to alleviate anxiety in cases where the outcome of an event is unknown. He did not agree with Frazer that magic is a pseudoscience, but saw it dying out as man's control over events increases. Those following the functionalism of Radcliffe-Brown have been preoccupied with the social functions of magical practices, such as social control and mediation of conflict. Whiting's (1950) work on Paiute sorcery represents such an approach to the study of North American shamanism.

Métraux (1941, 1944), who worked extensively on South American shamanism, reflects the confusion of the concepts. He called shamanism magico-religious and considered it more primitive than organized religions. However, he recognized that, outside the Andean area, religious life is centered on the shaman as mediator for the individual and the community with the supernatural world, and that the shaman has an important social role in influencing community plans and economic activities, and in maintaining tribal tradition and moral code. However, Métraux (1941, 588) denied the shaman a "primarily religious role" because, in his view, the shaman's efficacy is derived from his "magical" powers, which give him control over spirits, and also because his functions are primarily prophylactic or remedial and performed on behalf of individuals. The activities of applying magical techniques to ensure good luck, avert danger, cure or inflict diseases, and so forth, are less important than "more significant religious or social phenomena" (Métraux 1941, 580). However, since the shaman acts on the behalf of the community, and organizes and leads group ceremonies, Métraux concluded that there is no clear distinction between the shaman and the priest, and that there is a historical development from shaman (who acts in tribal societies through direct contact with spirits) to priest (who acts in state societies conducting routine propitiatory acts of adoration not marked by ecstasy and frenzy) (Métraux 1941, 586). As late as 1973, this evolutionary model of religion-as-adoration versus magic-as-instrumental, identifying the shaman as magician and mystical, and the priest as routine and socially legitimized, appears in the treatment of South American shamans (Weiss 1973). Hoppál's (1987, 93) review of shamanism in Russian anthropology demonstrates that this view has also been popular among studies of Siberian shamans.

These preoccupations with universal definitions of magic and religion, and the failure to recognize shamanism as a central expression of the worldview of a culture, as well as an institution with important sociological functions, did not lead to a productive understanding or to adequate models of shamanism. Moreover, the category of magic is a false category in the description of shamanic systems. As an analytic concept, it obscures any objective study in native practices and belief systems. Part of this is due to Western conceptions of magic, magicians, and witches, all terms that have been linked with shamanism. We treat magic as if it does not work. It is a separate isolated phenomenon. Magicians are tricksters, and witches are people who harm others. Implicit in the category of magic as developed in early anthropology is that it can be isolated as a separate trait in other cultures, that it is a valid cross-cultural category. In investigating shamanic techniques as magic and the shaman as magician, we have made the understanding of shamanism impossible, and we remain incredulous to its seriousness and persistence.

SYMBOLIC ANTHROPOLOGY AND SHAMANISM

During the same period of renewed interest in shamanism, a new interest in symbolic anthropology developed, and it has been the symbolic perspective that has offered the most satisfactory resolution to the study of shamanism.

Symbolic anthropology is concerned with symbolic representations in ideological systems and rituals as well as their relationship to society and human motivation (Dolgin et al. 1977; Geertz 1966; V. Turner 1966, 1967b, 1974, 1977). Magic and questions about health, so common in shamanic systems, are linked with the preoccupations of religion in expressing and explaining the order of the universe (Douglas 1966). Using Geertz's definition of religion, South American shamanism is a religious system. It contains ideas and practices about the world and its reproduction, the worldview and reflection of the world. As mentioned earlier, the work of Mary Douglas has demonstrated that magic is not a distinct phenomenon from religious sacraments in complex societies. Thus, the anthropologist no longer focuses on whether beliefs are magical or religious, but rather on the symbolic systems which organize the worldview and society of a culture (Baer 1984; Chaumeil 1983; Crocker 1985; Sullivan 1988).

Ritual is an important and necessary expression of a belief system. Considerations of its efficacy have moved from the positivistic problem of whether it "really works," to a consideration of the symbolic and expressive experience linked with human motivations and needs to understand the world. Ritual works because it expresses (Lévi-Strauss

1958). Its efficacy lies in its power as metaphor to express and alter the human experience by altering perception. This may, in turn, have observable social or physiological effects, but they are not the only proof of the efficacy of shamanic rituals (Munn 1973; V. Turner 1967a).

Within symbolic analysis, the shaman is central in ritual expression since he is the master of the ritual and its representations. His authority to conduct ritual comes from his position as mediator between various domains, the human and superhuman, the natural and the cultural. He is an ambiguous or liminal figure (Douglas 1966; Leach 1976). He is both animal and human, since he transforms into animals. He is neither inherently good nor evil, because he works for the benefit, as well as for the misfortune, of others. His power derives in part from his ambiguity, since he does not fit into the mutually exclusive categories that organize the world.

CONTRIBUTIONS OF THIS BOOK

The articles presented here are the result of papers and discussions from four international symposia on shamanism held from 1982 to 1985. The first, in Manchester, England, was organized by Joanna Overing Kaplan (1984), who called on the participants to view shamanism as a complex, rather than to focus on the shaman as an individual or on his particular magical feats. This perspective was maintained throughout the subsequent symposia and in the selections in this book. All of the contributors have been influenced by the symbolic perspective and are committed to the native view for understanding the phenomenon of shamanism. Such a perspective requires symbolic analysis, native interpretation of events and rituals, and the logic of belief systems within their cultural context.

Concomitantly, the articles also demonstrate the social aspects of shamanism. As a globalizing phenomenon shamanism "also functions on the sociological level as a true institution" which must be studied in its double dimension: religious and social (Chaumeil 1983, 21). One advantage of this volume is that, while paying attention to particular case studies, the selections also allow a comparative view of shamanism as a sociological institution throughout time and space. Eleven cultures are represented in our collection, coming from various culture areas in South America, as well as from different language families and states of acculturation. Thus, we are able to generalize about South American shamanism as an institution in spite of the differences.

The most striking characteristics of these various cultures is the similarity of worldview and logic of beliefs found in all. They share the idea of a multilayered cosmos, as well as a vision of two different realities composed of the extrahuman and the human. However, these two realities are linked through a general principle of energy to form an undivided universe in which all is related to the cycles of production and reproduction, life and death, growth and decay. The extrahuman domain exerts its energies and forces on the human. Through the shaman, the human, in turn, exercises forces on the extrahuman. Shamanism is a religious institution representing the culture's preoccupation with the flow of these energies as they affect human well-being. It attempts to make sense out of events and to possibly influence them. In its broadest sense, shamanism is preoccupied with the well-being of society and its individuals, with social harmony, and with growth and reproduction of the entire universe. It encompasses the supernatural, as well as the social and ecological. Thus shamanism is a central cultural institution, which, through ritual, ties together the mythic past and worldview, and projects them into daily life and activities.

Power

The key concept linking these shamanic systems is power. Although the first four articles of the book are dedicated primarily to the exploration of the native concept of power, all of the chapters make reference to it. The shaman is the possessor of power, and it is power that enables him to mediate between the extrahuman and human. This concept of power is intimately linked to the idea of energy forces, the manifestation of these forces in the soul, and the growth and development of humans. It can only be understood in its relation to this worldview—for the shaman's power interacts with the global energy system. In many groups, such as the Siona, Matsigenka, Shipibo-Conibo, or Kagwahiv, ordinary humans possess this power, which increases with adulthood. The goal of shamanic training is to increase it sufficiently in order to mediate with the supernatural. Among the Matsigenka and Shipibo-Conibo, power manifests itself as light or aura. Among the Siona and Peruvian mestizos, it manifests itself in song. The shaman gives light in ritual, which represents his communication with the spirits. The word *shinan* used for impersonal vital power among the Shipibo-Conibo connotes this aspect, for it means luminous.

Native concepts for power are polysemous and connote its various manifestations. Thus, the Siona use the word *dau* to speak of a shaman's power. They also use it when speaking of sickness caused by extrahuman agents, and of specific disease objects found in the body. *Halojk,* for the Toba, connotes the shaman's power and material objects of his power. *Wanülüü* is an equivalent term among the Guajiro; the Culina use the term *dori.* For the Kagwahiv it is expressed by the verb *ipají,* and the shaman is "possessed of power."

Kracke states that what is central to shamanism is not the shaman as a specific role, but the quality of power that the shaman has. Several articles clarify that there is not one kind of shaman, but various kinds of shamanic specialists, depending on the kind of power they possess. The Desana have three kinds of shamanic specialists: the jaguar shaman *ye* whose role of divination is strictly associated with the intake of hallucinogens; the *sakaka* shaman who travels in the aquatic realms of the universe; and the chanter whose principal task is to cure through the naming of spirits, animals, plants, and substances having direct connection with the source of sickness or with the restoring aspect of the cure. Hill also describes two different ritual specialists for the Wakuénai: the chant owner and the specialist who contacts the spirits through the ingestion of hallucinogens.

In most cases, the shaman employs his power in public ritual for the benefit of the community or for individuals. Through it he mediates with the spirits to cure illness, negotiates with the master spirits of animals and fish to gain food, and so on. However, he may also employ his power to cause harm to others, thus giving the shaman an ambiguous position in society. Generally, he employs power in negative ways when he wishes to direct it outside his group, but his potential to cause harm to his own people remains latent, and a reason to fear shamans. In only two cases presented do we find distinct categories for the good shaman and for a shaman or other person who only causes evil. The Toba employ a separate term for those who do harm. These "witches" are normally women and are considered to be of a different nature than shamans; they are secret with no public recognition. Nevertheless, shamans are viewed somewhat ambiguously among the Toba. The Matsigenka also distinguish between good and bad shamans (*seripi'gari* and *matsika'nari,* respectively). The Siona acknowledge that a shaman may become one who only tends to evil, but this is not normally the case since the shaman is seen as the protector of his group. In all cultures, identification of "witch" or "sorcerer" with shaman is incorrect.

Social Roles

The power attained by the shaman legitimizes his various social roles within the society. In his broadest exercise of power we find the shaman as the political-religious leader. For the Toba and Siona of the past, and for the present-day Matsigenka, he is called upon to mediate disputes, contribute to decisions regarding warfare, mobilize the group in communal activities, and direct the economic activities in the procurement of food. His ambiguity also serves as a mechanism of social control over the group in the absence of formal control systems. The extent of the shaman's role depends most often on the historical and cultural circumstances in which the role expands and contracts according to factors impinging upon the social organization of the group (Langdon 1985).

Depending on factors such as the existence of other leadership roles in the community and the presence of political or economic control by an external society such as the national government, shamanic roles expand and contract to organize the group, maintain native tradition, and serve as a major component of ethnic identity. Among the Wakuénai of the last century, the messianic leader Venancio Kamiko drew upon the shamanic metaphors of native society in order to protest against white invasion. Wright's and Hill's symbolic analysis of the movement demonstrates that it represented a historically situated praxis, in which key symbols were strategically employed to resist external imposition of alien political and economic systems. The Toba maintain the basic elements and symbols of their shamanic worldview in the face of advancing Christian influence, and have incorporated key aspects of shamanic worldview in their Protestant experience. The Sibundoy shaman's insertion in Colombian popular culture is not only a continuity of the shaman's role as mediator, but also an important inversion in which the low status of Indian assumes particular power among the popular healing systems. Finally, mestizo shamanism in Peru demonstrates how native cosmology and healing tradition continues even when the specific Indian identity is lost.

In all its expressions, the one role that is constant in these shamanic systems is that of healer. It is essential to all because health is viewed holistically. In the native perspective, it is intimately concerned with the energy forces that lie behind well-being, and well-being is not only the absence of sickness, but implies nutritional, economic, and social well-being for the community as well as for the individual. Illness is an expression of conflict, a disturbance of the psychosocial and ecological balance of the group. In the global conception of the world, these concerns cannot be separated from the extrahuman world that influences daily events. It is likely that the continuity of the holistic perspective among acculturated groups as well as among popular medical systems accounts, in part, for the fact that shamans as curers have survived and adapted to the various social and cultural changes occurring in native and mestizo societies.

Ecstatic Experience

The South American shaman is distinguished from the ordinary person in three ways which constitute his power: First, as master of the ecstatic experience; second, through the acquisition of auxiliary spirits via this experience; and third, through the acquisition of songs. It is the first of these, the mastering of the ecstatic experience, that makes possible the other two, for it is the ecstatic experience that enables him to meet his auxiliary spirits and to leave his body to explore the extrahuman domains. It is also through the visions and through the auxiliary spirits that the shaman learns his songs and chants. In all cases, control of the ecstatic experience is the essential criterion of this acquired power. The pursuit of such power is a never-ending endeavor in the life of the shaman, and among those qualified as shamans, some are considered stronger than others. We will also see that the shaman may lose his power through contamination, through the violation of taboos, or through the attack of a more powerful shaman. Shamanic battles are an inherent part of this hierarchical ordering among them. The result of the loss of power signals the inability of the shaman to control the ecstatic experience, which marks the loss of his auxiliary spirits, as well as the power of his songs, and most often brings sickness and, in some cases, even death for the shaman.

Techniques of Ecstasy

In the upper Amazon the use of psychedelics is the most common form for entering into trance, as can be seen by the descriptions of the Matsigenka, Shipibo-Conibo, Siona, Sibundoy, and of the mestizo shamanism of the region. *Ayahuasca* (*Banisteriopsis* sp.) is the most common substance used. In addition, many other drugs are applied as additives or used independently.

Although the use of hallucinogens constitutes the most common form of acquiring shamanic knowledge, we agree with Harner (1988, 12) that not all shamans rely on psychedelic drugs for their contact with the spirits or their journeys to the superhuman realms. In part, the use of hallucinogens depends upon the kind of shamanic specialist, for example the difference between chant owners and shamans who contact spirits through the ingestion of hallucinogens. There are also other techniques employed for the ecstatic experience, and several articles contribute to understanding them, as well as the nature of altered states of consciousness. Two of the common techniques examined are the use of tobacco, and the control of dreams.

The use of tobacco has long been recognized for its sacred role in native American shamanism and ritual (Mason 1926; Wilbert 1987). Wilbert (1987) has conducted the most extensive survey of "tobacco shamanism" and the possible pharmacological effects of tobacco on the neurohumors. He suggests that "there remains no doubt that through action on the central nervous systems, nicotine is apt to produce altered states of consciousness akin to hallucination" (Wilbert 1987, 148). In this volume, Perrin's article is particularly useful for its ethnographic account of "tobacco shamanism" among the Guajiro, who use it as their principal mechanism to achieve power. The Matsigenka shaman is "one intoxicated by tobacco." The Desana chant owners use it in training to concentrate and to memorize their chants. The Siona use it as a secondary mechanism for divining, and its use is evident in the curing rituals in almost all the groups described in this volume.

Two articles specifically address the link between dreams and trance. For both the Toba and the Kagwahiv, dreams are the primary mechanism for acquiring shamanic power, and they are employed for diverse ends. Kracke suggests that trances and dreaming are not of a different nature, and that a strict distinction between them should not be made. He supports Guss's idea (1980) that hallucinations and trances are conceptualized as a kind of dream, and that dreaming is the core of the shaman's power among the Kagwahiv, Makiritáre, Tapirapé, and others. Perrin's description of Guajiro shamanism shows this to be true for them also, in that they experience a kind of "waking dream."

Neither the Toba nor the Kagwahiv currently use hallucinogens, and it is not clear if the Toba did in the past. For both, dreaming is the central access to power and to influencing the world. Although the Guajiro use tobacco for inducing trances, dreaming is central to the shaman's power. The Siona novice receives his first call to drink *yagé* via a dream. Shamans use dreams to see the causes of illness or other misfortunes, to contact the animal spirits, and to cure. The dream realm is similar to the other realms of the spirits on the other side of reality.

Kracke suggests that hallucinogens are used to address more critical problems, while less critical life processes are resolved through dreams. The Siona data supports this conclusion. Also, it is possible to see, that in the face of change such as the Toba case, shamanic knowledge and power persist in dreams even when the use of hallucinogens is no longer practiced.

An intriguing area suggested by Kracke, and one that marks recent research on dreams, is the concept of the "lucid dream," or "waking dreams" (Price-Williams 1987; Tart 1969, 1977). Shamans control their dreams, as they do hallucinations. In the case of trances and dreams, we must concur with B. Tedlock (1987, 20) that "some cultures are much more interested in and sophisticated about alternative or altered states of consciousness than our own." The references to dreams and shamanism in this volume should make important contributions to this important research on dreams and native views, and the uses of dreaming.

Poetry and Art: Shamanic Creativity

Eliade tells us that the shaman is both singer and poet. In South America this creative aspect assumes special importance, for the shaman's songs and music are central to the notion of his power, ritual efficacy, and aesthetic expression.

Shamanic expressive culture has received increasing attention in the last ten years as interdisciplinary studies in literature, anthropology, and music have continued to grow. The translation of shamanic discourse, giving attention to poetic mechanisms and performance, has become important (Bidou and Perrin 1988; Sherzer and Urban 1986; Swann 1983). The relationship among hallucinogens, trances, and creative culture is another area of growing importance (Gebhart-Sayer 1985, 1986, 1987; Reichel-Dolmatoff 1978). And finally, the role of music in shamanic performance has been recognized as central to shamanic power (Sullivan 1988). A basic premise of our volume is that one of the best expressions of the dynamic quality of shamanism is found in the performance of shamanic ritual. We are pleased that several chapters in this book examine shamanic discourse, poetry, and music in the context of ritual performance.

Two articles, those of Luna and Hill, support Sullivan's analysis that sound is the source of shamanic power and that "music, rather than language, is the 'primary modeling system' organizing human bodies" (Hill 1989, 1073; Sullivan 1988, 439). Several others demonstrate that the acquisition of song is central to shamanic training and the native concepts of power. Buchillet discusses the acquisition of songs for the Desana shamans and shows that the aspect of naming in shamanic discourse is central to ritual efficacy. Both Luna and Hill present transcriptions of shamanic music. Hill's article is dually important, for not only does he discuss the importance of music in shamanic ritual, he also demonstrates how the efficacy of shamanic curing rituals comes from the musical, cosmological, social, psychological, medical, and economic nature of ritual performance. He clearly demonstrates that we cannot separate the objective from the subjective in shamanic ritual, as does Western rational thought.

None of the articles focus upon the formal components of performance as defined by Bauman (1977); yet those of Hill, Baer, Buchillet, and Pollock make important contributions to understanding shamanic performance. They demonstrate that shamanic ritual, in most cases, is a group event involving active participation of the various shamanic specialists, as well as the audience. Hill describes the efficacy of two kinds of ritual specialists interacting in curing rituals. Baer's analysis of the Matsigenka discourse not only makes clear the function of naming in shamanic song, but also the important role of women in shamanic séances. Few studies have dealt with this topic in masculine shamanic systems, yet the evidence presented by Pollock on the Culina, an Arawan group, indicates that the sex roles and audience participation in the performance of shamanic séances should be examined further. Buchillet's description of the Desana chanter's performance raises an important point with regard to the varieties of shamanic specialists and performances. As opposed to the public ceremony described for the Wakuénai, Matsigenka, Siona, and others, the curing ritual of the Desana chanter is a barely audible semiprivate performance between the patient and healing specialist. This is not to deny, however, that the Desana have other shamanic specialists who perform public rituals for other objectives.

FINAL CONSIDERATIONS

South American shamanism is an important institution which expresses the general preoccupations of societies whose worldview conceives of a multilayered universe that is a unity. Its central preoccupation is with the energy forces that are behind daily events. Through shamanic ritual these general conceptions of order are represented, made manifest, and re-created. The shaman draws upon this energy through the ecstatic experience, through dreams or through trances induced by drugs, and mediates between the human and extrahuman realms. The sources of the shaman's power are the sources of culture itself, and the knowledge he acquires is culture's content (Kaplan 1982). Through ritual he is central to the expression of the cultural system. His role as mediator extends into the sociological domain, where he plays an important role in curing, as well as in economic, political, and other social activities.

We believe this volume clearly demonstrates the new trends in research on shamanism from the cultural and sociological perspectives. We also believe that we have finally put to rest the previous concerns of magic in shamanism, of shamans as deviants, and of shamanism as an archaic form. Shamanism is an enduring institution that must be comprehended holistically. Those of us who have worked with shamanic systems and have participated in the intellectual discussion regarding shamanism have been deeply marked by its symbolic and sociological expressions and consequences. We hope that this book contributes further to the general comprehension of this important phenomenon.

Note

1. Examples of some of the monographs on South American shamanism that have appeared since 1980 include: Baer (1984); Chaumeil (1983); Crocker (1985); Degarrod (1989); Illius (1987); Luna (1986); Perrin (1986b); Taussig (1987); and Viveiros de Castro (1986). This is not considered an exhaustive list.

PART ONE

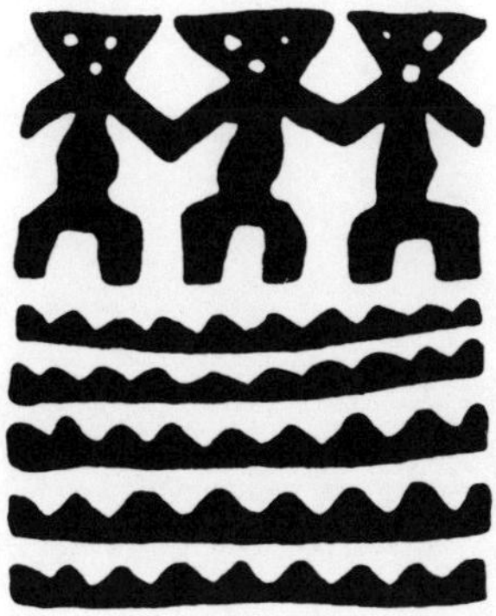

NATIVE CONCEPTIONS OF SHAMANS AND POWER

ONE

CULINA SHAMANISM

Gender, Power, and Knowledge

DONALD POLLOCK

The Culina Indians of western Brazil talk about shamanism as though it were an exclusively male institution: only men become shamans, only men are able to become shamans, and, at least in the past, all men became shamans. Becoming a shaman is a part of the process of becoming gendered as a Culina man, of acquiring—embodying—the special qualities and substances that equip men to act as particular kinds of persons in a gendered social world. Yet Culina shamanism requires the active participation of women, and shamanism invokes equally powerful and complementary female images. In this overview, I explore Culina shamanism as a form of gendered practice, as both a reflexive discourse on masculinity, and a mutually constituting dialogue between men and women, between the properties that comprise their innermost differentiating qualities and their public contributions to social life. Although shamanism among the Culina promotes especially visible constructions of the principal signs of maleness, it enrolls women in doing so; for a culture in which the focal properties of maleness and femaleness are viewed as complementary, rather than as hierarchically valued, shamanism offers one of many contexts in which the outlines of male and female define each other, and emerge more clearly in their interaction. Within this framework, the practice of Culina shamanism emerges as a special form of the social practice of masculinity.[1]

THE CULINA

The Culina are an Arawan-speaking group of perhaps two thousand individuals living in villages scattered along the major rivers of the Purus-Jurua region of western Amazonia. The majority of Culina live in Brazil, and a few villages are found in eastern Peru.[2] Culina are relatively recent migrants to the riverbanks, attracted in this century by easier access to the manufactured goods available from Brazilian and Peruvian rubber-tappers and sugarcane growers. Subsistence is based on the familiar pattern of slash-and-burn horticulture and hunting, supplemented with fishing and gathering. Local group size is quite variable, from single families of five to ten people, to larger villages of up to two hundred. Although there is considerable interaction and visiting among neighboring groups, each village conceives of itself as a group of kin sharing membership in a named category called *madiha,* or "people." The information presented here is based on research conducted in 1981 to 1982 among the roughly one hundred sixty Culina living in the village called Maronaua, situated along the upper Purus River in Brazil, near the frontier with Peru. The Culina at Maronaua distinguish themselves as *kurubu madiha,* the "*kurubu* fish people."[3]

SHAMANS

Shamanism is an active and vital institution in Maronaua. At the time of this research there were approximately ten shamans among the adult men in the village, and several adolescent boys were being initiated as shamans. All Culina shamans, *dzupinahe,* are men, and to be most effective as a village leader any headman must also be a shaman; indeed, it may be impossible to acquire sufficient power within a village to become a headman without also being a shaman. According to informants, in the past all Culina men were shamans, and even now only a few men deny shamanic ability.

Culina describe several overt roles performed by shamans. Only shamans have the ability to detect and treat two serious illnesses of mystical origin, the diagnosis and cure of which comprise an important aspect of the social control inherent in the shaman's role. Shamans are also able to see the movements of game animals in dreams, and are able to call game animals forth from the underground world where they live as spirits, so they may be hunted in the jungle. Shamans also lead rituals at birth and death that protect the community from the dangers posed by these events. Culina shamans, consequently, present the familiar boundary-maintaining image described elsewhere (e.g., Rivière 1970), controlling the entry of certain external beings—spirits, animals, and humans—into the village, and the exit of such beings out of the village. From the Culina point of view, the significance of these processes lies in the fact that they are all ultimately mystical in nature; their occurrence entails participation in and with the supernatural world represented by spirits generically called *tokorime*.

Shamans transform themselves into *tokorime* spirits, and they derive this ability, as well as their ability to control game animals and other processes, from the presence of a substance called *dori* in their bodies. *Dori* is said to permeate the flesh of shamans, where it is formless and insubstantial, though outside the shaman's body it is said to resemble a small stone. One shaman displayed his jar of pebbles, chips of quartz, and shards that he said were his *dori,* different colors being different types of *dori.*

The process of becoming a shaman is essentially one of acquiring a *dori.* Culina say adolescence is the ideal time to begin the training because sexual abstinence is imposed on the novice, and married men find it impossible to remain celibate for the necessary period. The process begins with the acquisition of two other substances, described as types of *dori: noma* is said to help the novice learn; *koronaha* is said to help the novice sing well. *Noma* is also required to prevent the novice from becoming ill from the *dori* he receives from his instructor shamans during his training. These shamans extract some of their *dori* and implant it into the novice's body. These is no loss of *dori* to these mentor shamans in this process, nor is their *dori* diminished by extraction for other purposes.

The Culina concern about the sexual activity of the novice provides an important clue about the nature of *dori.* Men, in contrast to women, are considered to be "wild," *wadita'i.* Men, for example, are hunters and are associated with the antisocial realm of the jungle and its inhabitants. Adolescent boys are especially wild: they have not yet been "tamed" or socialized by wives and marriage relations. The Culina view of the behavior of adolescent boys is predicated on this assumption; adolescents have considerable license for acting in ways that would be improper in children and adults, and they are assumed to take full advantage of this freedom. It is these wild youths who are initiated as shamans.

The relationship between the *dori* the adolescents acquire as shamans and their marked wildness is suggested by the prohibition of sexual intercourse during the training process. Adolescence, for males, begins with the development of semen and the sexual maturity it signals. Married adult men are tamed by wives through the social relations they enter into as husbands, an aspect of which is the controlled expulsion of semen in licit sexual relations. For adolescents, the loss of semen in illicit sexual encounters would entail the loss of the *dori* they acquire as novice shamans. That is, the seminal substance that renders adolescent boys wild is closely associated with the *dori* substance they may lose in coitus. *Dori* thus emerges as a kind of objectification of the wildness of men that is lost in improper adolescent sexual relations; this wildness is controlled by its incorporation into the body of a shaman. Adolescent illicit sexual relations are both improper displays of wild behavior and improper expulsion of a wild substance that must be controlled through sexual restraint; the loss of *dori* is a failure to control one's wildness. This is also suggested by the fact that the Culina say although today only some men possess *dori* (i.e., are shamans), in the past all men possessed *dori.* Also, any Culina man unknown to the members of a village may be considered a shaman.[4]

Acquisition of *dori,* of shamanic capacity, thus signals the regulation of the wildness exemplified by adolescent boys and metaphorized as illicit sexual relations. The taming or socializing process is one that all boys must undergo; consequently, Culina refer to a social ideology in which all men are shamans. Not surprisingly, the novice shaman is nearing the end of adolescence. *Dori* is also an aspect of the gendering of adolescents; it transforms their public wildness into sociability through internalizing the dangerous substance that renders them men, *mahi.* While it is not necessary to be a shaman to be an adult man, only shamans achieve the full potential of maleness: as village leaders, as masters of game animals, and as protectors of the village.

The concepts *dori, tokorime* (spirits), and *dzupinahe* (shaman) are closely related. The possession of *dori* is said to make one a *tokorime/dzupinahe,* and in most contexts the latter terms are, in fact, used synonymously. While "*tokorime*" may refer most narrowly to an insubstantial image, and "*dzupinahe*" may refer to the appropriate human or animal form adopted by *tokorime, dori* links human men as shamans both to the animals of the jungle—many of which are embodiments of spirits—and to the underground world of disembodied *tokorime.* And though human shamans may adopt the identities of many animal *tokorime* spirits, they may also be said to comprise their own category of *tokorime,* the *adzaba tokorime.*

Tobacco snuff is the means through which men possessing *dori* become transformed into shamans/spirits. The inhalation of tobacco snuff is a common theme in Culina myth, where its effect is to produce death followed by transformation into a *tokorime* spirit. The use of tobacco snuff by shamans in ritual has the similar effect of extinguishing human identity and transforming the individual shaman into a *tokorime* spirit.[5]

Culina recognize a wide variety of *tokorime* spirits, most of which are animal *tokorime,* the spirit forms of jungle animals. In addition, there are several types of *tokorime* that are human in form, said to be pure *tokorime. Tokorime* live in the underground worlds called *nami budi.* Shamans visit the *nami budi* in dreams or trance, and there they order the *tokorime* of animals to appear in the jungle for hunting, or to enter the village for curing.

Among this variety of *tokorime* spirits, two are of particular interest, the *hidzama tokorime,* or white-lipped peccary spirits, and the *dzumahe tokorime,* the jaguar spirit. These two serve as symbols opposing the qualities of sociability and wildness referred to above. In Culina ideology the peccary is a social, gregarious animal, which often appears in myth and ritual representing Culina themselves. The jaguar is a solitary animal, a dangerous hunter, quintessentially wild. Together the peccary and the jaguar define the limits of this critical axis of human life: the herbivorous peccary is associated with sociable women who form the core of households and contribute cultivated garden products to it, while the carnivorous jaguar is associated with the wild men who hunt in the jungle and contribute meat. Although the jaguar is a spirit, it has associations with the heavenly realm of Culina culture heroes. In this regard it also stands in opposition to the peçcary of the underground *nami budi:* the souls of the dead, if properly conducted to the *nami budi,* are eaten by and are transformed into peccaries, but those not properly conducted to the *nami budi* wander the earth and are ultimately eaten by jaguars. These *tokorime* thus represent two aspects of a cosmology that is played out in social life by the interaction of men and women. It is significant that, while each shaman calls on and is transformed into a unique set of *tokorime* spirits in ritual contexts, all shamans call on and become transformed into both the peccary and jaguar spirits.

The gendered contrast signified by the two *tokorime,* the peccary and the jaguar, is replicated in the contrast between *tokorime* and humans. For example, the *tokorime* are male, with perhaps only one exception. Of any animal species said to be *tokorime,* it is the males of the species that are referenced. These *tokorime* are consequently wild and dangerous, especially to women, and in particular to pregnant women whose fetuses may be harmed by an encounter with a *tokorime* in the jungle. One female *tokorime,* the *hohopade,* preserves this opposition by being excessively wild: it fails to cure, but chases women during curing rituals, and even kills shamans by hanging them from trees.

SHAMANISM AND ILLNESS

Culina shamans can use their *dori* to harm others, and in normal discourse the term most often refers to the intrusive illness-causing substance shamans throw or inject into the bodies of their victims. This *dori* substance is only detectable to other shamans. It is seen as a small lump in the flesh of the patient, and the illness produced is also called *dori.* A shaman cures *dori* illness by extracting the substance by sucking or by suction created with the hands. In the latter case, the hands are rubbed on the chest, so with either technique the shaman/curer takes the harmful *dori* into his own body and then vomits and spits it out. In cases of extreme illness, when death occurs or is felt to be imminent, a *dori* such as *dori makoko,* very red *dori,* may be diagnosed, a form that grows in the body faster than it can be extracted.

Shamans also diagnose and treat a second illness called *epetuka'i. Dori* afflicts adults and sometimes children, but never afflicts infants. Rather, infants contract *epetuka'i,* which is caused by parents who fail to obey the food prohibitions imposed on those who have newborn and infant children.[6] The curative sucking technique is also used for *epetuka'i.*

At the birth of a child, parents are nominally prohibited from eating the meat of certain animals. Identification of the exact species prohibited varies from individual to individual, as does the period of the most stringent taboos (some may even prohibit certain plants), but invariably it is the male of the species that is avoided. Eating these prohibited animals produces *epetuka'i* in the child, an illness said to be "like having a dung beetle in the abdomen." There are no exact symptoms, but *epetuka'i* may produce diarrhea, constipation, or vomiting, all signs of disrupted gastrointestinal processes, and signs consistent with the violation of food prohibitions or failure to perform food productive roles properly.

In reality, Culina consistently ignore these food prohibitions, or at least fail to observe them throughout the necessary period, which lasts, ideally, until the child is able to walk and communicate in a minimally competent manner. Moreover, infants regularly present symptoms that might be interpreted as *epetuka'i* without a diagnosis of the illness being made. *Epetuka'i* is diagnosed not so much as a condition of the child as a condition of its household.

The diagnosis normally follows a breach of proper standards of behavior among members of the child's household. A spouse's illicit extramarital affair that becomes too public, a son-in-law's consistent failure to produce enough game for his wife's parents' household, or excessive arguing between a husband and wife create conditions in which a child's illness will be diagnosed as *epetuka'i.* The explicit attribution of the illness to a violation of food prohibitions appropriately references an ideology of intrahousehold relations based on exchanges of types of food and mutual nurturance; a breakdown of relations within a household is metaphorically a failure to provide proper food, focused on the child that is created by and that itself creates these relations.

Adults do not contract *epetuka'i.* Rather, they become victims of witchcraft, of the penetration of *dori* into the body through the act of a hostile shaman. Not surprisingly, such witchcraft episodes signal various stresses and tensions in relations among local group members, particularly at the social level beyond that of individual households. Typically, such stresses take the form of open conflict between men in different households, often affines, but any overt display of anger, hostility, or violence may lead to the discovery of an illness that will be diagnosed as *dori.* In the context of such circumstances, and normally only in this context, virtually any sickness, no matter how apparently minor, may be diagnosed as *dori.* In the absence of intravillage hostility, sickness is never diagnosed as *dori,* except to account for fatal sickness.

The shaman's role in illness is not limited to the treatment of the *dori.* He also identifies the enemy shaman who is presumed to have caused the illness, normally (with nonfatal illnesses) a shaman from another village.[7] The diagnosis of the *dori* is a significant public sanction against the hostility that provoked it within the group, but the identification of the hostile shaman in another group also redirects the conflict outside of the village and reinforces the basic ideology of absolute harmony among the kin who comprise the village. Thus the curing of the *dori* equally marks a social consensus that the circumstances provoking the illness are ended. This aspect of the process is highlighted by a ritual that follows the successful treatment of illness. In this second ritual, held the night after the curing ritual per se, the entire village dances in a circle and sings songs directed by the headman, songs that have the general theme of proper order and beauty in the village.

If the successful cure of a *dori* symbolically represents the successful, if only temporary, resolution of intravillage tensions, the failure of treatment of a *dori* equally signals the presence of unregenerate hostility within the village. In such cases, as when the victim of witchcraft dies, the hostile shaman is identified within the group, and he is killed. Here again a shaman identifies the offender, normally a man in some peripheral social position, often a visitor not bound by the obligations of kinship to the members of the group. However, the politics of witchcraft are rarely so simple. For example, in two cases guilty witches had been allowed to flee and take up residence elsewhere; one perpetually moved back and forth between Maronaua and Santo Amaro, a closely linked Culina village several days downriver, while the other—whose crime had been committed in a village upriver in Peru—lived with his wife and children in a single isolated household half a day's canoe trip downriver from Maronaua.

Culina curing ritual essentially consists of the transformation of shamans into various *tokorime* spirits, which suck out the illness causing substances, either *dori* or *epetuka'i.* The curing ritual, itself called *tokorime,* takes place at night. The women of the village gather and call to the shamans/spirits, who then emerge one at a time from the forest, sing with the women, and attend to the patient. The shaman returns to the forest, and soon reappears as another *tokorime.* The ritual may last for several hours, not infrequently all night, and may extend for days in the case of serious illness. Men watch the proceedings but do not participate; they are said to be afraid of the *tokorime* spirits that cure the patient.

Several aspects of the curing ritual should be highlighted. The nighttime setting and the use of song in the ritual are related, inasmuch as the ritual is conducted largely through oral and aural media, enhanced by the darkness that obscures vision and the potentially false reality it displays. For Culina such oral performance has significant directive qualities. In speech one may order others to act; leaders are judged on their ability to use speech in this compelling manner—their power is indexed by the level of public compliance—and parents conceive of the education of their children as a process in which children hear and understand; knowledge is language and vice versa. Singing is a kind of heightened form of speech, a style that is especially compelling in its elocutionary force. The songs of the *tokorime* in curing rituals are perhaps the most powerful of Culina verbal performances; they are the maximally compelling medium for the creation of action, and, in this case, in the cure of illness caused by witchcraft. Shamans carefully prepare songs for use in curing ritual, and even stage mock curing ceremonies at which village women are taught the necessary refrains that they will sing with the shaman during the actual curing ritual.

The songs of curing rituals may be extremely simple, consisting almost entirely of the sounds characteristic of the animal whose *tokorime* is represented, or they may be complex in symbolic structure. A thorough analysis of such songs would be beyond the scope of this overview, but some of their common features should be mentioned.

A recurring theme of curing ritual song is the offering of food to the *tokorime* spirits that are called to the village to cure. Specifically, the food offered is *koidza,* a mildly fermented manioc beverage made of premasticated boiled manioc. This author has elsewhere considered *koidza* to be the quintessential female contribution to household subsistence, a kind of core symbol that condenses numerous significant aspects of femaleness for Culina (Pollock 1985). Manioc is the staple horticultural product produced and cooked by women. *Koidza* made from it, moreover, is doubly cooked and eaten because the tubers are boiled to soften them, are chewed to a pulpy mash, boiled again, and finally consumed communally by men. This cooking process and the exchange of proper foods—of which *koidza* is the preeminent female food—is a common Culina metaphor for the taming or socializing of men through marriage, men who were, as unmarried adolescents, wild.

The offering of *koidza* to the *tokorime* in curing ritual sets up a comparable minimal structure of exchange with several levels of significance. The outcome of the exchange, ideally, will be the taming of the male shaman/witch who has caused the illness, through the medium of the *tokorime* who control *dori,* and thus the cure of illness, both in the patient and the village. In somewhat different terms it is the wildness provoking the illness that is tamed in the transaction. In this symbolic exchange, *dori* again emerges as a representation of the maximally wild natures of men, which may be brought under control by the offering and consumption of an appropriate female substance.[8] Just as shamanic training signals the restraint of adolescent wildness, so too shamanic practice restrains the wildness of witchcraft. And just as shamanic training is a prelude to marriage, when the new husband is metaphorically socialized or tamed by his wife's *koidza,* so too shamanic practice metaphorically utilizes women's *koidza* to tame illness.

This dialogue of opposed qualities in curing ritual songs also appears among the *tokorime* that participate in the process. The first spirit to appear in the ritual is the *hidzama,* the white-lipped peccary spirit, while the final spirit to appear is the *dzumahe,* the jaguar spirit. As noted earlier, these two are opposed on at least two levels, representing Culina as sociable women versus wild men. The peccary spirit is said to cure; it appears and drinks the *koidza* offered in the ritual. The jaguar does not cure: it finds no *koidza* when the illness is cured by the end of the ritual.

The metaphors of food, including its consumption and expulsion, and the structures of exchange that inform and shape the curing ritual draw on the meanings and relations that also inform and structure the interactions of men and women in other contexts that constitute a kind of semiosis of maleness and femaleness for Culina. While shamans are normatively men and are conceptually the critical activators of ritual curing, the roles of women in shamanistic performance must also be underscored. Indeed, curing ritual is organized in a manner identical to other, secular, rituals in which the themes of male/female interactions are more explicit (Moore and Myerhoff 1977). For example, Culina curing ritual bears close similarities to the common ceremonial process in which women order men to hunt, called *dutse'e* (*bani*) *towi* or "order to get (meat)." In the *dutse'e towi,* village women collectively go from house to house, singing to the adult men in each to go hunting. The men do so, and at their return collectively drop their catch before the reassembled women. The women cook the meat and serve it to the men, along with the *koidza* manioc drink.[9] Processually the curing ritual and the *dutse'e towi* are virtually identical. In each, the village women collectively sing to men (shamans or hunters) ordering them either to remove a wild substance from the village (*dori* or *epetuka'i*) or to bring a wild substance into the village (meat). In both contexts the women reciprocate through the manioc *koidza,* provided either symbolically in curing ritual song, or actually in the meal prepared for the hunters' return. It should also be noted that Culina divide the annual cycle of activities into the dry season, when the *tokorime* curing ritual is held regularly but the *dutse'e towi* is rare, and the rainy season, when Culina say they do not perform the curing ritual (although it is occasionally performed), but when almost all adult male food gathering or hunting activities are initiated by women through the *dutse'e towi.* That is, the two rituals essentially replace each other as the seasons change.

In both curing ritual and hunting/ordering ritual women play a critical role in transforming wild attributes to tame or sociable ones. While men control the movement of wild things into and out of the village, women control the transformation of wild things into socially palatable things within the village. To the extent, then, that the illnesses represented by *dori* and *epetuka'i* are conceived as improper intrusions of antisocial wildness into the life of the village, the cure of illness requires the intervention of women who are able to tame or socialize such dangerous properties.

SHAMANISM, BIRTH, AND DEATH

Although shamans are active most often and most publicly in curing ritual, their participation is also crucial for the successful completion of birth, and for the proper disposition of the dead. Again, these processes are linked to the realm of the *tokorime* spirits to which shamans have access, and it is only through shamanistic intervention that they can be negotiated properly.

At the birth of a child the shaman/headman leads the village women in a short series of songs, sung at night, either during or immediately after the birth. Essentially, these songs refer to various *tokorime* that are called into the village to show that they harbor no witchcraft threat against the newborn infant, and, conversely, to witness that the child possesses no *dori* that could harm others. A fetus, and thus also the infant at birth, is said to be formed entirely of its father's semen, which is associated with *dori*. The newborn baby is consequently only half-formed, lacking the corporeal contribution that will be supplied by mother's milk. The baby is also in a vulnerable state because it as yet lacks a soul, a *tabari*. The Culina informants have no generally agreed on knowledge of when a child acquires its *tabari;* it is formed over the course of infancy. The *tabari* carries notions of social competence, and thus develops gradually over this period. Babies, *nono,* lack a soul, but a child, *ehedeni,* possesses this *tabari,* which is derived partly from mother's milk, a tame female counterpart and complement to semen, and later derived from eating the meat of animals who are the reincarnated spirits of dead Culina. The lack of a soul exposes the infant to the danger of *epetuka'i,* the harmful influence of parents who fail to observe food taboos: that is, of parents who act too wild, conceived symbolically as the improper consumption of male animal substance. The songs sung by shamans at the birth of a child protect it from such influences, represented in the songs as the danger posed by *tokorime* spirits, and their male animal counterparts.

The shaman's role in death is inverted: essentially the shaman must conduct the *tabari* of the deceased to the underground world, the *nami budi,* so that this disembodied soul will pose no threat to the living members of the village. Here again, the medium of performance is song, sung in a nighttime ritual conceived as a journey in which the shaman, transformed into a *tokorime,* conducts the deceased soul to the *nami budi,* where it arrives at the village of the *tokorime* spirits. A ritual is held for it there, of the general form of Culina rites of passage, at the end of which the soul is consumed by peccary spirits and is itself transformed into a peccary.

A shaman killed by members of a village, normally to avenge the death of a village co-member, is not accorded this eschatological privilege of access to the underground afterlife. His soul remains on the palpable earth, where it wanders for several days "looking for its hammock" (i.e., for a proper burial) or for red urucú facial paint (a sign of liminality and transformation), posing a temporary threat to village members who may even abandon the area in fear. After a few days the soul is said to be eaten by a jaguar spirit, transforming it into a jaguar.

These processes set up cycles of birth and death; in the normal cycle the souls, the *tabari,* of people are transformed after death into the peccaries that shamans call forth into the jungle for hunting. The consumed peccary meat, in turn, forms the bodies and souls of living people. The cycle is broken for shamans who are killed without proper burial; the jaguar is never eaten by humans, and is thus never retransformed into a Culina person when it dies.

Culina conceive of people and life itself as a balance and interaction of various complementary qualities or attributes. One such set, a gendered contrast is glossed herein as wildness and sociability, and this description could be expanded to include dimensions such as smell or social space. These sets are related paradigmatically, and they model others, such as meat and garden products, semen and milk, jungle and village, and so on.[10] Such complementary properties and substances engage in a kind of dialectic in which their synthesis or conjunction forms proper persons, while an overemphasis on either is improper or even dangerous.

Shamans intervene in circumstances understood as threatening the imbalances of such properties. The illnesses *dori* and *epetuka'i* may be viewed in this regard as the manifestations or unregulated intrusions of wild qualities associated with men, either without moderation by corresponding qualities associated with women, or to an excessive degree. In the former case, wildness subverts proper sociability, socially as conflict between village co-members, and conceptually as the anger of an evil shaman. This excessive wildness is signified by the male substance *dori.* In the latter case, too, the wildness of intrahousehold hostility is conceptualized as an inappropriate excess of male substance through the meat of male animals, symbolized as *epetuka'i.*

If the intrusion of excessive male qualities and substances is dangerous, so too is the intrusion of excessive female qualities, represented in the most extreme and dangerous form as menstrual blood. Menstruating women are not secluded, but do avoid cooking for and eating with their household members for fear of contaminating the food. The informants were unable to specify precisely the consequences of eating food contaminated in this way; the situation appears to fall into that class of events that simply do not happen. Instead, it is the inappropriate *retention* of menstrual blood and the corresponding inability to incorporate semen properly that is significant and produces infertility.

Infertility is understood as a woman's failure to conceive. It is always attributed to an intentional act of women, and is caused by a shaman who places a substance called *awabono* in the uterus. The *awabono* blocks the passage of semen into the womb and the flow of menstrual blood out of the womb. Infertility is thus a kind of inversion of normal illness: illness is an improper incorporation of a male substance, while infertility is an improper failure to incorporate a male substance. Infertility inverts illness in another sense as well; the contraceptive *awabono* is said to be requested by a woman herself, by a woman who no longer wishes to bear children. Those who contract illness are unwilling victims of a witch, but those who "contract" infertility are willing clients of a shaman. Nonetheless, illness and infertility share an important characteristic. Both are matters of social concern when they threaten the ability of people to fulfill appropriate social responsibilities, either the withdrawal from social life that accompanies illness, or the refusal to be socially fecund through infertility.[11]

Birth and death may be viewed in similar terms. Newborn babies are explicitly presocial for Culina, composed of male substance which requires the exclusive consumption of complementary female substances to produce a soul. At death, this soul threatens to be excessively and inappropriately sociable through its desire to remain in its human village, where it endangers its remaining kin by tempting the souls of the living to join it. Again, shamans intervene to insure that proper balances of these metaphorical qualities are created, protecting babies from the excessive wildness of male substance, protecting the village from the excessive sociability of the dead.

Culina, then, view shamanism as outward-looking. Shamans interact with the world beyond the village, with enemies in other groups, with the spirits which populate the forest in the form of animals, or with the mystical realm of the dead. The terms through which this cosmology is constructed, however, are those through which Culina conceive and understand the mundane society of village life. Shamanism emerges, then, as a means for creating and maintaining proper persons through the control that shamans exercise over the fundamental qualities of which these persons are composed, qualities that may become unbalanced at the beginning or end of life, or in relations with others.

NOTE ON TRANSCRIPTION (CULINA)

The Culina words in this text follow general phonetic notation with the following conventions:

ts: an aspirated "s"
kk: an aspirated "k"
all vowels have roughly the same qualities as their Spanish equivalents.
' is a glottal stop.

Notes

1. I am grateful to Jean Langdon for her comments on an earlier draft of this paper.

2. The Peruvian Culina are described by Adams (1962, 1963, 1971, 1976), Rüf (1972), and Townsend and Adams (1978).

3. About one-half of the *kurubu madiha* have now moved to an abandoned seringal, or rubber-tapping camp, downriver from Maronaua, a site known as the Sobral.

4. *Dori* bears similarities to *dau* among the Siona, which Langdon glosses as "power" in this volume. Although the gloss seems appropriate for *dori* also, I find the generic term "power" too broad to be meaningful. All Culina, shamans and nonshamans alike, possess "power" of various types; my interest here is in exploring what type of power *dori* represents.

5. Viveiros de Castro (1978) suggests that Culina shamans also use *ayahuasca,* but this was denied by my informants. Though *ayahuasca* was taken regularly, it was not used in shamanic performance during my research. Note that local Panoan shamans, for example among the Cashinahua and Sharanahua, do use *ayahuasca* (Kensinger 1973; Siskind 1973a).

6. It should be noted that shamans treat only those illnesses that occur "inside" the body, and do not treat the broad category of illnesses that occur on the "outside" of the body, especially on the skin (see Pollock 1988).

7. Culina do not distinguish shamans and sorcerers terminologically: both are *dzupinahe.* However, Culina do use Portuguese terms such as "bruxo" and "feitiçaria" when translating the antisocial aspect of shamans.

8. *Epetuka'i* is similar, being derived also from males—male animals. In

this case, however, the exchange themes referenced also include semen/mother's milk, the former creating the fetus, the latter creating the child following birth.

9. Rüf (1972) has described the *dutse'e towi* among the Peruvian Culina in detail. Siskind describes a similar process among the Sharanahua, neighbors of the Peruvian Culina (1973b, 96–104).

10. The logically simple structure of oppositions simplifies what is more correctly an elaborate semiotic calculus. My paper on food and sexual identity explores some of these relations further (Pollock 1985).

11. It may be objected that barrenness is not perfectly comparable to illness, as only women become barren, while both men and women contract *dori*. However, I believe it is consistent with Culina views to suggest that a woman's infertility affects her husband, who is also denied children: thus, both sexes become "barren," at least socially.

TWO

DAU

Shamanic Power in Siona Religion and Medicine

E. JEAN MATTESON LANGDON

Reichel-Dolmatoff (1975) has described a shaman-jaguar complex found among many indigenous groups of Central and South America, and in particular among those of Colombia. The central characteristic of this complex is the association of shamans with jaguars and the belief that shamans have the power to transform into jaguars. Through an extensive review of archaeological, ethnohistorical, and ethnological literature of Colombia, he documents this association among highland groups such as the ancient Muisca (Chibcha), and among the living Paez and Kogi; among Pacific lowland groups from Panama to Ecuador, including the Noanama and Embera; and in the Amazonian lowlands where it is nearly universal for all groups. In the Amazon, it is linked with the use of hallucinogenic snuffs or the infusion of *yagé* made from species of the *Banisteriopsis* sp. vine. Shamans use hallucinogens not only to transform into jaguars, but also to divine the future, to adjudicate quarrels, to perform sorcery, to identify hunting and fishing areas, and to heal illness (Reichel-Dolmatoff 1975, 28).

Regardless of the linguistic family or cultural subdivision to which the group belongs, similar conceptions and use of hallucinogens to establish a direct contact with the supernatural sphere are found. In the northwest Amazon, one center of this complex is the Putumayo-Caquetá area, where *yagé* is used as the principal hallucinogen (Reichel-Dolmatoff 1975, 36). The Siona, a Western Tukanoan group living along the Putumayo River, consider themselves to be specialists in the use of this and other hallucinogenic drugs. Siona shamans have been famous throughout the region for their powers, and have served as teachers to novices from highland as well as lowland groups (Langdon 1981).

The focus here is on the shamanistic complex as it is manifested among the Siona Indians. It includes exploration of the Siona conceptions of the universe, of the forces that make for well-being or ill health, and of the nature and source of shamanic power.

Power, expressed in the Siona term *dau,* is perhaps the most central concept to be examined here, for it is through possessing *dau* that a shaman is able to understand and influence the forces responsible for well-being. The Siona are ultimately concerned with knowing what is going on in their universe and its implications for daily life. In an important way, shamanism is a quest for knowledge, and knowledge of the sort they seek is power.[1]

THE SIONA UNIVERSE

The Siona universe consists of five levels organized hierarchically. In ascending order they are called "beneath the earth," "first heaven," "second heaven," "third heaven," and "little metal heaven." These levels are flat discs conceived of as similar to the cassava grill. The first level, that of beneath the earth, rests on three "fire dogs," the South American clay cylinders that support the cassava grill over the cooking hearth. The first three levels replicate each other in that they are divided into realms belonging to different beings, spirit, human, or animal, and in that these beings live similar life-styles. Their social organization, material goods, houses, clothing, and customs reflect each other. Countless supernatural forces inhabit all levels. These supernatural forces, embodied in spirits and living as humans do, give life and power to reality.

The surface of the earth, called the first heaven, is the dwelling place of humans and animals. In ordinary everyday reality the forces that influence events are hidden, but the Siona know of another reality in which the embodied forces are visible. They speak of these two realities as "two sides." "This side" is that in which we normally operate. It is characterized by three principal habitats—the jungle, the river, and the homesteads—each with its distinctive inhabitants. The jungle is the home of the wild animals. The jaguar with its power and strength is the dominating figure of the jungle. The river is the domain of the water animals and fish; the anaconda is ruler there. The homesteads belong, of course, to the Siona with their domesticated animals and plants; the shaman is leader of this realm. When looking upward, this side stretches as far as the eye can ordinarily see, and its boundary is marked by the Sun's Heaven River that cuts across the sky dividing the first heaven from the second heaven.

The "other side" is a world of spirits and forces operating in non-ordinary space and time, not only on the earth's surface, but also on the other levels. All aspects of existence on "this side" are influenced by these forces. In the second heaven, activities of the Sun, Rain People, and Thunder are responsible for the weather and the seasonal cycles on earth, and, consequently, for success in harvests, as well as the annual cycles of the plants, animals, and fish. In the jungle, the animals have a master spirit who dictates the size of the group and where the animals roam in the forest. Thus, if one wishes to have weather favorable for the crops, to find game in the jungle, and so on, the proper spirits must be contacted and persuaded to cooperate in order that the normal rhythm of life continues. However, these supernatural forces may also cause disruption of the normal routine and present dangers to the security of life.

The Siona's relationship with the spirits could be characterized as fearful as well as dependent. They see the world full of dangerous spirits ready to attack the unaware victim. The general concern is that these spirits will cause serious illness, although they may cause other dangerous abnormalities, such as scarcity of food, behavioral deviations, floods, or earthquakes. Certain hours of the day, as well as certain seasons, are believed to be high activity periods of illness bearing spirits. Thus, the river is dangerous for bathing during certain hours, and the air is believed to be full of spirits causing flu and boils during the dry season. A person may also become a victim of a spirit attack by breaking a taboo or approaching a location known to be occupied by a malevolent spirit. Thus, one should not kill a deer, walk near the silk-cotton tree, nor pass by the graveyard alone. A woman should never bathe in the river during menstruation, for her odor will attract malevolent spirits. Small children, particularly infants, are considered the most vulnerable of all and suffer the greatest danger of random spirit attack. Adults, on the other hand, are more often victim of spirit attacks motivated by sorcery. Hence, to live and prosper in this world, to insure one's security, and to counteract dangers, it is necessary to understand and to learn how to influence these ultimate forces. The central quest of the Siona shaman is to discover the forces on the other side in order to understand and influence events on this side.

LIVING AND DYING

Successful well-being for living organisms is a result of the balance between the living and dying forces that affect them and make up the general cycle of life. When a Siona greets another in the traditional manner, he inquires, "Are you *wahɨ?*" Translating this into Spanish, they ask, "¿Esta viva?" ("Are you fully living?"). Although we might be inclined to translate this phrase into, "Are you well?" the word living seems more appropriate if we consider the replies to this greeting. Generally, one would reply, "I am alive," but if sick, one would say, "I am *hũ'i,*" or I am dying. *Wahɨ* is the opposite of *hũ'i,* to be dying, and its most appropriate meaning in this greeting is "to be living." Neither living nor dying is a static state, but represents the process of growth or death of the organism.

Wahɨ is a key symbol that conveys the characteristics attributed to well-being and growing life forces. It is used both as a verb stem, as well as an adjective. It has several meanings, particularly in its adjective form, and thus cannot be given justice by a single English term. For instance, *wahɨ* is used to describe someone who is fat. The quality of fatness is considered to be a sign of good health. In fact, the fatness of good health is epitomized in the plumpness exhibited by healthy babies. *Wahɨ* also means to be immature, fresh, young, or tender. Light shades of the color green, such as those we might associate with spring, are also called *wahɨ*. Thus, from these various meanings, there emerges a sense of what it means for the Siona to be fully living or healthy. *Wahɨ* implies the concept of a state of youth and plumpness with the promise of further growth. This concept is made concrete through the different qualities associated with *wahɨ*.

This conception of good health becomes even clearer if we consider the qualities attributed to the state of dying. Lévi-Strauss (1963) has demonstrated that Amazonian Indians tend to order their worldview along a series of binary opposites, such as raw and cooked, nature and culture, jungle and river, and so forth. The Siona exemplify this kind of thinking, particularly with reference to the qualities associated with the state of health. While *wahɨ* is one term with several meanings, there is not one comprehensive term that serves to signify all the oppositions. Instead, there are several terms that stand in opposition to each of the various meanings of *wahɨ*. *Hũ'i,* to be dying, is the opposite verb. The key adjective is "rotten," with the closely linked terms meaning hot, dirty, old, dark, and emaciated. Each of these are qualities indicating the dying or death forces, and the full set of oppositions is as follows:

living	dying
immature	rotten
new, clean	dirty, rotten
fresh (cool)	hot
young	old
green	black, dark colors
fat	thin, emaciated
raw	cooked

The Siona associate the qualities of thinness with old age and sickness, black and dirty objects with rottenness, and heat with sickness and aging. Living is a positive state. It is a time of growth and youth, in which one is plump and fresh. When extended to mean good health for the community, it means that there is sufficient food for all. There is success in hunting and fishing. The crops are growing well with proper sun and rain, and everyone is performing their duties and responsibilities. This state of living is contrasted with dying, in which one is old, skinny, and past the peak of growth. For the community that means a scarcity of food or dissention among the people. In other words, *wahɨ* is associated with the waxing forces of life, those that help maintain good health and growth. *Hũ'i,* on the other hand, is associated with the waning forces, those of aging, sickness, and destruction. The tendency toward life or death predominates, depending upon the disposition of the supernatural forces and the shaman's ability to control them.

MEDICINE

When the Siona wish to contact the supernatural agents which give life and power to this reality, they gather with a shaman to ingest *yagé.* The Siona term for *yagé* is *'ɨko,* which signifies medicine. The *Banisteriopsis* sp. vine and its products are not the only substances designated as medicine among the Siona. The term *'ɨko* refers to a very large number of plants, animals, insects, and their preparations that are used in dealing with illness and welfare. The term medicine has a more general use and meaning than what we connote by the term. A medicine may be used to insure that an event or person will mature properly, to insure continuation of a healthy state of being, to prevent danger or disruption of normality, or to return an unsatisfactory situation to its normal state, such as curing illness. Most of these medicines are nonhallucinogenic. However, all classes of medicine derive their meaning, use, and power from the principal medicine, *yagé.*

The main use of *yagé* is as a divinatory aid to understand the activities of the spirits in order to maintain or restore the well-being, either of the community as a whole, or of its individual members. It is the bridge between this world and the "other" realities or realms. In the past, when there were master shamans in all Siona communities, the members of the community gathered weekly to participate in a ceremony led by one of them. He directed the ceremony to the game spirits, weather spirits, river spirits, or others, depending on the season and needs of the community. In addition to these weekly ceremonies conducted for the well-being of all, there were special sessions for cases of severe illness, or emergency situations requiring immediate divination of the supernatural forces operating behind the event. Today, when master shamans are not readily available, these special sessions are the ones most commonly held. They generally involve the affected individuals, their families, and others who wish to participate.

Yagé, as medicine, does not imply a substance with curing powers. More appropriately, it empowers shamans with knowledge, and the knowledge they gain allows them to control and influence events in both sides of reality. The relationship between *yagé* and other medicines demonstrates this quality of empowering through knowledge. The Siona say that all nonhallucinogenic medicines have been discovered through *yagé* visions. When a shaman has reached a certain level of knowledge, he travels to the house of God, where he is shown a book with all the medicines in it, and it is from this that he begins his career in healing illnesses. *Yagé* empowers in a second way. The knowledge *yagé* gives to a shaman forms a substance that grows in a man as he continues to ingest the drug. This substance, called *dau,* is the root of the shaman's power. It is the shaman's *dau* that imparts healing capacity to medicines. Ideally, the shaman should sing over all medicinal substances, and it is his songs that activate the healing properties of plants and other substances.

DAU

We shall now consider the final, and perhaps most important, term in Siona shamanism: *dau.* Previously we have explored the meanings of *wahɨ* as aspects of a general conception of health, and of *'ɨko,* which enables the shaman to transcend everyday reality. The concept *dau* completes the set, for it is an essential element in both the curing and causation of illness, and it is the basis of the shaman's power. Translating *dau* into an English term is difficult, for several different and often seemingly contradictory usages are attached to it. There are three different and specific usages of *dau:* (1) *dau* as a substance that grows within the shaman's body and embodies his knowledge and power, (2) *dau* as a concrete witchcraft substance, and (3) *dau* as sickness. Following this discussion, an interpretation of the word in its most general and abstract meaning is suggested.

When a man begins to drink *yagé,* it is said that a substance grows inside of him. This substance, called *dau,* embodies the knowledge and power gained from his experiences with the hallucinogen. It enables him to travel to the different realms of reality in order to contact and influence the spirits. Later, when he becomes a shaman, his accumulated *dau* gives him power to cure or to cause misfortune to others. From it comes the shaman's ability to induce visionary states with lesser stimulants, or to induce curing powers from the state of sweating. Without *dau,* he is "only a man."

There is no one particular location or structure of *dau* inside a person's body, rather it is dispersed throughout. However, a shaman's *dau,* at least part of it, may leave his body, and when it does it takes a particular material form, most commonly that of a dart, a stone, or a snake's tooth. Other forms include a "rotting substance," or a "black butterfly." When a shaman teaches an apprentice his visions and songs, he imparts some of his *dau* to him through showing the visions he knows.[2]

While the accumulation of *dau* means knowledge, and consequently power, it also means that the recipient must now be ever alert to protect himself against influences that could damage his *dau*. *Dau* is very sensitive or vulnerable and can easily be "damaged," which results in loss of knowledge. For this reason, the Siona often employ the term "delicate" to indicate that a man has reached the level of "one who leaves."

A man's *dau* may be damaged in several ways. Any woman who is menstruating, pregnant, or has given birth during the last three to five months has an odor that can damage his *dau*. If he passes near such a woman, or receives food prepared by her, he may suffer from headaches and body aches, and when he drinks *yagé,* he is likely to have a bad journey. Many Siona customs, including the menstrual hut and period of isolation of the parents during and after pregnancy, have the effect of protecting the men of the community possessing *dau*. *Dau* can also be damaged when one experiences a bad journey on *yagé* caused by other contamination or sorcery. The Siona who described such personal experiences said these were always followed by serious illness; treatment involved extirpation of their corrupted *dau,* and thus, a loss of knowledge. Finally, *dau* may also be damaged by a surprise encounter with a spirit while not under influence of the drug. One Siona elder has had several such experiences. In one, he was hunting in the jungle and heard a baby cry underneath the ground. He became deathly afraid, and returned home, unable to speak. That night he had an intensely high fever that made him delirious. His brother, a shaman, performed a curing ritual. He first chanted over several remedies, took the stimulant *yoco,* and performed a blowing ceremony designed to cleanse the patient's body of evil spirits.[3] When the ritual failed as a cure, the shaman drank the more efficacious *yagé*. Its vision revealed that a shaman from a neighboring group had sent the spirit to destroy the victim's *dau* in order to prevent him from becoming a great shaman. When the victim was cured by his brother, his *dau* was removed. The next time he drank *yagé,* all he saw was darkness, and he had to start from the beginning again to accumulate knowledge.

This case helps to explain why only a few men ever reach the level of master shaman. Journeys into the visionary realms might involve physical or mental accidents. Most bad journeys, and also frightening encounters with spirits, are followed by physical sickness. Moreover, the individual is haunted by painful memories. When "traveling," one may be plunged into the deep darkness of a moonless night. Evil spirits with long tongues and big ears approach the victim and attempt to tie him up. There is a struggle. If the spirits succeed, the victim will stay forever on the other side. He will die. In addition to such bad journeys, Siona men have had unsolicited spirit encounters, such as the one described in the previous paragraph, when walking in the jungle not under the influence of drugs. The jungle changes from this familiar reality to that of the spirit realm on the other side. Menacing spirits appear and try to trick the individual into eating rotten honey or drinking native beer so that he will never return to ordinary reality. Such occasions are described as extremely threatening to one's health and life. Listening to so many accounts of this kind, one wonders if these noninduced visionary experiences are perhaps a residual effect of frequent ingestion of hallucinogens. This would suggest that those who become master shamans are of a mental stability and strength of character that can withstand constant hallucinogenic experiences with no detrimental effects, while the others succumb in fright to the visionary experience. The master shaman maintains a sense of control on both sides of reality.

Dau not only gives the shaman the ability to contact the spirits for beneficial purposes, but also the power to do the opposite, to injure people. The shaman's *dau* enables him to "think ugly" of someone, causing some misfortune to befall the individual. This is due to the fact that the *dau,* which builds up in the shaman, has an existence somewhat independent of the intent and will of its possessor. The substance is only partially under conscious control and can cause harm without the shaman actually intending to act upon his angry thoughts. This is the double-edged aspect of *dau* that makes its possessor both respected and feared. *Dau* enables him to cure sickness and influence forces for the welfare of his people; it also empowers him to harm them, either consciously or unconsciously. One Siona narrative gives an account of a good shaman who would never look directly at people, for if he did, they might die. Although he did not wish to harm them, his *dau* was so powerful that it caused injury just by his glance. *Dau* may sometimes be so independent that it turns on its owner and strikes him. Thus, there is even a sadder story of another shaman who was very good to his people, but who unintentionally caused his father-in-law's death. In his attempt to find and punish the culprit through magical means, he unwittingly caused his own death. Because of this independent quality of *dau,* when a shaman dies it remains potent and continues to cause harm. Therefore, the *dau* should be removed from his body and sealed in a tree hole with beeswax, so that it does not remain at large, dangerous to the living.

When speaking about *dau* in its special sense as a witchcraft object, the Siona conceive of it as a physical object, which may be inside the shaman, flying toward the victim, or in the victim. When inside the shaman, the *dau* appears in the form of darts like those of the blowgun. His lower left arm serves as the "dart holder," and he shoots the darts at the victim through his middle finger. When he prepares a witchcraft weapon from the *dau* dispersed in his body, the Siona call it "working" or "weaving" the *dau.* He works it and throws it at the intended victim. Instead of a dart, the *dau* may become a rock, a rotting substance, a snake's tooth, or a black butterfly. When someone is suffering from a sickness caused by witchcraft, the *dau* then penetrates the victim in any of these concrete forms. Often the Siona conceive of the *dau* as sucking the blood of the victim. It may also be cooking the blood, or rotting the victim. If the individual is to be cured, the *dau* must be removed by a shaman.

The third meaning of *dau* is illness. In reply to the greeting, "Are you living?" a sick person will say, "I am dying of a *dau.*" In the beginning, a physical symptom or ailment may not be considered serious enough to be recognized as *dau.* It may only be regarded as some minor discomfort. Thus, the Siona recognize a class of ailments not considered *dau.* They are described by simply giving the location and predominant sympton, such as "it burns" for infections, "it hurts" for pains and cuts, and "it itches" for rashes. If the ailment does not disappear, or if it begins to take on the symptoms of a recognized sickness, then the Siona begin to speak of "dying from a *dau.*" This usage of *dau* does not necessarily refer to the magical substance inside the individual that is causing the condition. At first, *dau* is used in a loose metaphorical sense. However, within it is the implication that there may be a supernatural cause, and if so, there is a substance *dau* in the patient that must be removed if he is to recover. The usage of *dau* in this metaphorical sense to mean sickness, or in a specific sense to mean a supernatural substance, depends on the history of the illness and its response to treatment.

Supernatural causation may be immediately suspected in certain cases. Some named syndromes are associated with spirits, such as the "cough spirit," "flu spirit," and so forth. Also, severe or unusual symptoms, or illnesses marked by sudden onset, are indicative of supernatural causation. In such cases, a shaman is immediately contacted to perform a curing ritual with *yagé.* In most cases, however, the Siona will begin to administer nonhallucinogenic medicines that they believe will cure the illness. They may ask a shaman to chant over the preparation. If there is no response to treatment, then supernatural causation is suspected. First, *yoco* may be used in a ritual to divine the cause and cleanse the patient. If the supernatural cause is not strong, it is believed that this may be sufficient. If not, a shaman will be requested to perform a *yagé* ritual. Then specific medicines aimed at treating the physical symptoms will be administered again. If the disease does not respond, more *yagé* ceremonies are performed by shamans, several of whom might be consulted. Such treatments last for a month or more under each shaman. Treatments from other tribes may be resorted to, depending on the success or failure of the ones within the community.

When an illness has reached this stage, the term *dau* refers to a specific malevolent substance within the individual. The *dau* may come from a spirit or a shaman. In both cases, it is believed that the *dau* is eating the victim, causing rottenness inside. The *dau,* as a physical substance, must be removed from the patient if he is to be cured. Not every shaman can remove all kinds of *dau.* It is required that he possess sufficient *dau* to be able to see the mystical cause of the sickness *dau* and to overcome it, be it a spirit or a shaman. If it is a spirit, he must know the spirit's song and vision in order to bargain with him. If it is a shaman, he must possess more *dau* that the aggressor.

The Siona say that when the *dau* is removed, the shaman does so by sucking it out. They indicated that this *dau* is invisible to the normal person, but the shaman can see it. He examines it for the prognosis of the patient. If the *dau* is in the form of a rock or spine, he will determine how much is clear and how much is dark or rotten. The dark represents the victim's blood and rottenness. If the object is totally dark, it indicates that the victim will die. If only partially dark, the victim will live. (One informant made an analogy to my plastic ballpoint pen in which the clear sides allow one to see the dark line of ink inside. In *dau,* the dark line is the blood of the victim and the plastic the clear parts, indicating that the patient will live.) The *dau* in this form is a concrete manifestation of the dying force in the victim. It brings about the sickness and rottenness with which the hostile spirit or sorcerer intends to afflict the patient. It is not uncommon and is considered acceptable when the shaman says that the *dau* has been in the patient too long for him to survive the damage. To cure the patient, the Siona speak of "returning the *dau* to where it came from."

Although three different meanings of *dau* have been outlined here, it should not be implied that they are totally distinct in the minds of the Siona. *Dau* is knowledge, but not knowledge in its limited use in Western culture. It is knowledge that enables its possessor to influence the forces of the universe. Its most central manifestation is the shaman himself, the possessor of *dau,* who is able to travel in the other side of reality and show it to others. It is manifested in the curing power of medicine, used in its widest sense, and also as the *dau* of sickness. The various uses of the term indicate that *dau* is a key symbol for an important general conception of energy or power (Ortner 1973). The conception lying within the meanings of *dau* implies the potential energy source that powers the dynamic states of being, living, and dying. It is manifested in the shaman, in sorcery objects, or in sickness, and activated by *yagé.* The manner in which it becomes manifest and operative depends on various circumstantial factors, such as the knowledge, experience, and intentions of the shamans, the intentions of the spirits, and the compliance or noncompliance with mores involving pollution and purity.

THE QUEST FOR KNOWLEDGE

The shaman is the "master" in *yagé* visions, having superior knowledge and experience to lead the rest. However, the Siona elders consider it the duty of every man to learn as much as possible of the teachings of *yagé* in order to fulfill his duties as provider and protector of his family. To be a man is to be strong, and it is necessary to be strong to face the fears and dangers of the hallucinogen. Thus, in the past, most young men served as apprentices to shamans during their youth and attempted to learn as much as they could. Although women drink *yagé,* they do not have this obligation, since their primary responsibility is to give birth and to care for the family. The Siona say that although a woman actually learns faster than a man, the ingestion of large amounts of *yagé* by her on a regular and intense basis will cause sterility. The one woman shaman remembered by the elders is said to have begun her career after she had raised her family.

The knowledge gained by the drug is not definite and circumscribed, nor a single stage of enlightenment. If the comparison can be made, it is more like the aims of our educational system, with a series of subjects one may master, perhaps specializing in one or more. For the Siona shaman the subject matter to be mastered embraces visions, "designs," and songs. All the spirits have their own design, as well as songs, which they teach to the drinker once he sees them. Each apprentice attempts to know as many visions and songs as possible, for as he enlarges his repertoire, so he increases his power with the spirits he knows and can deal with.

Along the scale of knowledge, three classes of men are recognized: "Only a man," "one who has left," and "seer," reflecting three ascending stages of knowledge. "Only a man" is the ordinary individual or novice who has had little experience with the drug. "One who has left" has had the experience of leaving his body and of seeing some of the visions on the other side; he is also known as "singer." The "seer" or "one who sees" is the master shaman. Other designations for the master shaman include "jaguar" and "one who drinks." At each stage of knowledge, the individual is expected to go through a set of culturally anticipated visions (Langdon 1979b). The *yagé* experience is not one of individual random visions or free association of the unconscious while under the drug's influence. It is, rather, an ordering of the induced visions into culturally meaningful symbols and experiences, thus gaining increasing control over the visions and events occurring. The anticipated visions are well-known to the novice. Descriptions of them are part of traditional oral literature and are common conversational subjects among the Siona. Also, during the sessions, the participants are guided by the shaman in various ways. He indicates what will be seen by the class of *yagé* chosen for the preparation. When he "arranges" the *yagé,* he sings of the visions they are going to see. After he "tests" the brew, he continues to lead them through his songs. The songs are rather detailed. They include not only naming the spirits and places seen, but also

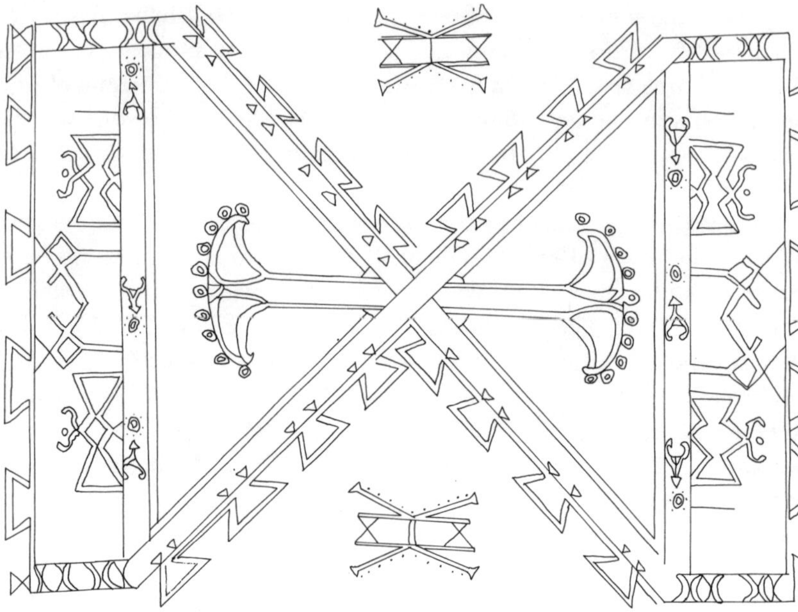

FIGURE 2.1. Siona design inspired by *yagé*. The original was drawn in twenty-four colors by Estanislao Yaiguaje.

naming the various abstract motifs and colors associated with each spirit (Langdon, in press). In the visions, these designs adorn the spirits' benches, cups, clothing, faces, and houses. In this reality, they appear on the painted faces of the elders, on pottery (particularly on that used during the *yagé* ceremony), and on other decorated artifacts. Thus, the motifs are familiar to all the Siona. The colors are those of the brightly colored plants, birds, insects, and animals of the jungle, although they maintain that no natural colors approach the brilliance of the hues in the visions. This is not to say that the shaman describes all details; according to the informants, he gives an outline of the significant features he is seeing, and each individual then elaborates variations depending on the extent to which he is being affected by the drug and the knowledge that he has of the visions.

The culturally anticipated visions do not come automatically, nor

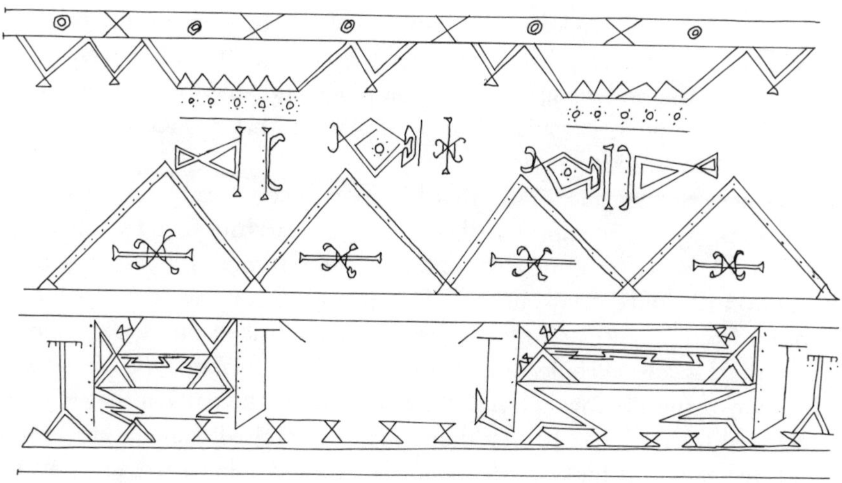

FIGURE 2.2. *Yagé*-inspired design. The original was also drawn in twenty-four colors by Estanislao Yaiguaje.

without suffering. The serious novice must devote several months of preparation in order to change his status from "only a man" to "one who has left." As early as ten or younger he may have ingested *yagé*, but such occasions are considered only as preliminary for the period of rigorous and intensive apprenticeship. Sometime between puberty and the early twenties, before beginning sexual relations, the youth contacts a shaman he trusts and requests that he show him his "designs." The shaman then instructs him in the proper way to prepare himself. The youth isolates himself in the jungle with three or four companions who are also ready to begin. They are not allowed to enter the populated areas of the community, mainly due to the risk of contamination from women. Sexual relations are prohibited. Only the mother can serve food to her son, while he cleanses himself through a special diet and a series of emetics, purges, and baths. The diet consists of green plantains, small fish, and the meat of certain birds. Sweets, ripe plantains (which are sweet), and most meats are prohibited. The novice takes emetics daily for a month or more. The Siona use *yagé* leaves as their principal emetic, although they know of others used by closely related tribes. One purpose of the emetics is to cleanse the body so that when one finally drinks *yagé,* he "leaves" immediately and sees the visions. As explained by one informant, the body is lighter after the purge and able to travel farther. Also, one eliminates contaminating substances that attract the wrong spirits when drinking *yagé.*

When the shaman decides that his apprentice is ready, he begins to give him *yagé.* It is expected that during at least the first two nights, which the Siona speak of as "two houses," the novice will pass through a period of "only drunkenness." This period, according to Siona lore, comes from preancestral times when the stars walked the earth as men and the Pleiades People first drank *yagé* on this earth. The youngest brother of the Pleiades, playing the trickster, set the pattern that is still followed today. When he first drank *yagé,* he vomited, fainted, urinated, and defecated on himself. He "went crazy" and rubbed the feces over his head and clothes, finally fainting from dizziness.[4] The Moon also went through a similar experience when he learned from the Sun, his grandfather. And thus it is expected of man. The Siona must also cry out, vomit, fall out of their hammocks, and soil themselves if they wish to learn from *yagé.* The novice must be willing, and have the strength to endure this unpleasantness.

It is expected that by the third night the apprentice will pass through the craziness stage and begin to see the visions. The principal characteristic of this stage is one of fear. It serves as a test to the novice, to see if he is strong enough to travel in the spirit world. One must be "strong" to drink *yagé.* Many do not pass this test. In the first visions encountered, there is a pervasive fear of death and destruction. All of the informants have described the following experience with a few individual variations.

First, the novice sees a huge fire burning everything in its path. It moves toward him, threatening to consume him also. The *'ɨko* People begin to descend, crying and telling him that he is going to die. The fire then becomes a huge grinding machine that grinds everything in sight as it moves toward the person. The novice even sees himself ground up and thrown out in pieces. Snakes appear and wrap around him. At any point, the apprentice may succumb to these fearful sights and "go crazy," screaming and crying since he cannot face the fear of death. The shaman will chant over him, blow tobacco smoke, and bring him back to this side. If he faces the frightening visions, a tall woman dressed in white with large drooping breasts appears. She is the Jaguar Mother, mother of all creatures considered to be jaguars, including the shamans. She is also called the *Yagé* Mother. She gathers the apprentice up in her arms as he becomes a small baby. She wraps a long cloth with beautiful designs around and around him and gives her breast for him to suck. The novice sucks, but suddenly he is thrown out by her and, once again, faced with death. She begins to cry and tell him that he is going to die. "Why did you drink the *yagé?*" she asks, "For now you are going to die. Look, there is your coffin. There are all your things arranged for your death, your beads, the *chambira* you were weaving for a hammock. You will never see your family again." Hundreds of small snakes appear, which the Siona say are the leaves of the *yagé* vine on this side. These snakes then merge into one, the Drinking Stick Snake, which is designated as the "owner" of the *yagé.*[5] Since the shaman is also considered the owner, the snake is perhaps considered a transformation of the shaman. At first he is very sinuous, and may wrap all around the person, causing again the fear of death. But the snake straightens out and takes the apprentice into the other realms. With this vision, the apprentice has passed the initial test and will now begin to travel to the other realms. He is now "one who has left." Through the mystical death, he has been transformed from "only a man" to a child of the Jaguar Mother, spirit parent of all shamans.

The apprentice is now ready to learn all that the shaman has to show him, provided no bad experiences occur during his training. He remains with the shaman, isolated in the forest for two to four months, drinking *yagé* almost continuously. They drink three to four nights consecutively until the apprentice learns to see the particular visionary realm and spirits the shaman wishes to show. After a rest of a night or so, they resume drinking to see another realm and other beings. It generally takes two to three "houses" or nights for the apprentice to see the designated visions clearly, to arrive at the house of the spirits, and to learn the accompanying songs. Through a sequence of journeys, the apprentice hopes to arrive at the house of God and become a master shaman. The following is a summary of a number of such visions as seen by those traveling on the "other side."

Once the *yagé* snake begins to straighten out, he moves forward in a slow rhythmic motion with the drone of a heavy motor. The apprentice mounts the snake so that he can be carried to the other realms. The snake first takes him inside the river. The *Yagé* People accompany him and explain each scene as it slowly passes. The voyager visits the house of the Anaconda, the houses of the River People, and the houses of other spirits and beings there. During the journey, the *Yagé* People continue to explain all that he is seeing. Later, in other sessions, the snake will take him to the end of the world, where the great water tube connects the first heaven with the second heaven. If he is progressing in his knowledge, the apprentice will journey up that tube into heaven. One informant reported that when he arrived at the water tube, the Metal Saint People told him that he had to take out his intestines to go up in the tube. When asked how he responded he replied, "Half thinking, there were my intestines floating in the lake, and I went up." In the visionary realm, he easily left his innards to travel to the next level. When arriving in heaven, one sees the Sun People dancing around their "maypole." They introduce themselves to the Siona as the Tender (*wahɨ*) Sun People. The voyager may be asked to clean the Sun's huge mirror, which is all dirty and clouded over with the excrement of the cicada that comes in the summer of August. They give him cotton and the milky sap used in the *yagé* ritual to clean the mirror. The voyager cleans the mirror, a process which turns winter into summer on earth.

During other nights of visions, the apprentice journeys to other "house sites" in the different realms of heaven, always being led by the shaman who "knows the vision" and is willing to show him. He may go to the house of the Thunder Being, to the Earthquake Tapir, to the houses of the animals, or to other places. He is instructed in different curing visions when he visits the spirits of different illnesses. When he journeys to the house of the Jaguar, the Jaguar Women appear, resembling beautifully painted human women. They call the master shaman "husband" and treat him as master of their house, giving him and the novice food and drink as they rest in hammocks.

After the initial period of training and isolation, the apprentice returns to his home, but maintains sexual abstinence for a year or more. He often serves as one of the shaman's assistants in the ceremonies and continues his study as far as he wishes or is able. He may also visit other shamans, including those of other tribes, so that his knowledge grows beyond that of the original teacher. Generally the period of apprenticeship lasts from one to two years.

The visions form a graduated series in which some are more difficult to achieve than others. For instance, only the most advanced shaman can go to the Moon. One informant told me that he saw it "from a distance," but that he did not have the ability to get close. Only the most advanced may enter the house of dead shamans. The less advanced will never return to this side after entering. Also, the top layer of the heaven, the little metal heaven, is only visited by the most learned. Like any true learning process, it never ends for a shaman as he tries to continually enhance his power and knowledge. Thus, not every shaman has the same knowledge. Individual shamans specialize in different aspects of the art. For instance, some shamans specialize in the visions of hunting and contacting the spirits of animals. Others specialize in seeing certain beings in the heavens, such as Thunder, Sun, or Moon, and others in curing sickness. In the field of curing, there is also specialization. A shaman is capable of curing those diseases for which he knows the responsible spirits and the proper songs. Of course, all apprentices seek to go as far as possible with their knowledge, but they do not all have the same opportunities, abilities, or strength.

The discussion here has focused upon Siona cosmogony and their quest to discover and influence the ultimate forces of the universe. Shamanism has been described as a quest for knowledge, and knowledge has been described as power.

In this description, the shaman is a living embodiment of power, for he possesses *dau,* and uses it for the benefit and detriment of others. He is the central figure in the quest for meaning, for he mediates between ordinary humans and the ultimate forces. In particular, his importance as mediator is underscored through his leadership of communal rituals. Because of the dangers that journeys to the other side pose, all rituals require the presence and leadership of a master shaman. In the past, Siona rituals were held regularly for the benefit of the entire community. Even though they are now only performed sporadically, they are still viewed as essential for continued well-being. The rituals fulfill the functions as elaborated upon by Geertz (1966, 1973b). They are a dramatic symbolic presentation of the key conceptions of Siona religion, and the use of hallucinogens makes them a particularly powerful experience, fusing the imagined and commonsense realities of the Siona worldview. Under the effects of the hallucinogen, what happens on this side of reality is a pale reflection of what is seen on the other side. This visionary

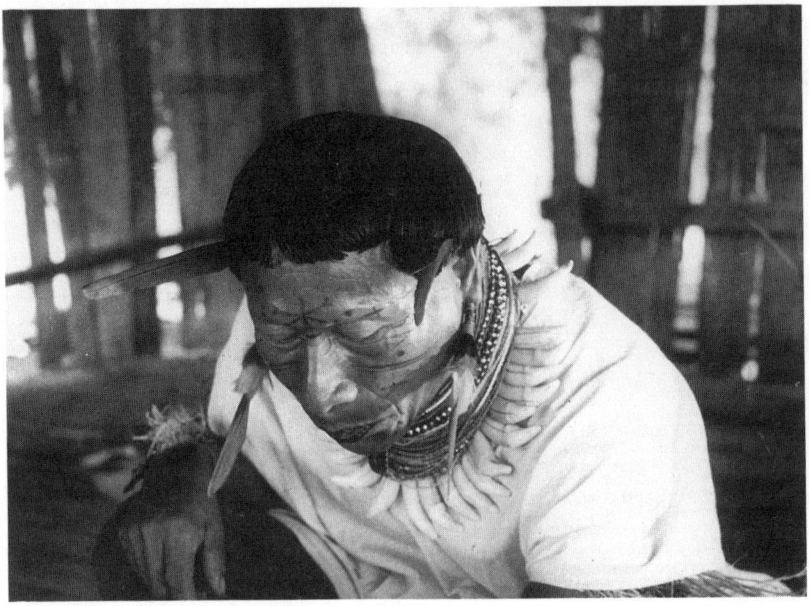

FIGURE 2.3. Siona shaman performing a curing ceremony. (Photograph by Carlos Garibello Aldana)

reality is experienced with the "aura of factuality" Geertz describes as essential to the ritual experience (Langdon 1979a).

Although not discussed here, the presence of master shamans, and the continual performance of ritual throughout three hundred years of contact with missionaries and traders, enabled the Siona to maintain their distinct identity and worldview. In addition, the shaman as a human embodiment of power, and as mediator between the two realities, emerged as the key figure in Siona social organization (Langdon 1985). After initial contact with the Spanish, the Siona experienced significant depopulation and social disorganization. From this, the shaman emerged not only as the religious leader, but also as the political leader of the community. Other leadership roles that might have existed prior to the conquest and been documented for the Eastern Tukanoans disappeared

(S. Hugh-Jones 1979). The shaman became the leader in all aspects of sacred and secular life, with no other leadership role to rival his until permanent occupation of Siona territory by whites.

NOTE ON TRANSCRIPTION (SIONA)

The sign ɨ represents a central closed vowel situated between *i* and *u*. ' represents the voiceless glottal consonant. Nasalization is represented with a ~ disposed over the vowels.

Notes

1. The data on which this work is based were gathered during twenty-two months of fieldwork in Colombia from 1970–1973, and the summer of 1980. The study was supported in part by the Tulane University International Center for Medical Research grant A1–10050 from NIAID, NIH, U.S. Public Health Service, and in part by a traineeship from USPHS, Grant 5 T01 MH–08554 with Dr. J. L. Fischer, Director.

2. Harner (1972, 119–21) indicates that the Jivaro have a similar concept of *dau,* which they call *tsentsak.* During the apprenticeship, the shaman actually passes from his mouth into that of the apprentice an object that is said to be the *tsentsak* and a symbol of his knowledge and power. For the Jivaro this object is in limited quantity within the shaman's body, and thus, in imparting it to the novice, he reduces his own knowledge and power, which must be rebuilt. This does not seem to be the case for the Siona. I have no evidence that they consider the quantity to be reduced when the shaman imparts his knowledge.

3. *Yoco* is a mild stimulant that is believed to yield visions for a shaman, although not for nonshamans. It is often used in minor healing ceremonies before *yagé* is employed.

4. One cannot help but note the similarity between this old Siona myth and Carlos Castaneda's first encounter with peyote (1968).

5. Siskind (1973b, 140) describes the small snakes and the large snake, symbolic of the vine, as part of the early Sharanahua visions. See Mallol de Recasens (1963) and Mallol de Recasens and de Recasens (1964–65) for other accounts about Siona visions and the presence of snakes.

THREE

THE CONCEPT OF NIHUE AMONG THE SHIPIBO-CONIBO OF EASTERN PERU

BRUNO ILLIUS

When dealing with health, the Shipibo-Conibo of eastern Peru are principally concerned with *nihue,* the individual essence of an animal or plant. It is cited as the most common cause of illness and is of central concern to all medical practitioners. These include the shamans, called vine drinkers, or healers, as well as *vegetalistas,* and bone-setters who apply massages and hot baths. In Caimito, where this research was conducted, there are three major shamans who drink the hallucinogen *ayahuasca* (*Banisteriopsis* sp.).[1] The visions and songs quoted in this work were made by them.

Nihue is a complex concept involving the native theory of individual essences and cannot be easily translated. It means "wind" in everyday usage. The ethnographic literature translates names for similar phenomena in other Latin American societies as bad air (*mal aire*), or evil winds (*vientos maléficos*). "Individual essence" is a term coined by Arbmann (1931, 365) and most aptly chosen by Fischer (1965, 309, 310) to replace "soul substance," "soul stuff," and similar vague and unsatisfactory names. "Individual essence" prevents confusion or unjustified connections with concepts of soul, and, more appropriate in our case, avoids misleading associations with weather phenomena, which are its cause or transmitter in only a few cases. Furthermore, it does not imply any inappropriate moral judgments.

Under the influence of *ayahuasca,* the Shipibo shaman sees *nete,* a "thin hull of light," around living beings. With plants and animals this luminous hull or aura is always called *nihue* and has a specifically identified individual quality, such as color, smell, consistency, and so forth. In the case of humans, it is referred to by two terms, the above mentioned *nete,* and *shinan.* Although seemingly interchangeable, each term has its own specific meaning.

Nete alludes to the aura's shining quality. This quality is initially colorless or neutral but is always influenced or colored by the properties of substances or beings that its bearer approaches or contacts through touching, inhaling, or ingestion. When the amount of those alien essences is limited in a human's body and their qualities are in balance (neutralizing their powers), their bearer is in a state of equilibrium, or health.

Shinan in daily use means thought, reason, idea, or will. With reference to health, it connotes a being's share of an "impersonal vital power" (Fischer 1965, 314). Designating both physical and mental power of a human, it can be judged from the intensity of the being's *nete.* With healthy and strong individuals, it may culminate in a crown, which is a nimbus, indicating the bearer's *shinan* (power) by its size and brightness. Thus, *nete* (light) and *shinan* (power) cannot be thought of without each other. Together with different *nihues* in a being, they constitute what could tentatively be called the "accumulated essence of man."

Nihue (individual essence) is also a cause of serious illnesses attributable to witchcraft. When a shaman is offended, he indirectly sends harm to his intended victim by sending his spirit helpers to cast their *nihue* on him. Such shamans are acting as sorcerers and are called *yotomis* "ones who use to bewitch." When we indiscreetly ask a shaman the cause and nature of a particular case of illness, he most often answers, "He's caught bad *nihue!*" or, "It comes from *nihue,*" without identifying the source. This information is as precise as, "He got infected." One shaman, in fact, tried to help convey the meaning of the term *nihue* by comparing it with a "cloud of bacteria."

Since *nihue* has a variety of origins, qualities, intensities, and effects, its particular source must be diagnosed by a shaman. Based on his knowledge of the case history and circumstances of the sickness, he discovers the particular *nihue* causing the illness through *ayahuasca*-induced visions. As one shaman said, "The spirit of the *ayahuasca* vine shows me which spirt (*yoshin*) has poisoned the patient, and he tells me how to fight it." Through *ayahuasca,* the shaman sees the *nihue,* the qualities of which indicate its origin and proper treatment.

Although anyone may drink *ayahuasca,* it is necessary to train for a year or so in order to obtain visions for curing purposes. The training, or *dieta,* lasts at least a year and involves isolation, food taboos, prescriptions for bathing, celibacy, and other norms. The novice drinks *ayahuasca* and tobacco mixed with at least one other plant, normally a hallucinogen. The spirit of the *ayahuasca* vine serves as one of his advisers, and the apprentice is considered the master of tobacco. The third plant provides an additional auxiliary spirit.

As is common to many shamanic systems of this region, the training also involves the passing and accumulation of a substance that symbolizes knowledge gained through visions and training. For the Shipibo-Conibo, this substance is called *quenyon,* and it is materialized in phlegm. It is passed from the master shaman to the novice a few weeks after the training is initiated. The beginner sucks phlegm from the mouth of his master who has swallowed a great deal of tobacco smoke to bring it up from where it is accumulated in his chest. The novice does this nightly for a week. The phlegm first accumulates in the novice's stomach, where it is believed to be potentially harmful. To make it rise to the chest and remain there, he drinks tobacco water and swallows tobacco smoke. If the phlegm rises to the mouth, the novice must swallow it. Several precautions are taken to retain the phlegm within the novice, not allowing it to leave his mouth, nor to pass through other orifices. Thus, the education is centered around the handing over and preservation of pure and strong *quenyon,* or phlegm. It is said to be a sticky substance (sometimes a paste, or dough), and is thought to absorb and store *nihue.* It thus constitutes a kind of temporary container and carrier for *nihue.* In the case of sorcerers, their phlegm is said to be embedded with little arrows or chonta palm thorns, which are loaded in the phlegm with the *nihue* of diseases.

Also important to curing is the learning of songs, called *huehua, mashá,* or *icaros* (see Luna, chapter 10, this volume). These melodies paint beautiful linear designs, called *quené,* on the entire surface of the patient's body in order to restore health. The sick person's designs are distorted and must be restored to return to health. These songs, which are alleged to have healing powers themselves, provide reliable data for the shaman's covert performance and the meanings of his overt performance. During the curing sessions, he sings a number of these songs and undertakes a number of measures that aim to free his client from harmful *nihue* (see table 3.1). The shaman strives to ultimately strengthen his client's *shinan,* thus enabling him to hold a dream ego, called *caya,* whose final loss would result in death.[2]

Techniques are also performed to suck out illness, which, at times, involves the production of phlegm by the shaman. However, this technique is not central to our discussion here.

The following curing vision related by a Caimito shaman illustrates how they identify the *nihue* responsible for the illness. The curing song that follows was sung by another shaman; the song describes the *nihue* and how it should be treated.[3]

> What I saw last night was quite common, just a normal vision one could say. This is how it was: When I drink *ayahuasca,* the dangerous spirits (*yoshinbo*) come and try to kill me with their weapons. They have spears, arrows, and pistols, and I have to run and hide. I am always quite scared. They are numerous and have many weapons. But after a while, I can call my jaguars, which chase away the dangerous spirits.[4] I have a fast fire, too, which is burning like spilt kerosene, when I light it with my pipe. As the *yoshinbo* all prefer the cold, you can easily deter them with burns. Many doctors come to me, *sanitarios,* bringing many medicines. Beautiful white women come, nurses.[5] I hear *yoshinbo* sing, I also sing, I sing along with them.[6] Just like the father and the husband of Ronin Samé [the main patient of the night before] have sung with me, I usually sing with my (helper) *yoshinbo.* My singing is keeping away (dangerous) *yoshinbo,* as a weapon would. While I sing, they don't approach. (This is why one must not interrupt singing for too long a time.) The doctors are the men of the *ayahuasca* vine, they tell me everything. The *yoshinbo* of the trees I drank in my *dieta* also come and tell me by whom and why my patient has been attacked.[7] Sometimes the very *yoshin* who made him sick appears and he has to tell me everything. When I see a white *nihue,* the *yoshin* of the lupuna tree comes and speaks: "This man has urinated on my stem, so I couldn't do other than lay my *nihue* upon him." Or maybe he will say, "This man was leaning against a lupuna, so the lupuna *nihue* is sticking to him." But you don't

TABLE 3.1. Fifteen Treatments of *Nihue* According to Thirty Curing Songs.

Treatment Number	Frequency of Appearance	Shipibo Term[a] for the Shaman's[b] Action	Meaning in Respect to the Nihue[c]	Word Number and Meaning from von den Steinen's 1904 Dictionary[d]
1	39	choro-ti	to loosen to untie to unwind	3610: Churuqui—Desatar, Desplegar
2	33	soa-ti	to wipe away to rub off to wipe clean	4985: Suai—Rascar Suati—Ynstrumento para rascarse
3	28	queyó-ti	to put an end to something by distributing it or scattering it	4654: Queyoqui—Acabarse de consumir ó distribuir algo
4	14	bota-ti	to throw away	4542: Putaqui—Botar
5	8	matso-ti	to sweep away to sweep out	4069: Madzuqui—Barrer 4070: Madzuti—Escoba
6	5	toe-ti	to break into pieces to crack	5170: Tuequi—Rajar 5174: Tueyamaue—No lo rajes ó quiebras
7	4	bo-ti	to carry away	3348: Buqui, buai—Llevar
8	3	choqué-ti	to wash off	3595: Chuquequi—Lavar todo lo que no es ropa
9	3	quepen-ti	to open	4613: Quepuenqui—Abrir puerta
10	3	queyá ati	to lift to throw up high	4574: Queyá—Alto, altura
11	2	nacho-ti	to cleanse the inside of something from	4194: Nachuqui—Lavar basija por dentro
12	2	paque ati	to make something fall down	4397: Paquete, paquetai—Caer de alto
13	2	pishá-ti	to loosen to detach	4458: Pisaqui—Despegar algo
14	2	reene-ti	to grind	4776: Rennequi—Moler en batan
15	2	shete-ti	to break off	4912: Secquequi—Quebrarse, quebrar palo ó hierro

a—"predicate"
b—the "subject's"
c—"object"
d—The discrepancy between my translation and that of the Franciscan friar, whose manuscripts are the basis of von den Steinen's *Diccionario sipibo* may be because it was not easy to distinguish transitive from intransitive verbs definitively in the 1880s. This is not a problem today due to the excellent work of Norma Faust (1973).

need to touch *nihue.* There is the *nihue* of the Great Boa for example, which is magnetic and can be caught from a distance.[8] There are more *yoshinbo* present, but they don't act or speak, nor do they disturb me. When a patient has been bewitched by one who has studied black magic from a book, I see books and many papers falling from heaven, like leaves in a storm.[9] But all that is visible for short moments only, just like the pictures of a movie in the Pucallpa cinema. During all that, the sick man is lying in front of me in a circle of light (*nete*), as if he was illuminated by a big lamp. I feel safe and strong, since the smoke and my crown protect me. In the end, all gets weaker and fades, like a passing drunkenness from beer. Then I sing aloud . . . *mashá, huehua* . . .

A mashá curing song

1. The *nihue* of the lupuna *yoshin,*
2. I surely shall loosen it.
3. Its plant-like smelling *nihue,*
4. its saliva-like *nihue,* its white saliva *nihue,*
5. its whirling *nihue,*
6. its hot *nihue,*
7. I shall carry it away right now.

In reference to the curing song, the lupuna tree has one of the mightiest and thus most dangerous spirits known to the Shipibo. Many serious sicknesses are traced back to one or a few of its pathogenic *nihues.* One of those *nihues* is perceived by and named after its smell (line 3), another one by its color and consistency (line 4), one by its movement (line 5), and a last one according to its temperature (line 6).

Most songs, like the previous one, contain information about the dangerous spirit of a plant or animal and its *nihue* responsible for the sickness, as well as information about the *nihue*'s appearance and its treatment. We could also say that the songs supply information about an examination of the patient, the shaman's diagnosis (given here in lines 1 and 3 through 6), and a therapy (hinted at in verses 2 and 7).[10]

To get a better impression of the shaman's analysis let us look at another example made by a shaman as to how he sees *nihue:*

> [Having drunk *ayahuasca,* sitting in front of a patient] . . . it will be different, depending upon the case: If, for example, the [sick person's] body is all yellow, he has been poisoned by the air, coming from the bubbles in the mud on the shore. If there is black smoke ascending, as if

> oil was burned, then a death spirit has attacked. If the body appears whitish-yellowy, and the person has a whitish stool looking like dirty soapy water, then I know that a dolphin has poisoned my patient.[11] I'll blow smoke upon the crown of his head where it will enter and drive out the bad *nihue* at his other end. Sometimes you can hear it: a fart. When the Great Boa's *nihue* has struck the patient, it is seen as the snake itself wound around his body, its head lying upon the belly with a quivering tongue, wanting to scare me. It has cold *nihue,* caracho! All snakes, turtles and water spirits have this; in such a case I'll sing of water. Sometimes, a tree has poisoned a child; in most cases it's the lupuna tree. White smoke appears, the *shono josho nihue*. But a lupuna is damn dangerous: it also has three more *nihues.* So strong it is! Trees always come personally (their spirits look like "little men"). They are standing besides the sick, and I see (in the case of lupuna) white smoke floating down upon the child. . .

Table 3.2 lists and classifies the most frequently diagnosed *nihues* according to their properties.

Generally, *nihues* are not harmful under all circumstances, although a few are always harmful. Most only become pathogenic in a high dosage, or when one is in contact with them or exposed to them for a certain length of time. Age, constitution, and nutrition may make a person more or less resistant or prone to *nihue.* Pork is quite *itsa* but a small quantity won't harm a healthy adult, whereas the cayman's strong *itsa nihue* is dangerous to anybody. The *itsa nihue* of onions, tobacco, or kerosene (which can be administered in small dosages) are carefully applied as medicines.

A person may carry less pathogenic *nihues* within himself: the plant *nihue* of a melon he has just eaten, the *itsa nihue* from his own sweat or the tobacco he smoked, or some hot or cold *nihue,* depending on whether he has just come back from a fishing trip or has been idly lying in his house.

During his education and before every healing session a shaman tries to get rid of those various *nihues* by proscribed conduct and nutrition. A strong *nihue* might weaken his *shinan* or repel one of his spirit helpers. One exception is the *nihue* of tobacco, which pleases all potentially helpful spirits and can be used against any harmful *nihue.*

Seeing a *nihue* is similar for all shamans: the *nihue* of the lupuna tree is always described as white, the *nihue* of the catahua tree as yellow, and so on. The simultaneous appearance of the tree's anthropomorphous

TABLE 3.2. *Nihue* Sources and Classification of *Nihue* Properties.

Consistency		Smell				Light, Colors					Motion		Temperature		Preliminary categories
resin-like *bepon*	saliva-like *huishton*	putrid *pisi*	blood-like *bia*	plant-like *jansho*	earthy/fiery *itsa*	black *huiso*	red *joshin*	yellow *panshin*	blue *yancon*	white *josho*	glistening *sahui*	whirling *maya*	hot *shana*	cold *matsi*	Name of the *nihue* / *Nihue* sources
		X												X	papaya (*Carica papaya*)
				X										X	juicy fruits
					X										onions
	X			X	X					X		X	X		lupuna (*Ceiba pentandra*)
X								X			X		X		catahua tree
		X													rotten plants
		X	X												white heron (*Casm. alb.*)
		X			X										vulture (*Coragyps atr.*)
				X									X		tapirs (*terr. et pinch.*)
				X									X		cow
					X										pigs
				X										X	manati (*Trichechus m.*)
			X	X	X										cayman
			X			X								X	nutria (*Myocastor c.*)
			X	X											dolphin (*Inia geofro.*)
														X	turtles
														X	snakes
			X								X	X		X	Great Boa (Spirit Anaconda)
			X												fish of prey
			X												stingray
		X	X												dead animals
				X											sperm
		X		X											newborns
		X	X												menstrual blood
				X											mother's milk
		X		X											farts, feces
		X													rotten flesh
					X	X								X	death spirit
								X							shore bubbles
												X		X	water spirits
												X		X	river *pozos*
												X		X	whirlwinds
														X	night air
X							X	X	X	X			X		rainbow
					X										kerosene

spirit differs from shaman to shaman. The spirit of a plant or animal acts as an individual, as does a man's dream ego. This is one reason why one could say that *nihue* must have some physical basis; however, its "dramatization" may be a different one with each shaman. Some shamans see certain spirits dressed and acting like Indians, whereas others see the same spirits as "viracochas," white men. In one session for example, both shamans first perceived the *nihue* of a cayman by its smells, and then each dramatized it individually; one saw a cayman lying upon the patient's body; the other saw the tail of a cayman protruding from the patient's mouth.

Reports of *ayahuasca* visions indicate that a vision has fixed elements, which are chemically stimulated and, to a fairly high degree, culturally conditioned. A vision also has a variable part, the "dramatization," which is mostly culturally conditioned, and which includes the shaman's individual explanations and embellishment of his adventures.

The previously mentioned song of the lupuna tree gives two hints at a therapy for *nihue:* to "loosen it" and to "carry it away." In thirty songs, some of them consisting of nearly a hundred verses, fifteen ways are mentioned showing how the shaman can treat *nihues.* These are presented in table 3.1 with their frequencies of occurrence.

What is easily noticed, and seems most significant, is that none of these treatment terms describes a final annihilation of *nihue;* it is only "taken away" from the sick body. The term *queyó-ti* (3) is doubtlessly the most revealing one, since it also relates what happens to the *nihue* after it has been removed: it is scattered or distributed. Often *queyó-ti* is combined with one or two of the other terms, such as, ". . . having loosened (1) it [the *nihue*], I shall put an end to it by distributing it. . ." Or, "I shall break it off (15), and then put an end to it by distributing it. . ." [And,] "Right now, I shall grind it (14), and then put an end to it, scattering it. . ."

Through his visible and invisible paraphernalia and auxiliary spirits, the shaman treats *nihue* and restores the distorted ornaments or designs of the sick body. The meaning of the first treatment term, *choro-ti,* "to unwind," refers to the shaman's treatment of the distorted ornaments. These actions of the treatment of *nihue,* and the restoring of body designs are described throughout the healing songs, and this is further demonstrated by the excerpts that follow. Beginning this sampling is one shaman's standard stanza, which contains the three terms used most often. It is usually sung in the beginning of a session and is sometimes inserted into other songs with only slight variations.

1. With my great power, [original text: *podero*]
2. with my great *shinan,* [shaman: "this is my *podero*"]
3. I shall soon put an end to the spirit *nihue* by distributing it. [term (3)]
4. With the power of God, [original text: *dios-en podero*]
5. I shall heal this body right now.
6. With my great medicine [shaman: ". . . my medicine is *ayahuasca* and my *shinan*"]
7. I shall loosen the *nihue* [term (1)] from the culminating points of the body.
8. Blowing vigorously with my great tobacco,
9. I am putting an end to it, scattering it. [term (3)]
10. Then I shall wipe the body clean. [term (2)]

To punctuate his singing, the shaman rhythmically shakes a bundle of leaves like a rattle. It is his "drum," and at the same time it is counteracting bad *nihue* with its scents. The bundle is made with the leaves of a fragrant shrub, *huiroro* (*Ocimum micranthum* W.), or of a nettle, *ishanka* (*Urea caracasanum,* or *Laportea* sp.). The nettle has an additional effect, as the following song demonstrates:

> With its sharp and pointed teeth, with its many little hooks, it will grasp the *nihue* and throw it away; oh it is good at throwing, my *ishanka,* my medicine *ishanka!*

The shaman may brush the bundle slightly against the patient. Sometimes he stretches his arm over the patient's body and wags his hand to the right and left, singing:

> My staff with the boa designs, I'm swinging it. I give out blows like lightning, and then can wipe away the strong *nihue.*[12]
>
> With my mighty metal broom, my broom with golden stripes of designs, my hissing broom, I shall put a thorough end to the *nihue* in this body, scattering it all, and my good songs, my mighty songs, they will straighten out the designs on the body.

After two or three songs, the shaman clasps his hands around the patient's arms, legs, and body and performs pulling movements, as if he was stripping pieces of cloth from the limbs. Then he slaps his hands together, while turning his back to the patient. One shaman at the edge of the house platform was seen sweeping his garment with the bundle of leaves, singing:

> With the glistening *nihue* broom, the ayahuasca *nihue* broom, we [he and his auxiliary spirits] shall sweep, sweep, sweep. . . Sweeping, let's put an end to the sickness, scattering it.

After the song he stood in front of the patient, and, holding the corners of his clothing, he vehemently fanned the entire group present. He later explained that he was "fanning all detached *nihue* away."

The Caimitoan shamans have spirit helpers known as the Inca People, who are said to inhabit one of several towns above the clouds, where shamans receive advice and medicines and can recharge power (*shinan*) by absorbing some of the abundant light (*nete*) there. They possess impressive equipment and weaponry, such as metal tools, machine guns (referred to as cannons), and other modern machinery, which they use for the benefit of the Shipibo. There are also chiliastic expectations to be noticed among the Shipibo, wherein the Inca play a leading role. The Inca's aid and weaponry permeate many curing songs.

> My Inca king, with his million people, slowly approaches while we sing. From his big cannon, from the mouth of his cannon, come fiery balls, wiping away everything.
>
> The spirit's songs, the songs of the witch doctor's bird *shane,* I'll loosen them; I really will. Their strongest songs, I'll crack them with the Inca's steel.

In the latter passage, the shaman identifies the sorcerer as a mestizo by referring to the bird *shane,* which is used as a euphemism for mestizo people. Just as the shaman's songs are painting a beautiful, good ornament on the patient's body, the spirits' songs are destroying the ornament by entangling the body and applying bad *nihue.*

Another method to take away the body ornaments ruined by spirit songs and *nihue* is described in the following:

> I shall take them [the ornaments] away with my *torno*.
>
> I shall unwind them from the body and wind them up on the *torno*. Unwind them and wind them up, unwind them. . .

The *torno* is a rotating rope-making device, twisting together three cords or more and reeling up the produced rope.

Shamans also employ modern weapons:

> I just put my dynamite there and make it blow up the *nihue*.
>
> Tiri! Tsarara! It is breaking to pieces the most serious *nihue*.

The *nihue* of the Great Boa has, among other qualities, electrifying and magnetizing power. Singing for patients struck by such *nihues,* two shamans were quick to make the tape recorder a means to their ends and sang:

> Those *nihue,* whirling mightily inside [the patient's body], this big machine is taking them away right now.
>
> With the electric power of the mighty machine, I shall loosen the *nihue*. With the steel, curving shiningly [i.e., the tape spools] I shall loosen it.

"Electricity" and "electric" are sometimes rendered in Spanish, but mostly the syllable *rin* is used to represent the sound of electricity, which is said to be heard when it is released from somewhere. Two Caimito shamans command a boa, who assists them with this kind of energy:

> I can break the *nihue* with my steel, while it [my boa] is making *rin,* my metal boa, making a sudden *rin,* while winding itself.
>
> It is lying in the town of the Inca, the metal boa is lying there. I make her give out a sparkling *rin,* and we put a thorough end to the *nihue,* scattering it.

There is one more boa competent for *nihue:*

> The bamboo boa, having little teeth on its tongue, it makes *re-re-re-re-re,* while meandering over the body. Making this, it is grinding the *nihue,* and we put an end to it. Let me sweep it away. . .

The constant singing and rattling with leaves is sometimes interrupted to blow tobacco smoke over the sick person's head or whole body:

> The *nihue* he has brought here, the *nihue* the spirit has brought, I'll put an end to it by distributing it. Right now, I'll do that with my thick tobacco smoke.

Covering the patient all over with a protecting veil of tobacco smoke (i.e., a final fumigation with good *nihue*) usually signals the end of a session.

Asking for the place where *nihue* is sent (distributed), is a serious breach of etiquette, or at least, a most awkward and embarrassing question. The question is ignored, evaded, or at best, answered very vaguely: "anywhere else!" or "just away!" or "anywhere!" The answer is never "to where it comes from!" since the spirit of the *nihue*'s plant or animal source may have helped the shaman remove it from his client, tacitly implying that the shaman will find another person in whom the *nihue* can stay. *Nihue* itself (which can be moved with the power *shinan*) has a certain amount of inherent energy; this energy seems to require a material carrier or dwelling place.

In sum, humans have a dream ego and an amount of impersonal vital power (*shinan*), which with healthy and strong individuals produce a crown of light (*nete*) around the head.

Their bodies are decorated with lineal ornaments. The condition of the aura and the crown, both visible through their light and the state of the body ornaments, may be influenced by spirits with the individual essences (*nihues*) they control. The *yoshinbo* might be called counterparts of human dream egos because the shaman's dream ego negotiates with them as co-equals.

The spirit's *nihue,* having a certain amount of energy and an individual smell, color, temperature, or consistency, seems to be analogous to a man's aura (which is produced by his *shinan,* seen as light [*nete*]) and his individual body ornaments.

During his apprenticeship the shaman trains his dream ego to leave his body at will and accumulates a surplus of *shinan* enabling him to be effective.

The shaman is able to remove *nihue* from a sick body, but he cannot destroy it. If he doesn't want the *nihue* to stay in his immediate environment or on himself, he has to cast it on another living being who doesn't possess enough *shinan* to repulse it. Thus, in curing one, he is always bewitching another. Since he normally choses a victim in a distant social unit (and preferably one without a powerful shaman on its side), he is a kind of politician, deciding and working for his group, and he is, accordingly, a sorcerer for any other group, as the inhabitants of the next village will readily confirm.

Of course, it is easiest to send the *nihue* just taken from a patient to someone living nearby. That is why people are aware of a constant threat from their own shaman. They know the shaman is not beyond good and evil, nor in between; he is both good and evil. *Nihue,* which is only to be moved by a person with excessive *shinan,* can neither be destroyed nor permanently exist without being attached to a living being. Thus the shaman, as manipulator of energies, sees his world, with respect to the sum total of *nihue* and *shinan,* as a closed system. In this sytem his role is that of a strategist who is, by means of his *shinan,* distributing and redistributing *nihue.*

Notes

1. The present paper is based on nine months of fieldwork in Caimito (1981). I have described life in Caimito and the shaman's world in more detail in my 1987 thesis *Ani shinan: Schamanismus bei den Shipibo-Conibo (Ost-Peru)* (Tübingen, Verlag S&F). In the following, Shipibo stands for Shipibo-Conibo, since the tribes have merged and are usually treated as one in recent ethnographic literature. People still are able to trace back their lineage to either Shipibo or Conibo, but, to the best of my knowledge, there are no noteworthy differences relevant for our topic.

2. "Dream ego" is preferred by Fischer (1965, 243) to the established term "free soul." He uses dream ego as a principle of consciousness. This dream ego may temporarily leave the body (as in dreams, unconsciousness, and ecstasy). In addition it has some functions of a *Doppelgänger,* but it is *not* a soul. Fischer's criteria coincide well with an explication of the Shipibo conceptions.

3. A middle-aged shaman related the vision in Spanish with occasional Shipibo terms. Additional comments made by the shaman the next day are placed in parentheses. The other shaman sang the curing song in the native language and it was translated by him and another Shipibo.

4. All shamans have jaguars as their helpers. In Caimito, however, only one claimed (and mentioned in his songs) that he was able to transform himself into a jaguar.

5. During his military service and a few visits to Pucallpa, the shaman became acquainted with hospitals and pharmacies.

6. The singing "in chorus" reminds me somewhat of the ancient Greek "poeta," singing along with the muses. Caimitoan shamans do not claim authorship of their songs but attribute the words to the spirits.

7. This refers to the extracts of plants that were consumed together with *ayahuasca* and tobacco.

8. "Ronin" is the Great Boa; one lives in each river and laguna, at times giving birth to a new generation of fish through a rumbling sound. The syllable "ron" is the sound of thunder; "nin" is a suffix for words with an uneven number of syllables meaning "with."

9. In the Pucallpa market one can buy cheap manuals on all kinds of magic. Those on black magic are sold in sealed covers.

10. The examination may include an inquiry of the shaman's helper spirits, of the spirit of the plant having poisoned the sick, and, rarely, of the patient himself.

11. External symptoms of many diseases are well recognized and evaluated in the diagnosis. In this context, I shall not take them into consideration.

12. Light (*nete*) is the most obvious and immediate manifestation of power (*shinan*). The ability to release excessive power as flashes of lightning is usually conceded only to the Great Boa and to an electric eel.

FOUR

THE ONE INTOXICATED BY TOBACCO

Matsigenka Shamanism

GERHARD BAER

In order to describe some important elements of Matsigenka shamanism, it is advantageous to look particularly at the functions and roles that, in the Matsigenka view, are characteristic of the curing shaman, or *seripi'gari,* "the one intoxicated by tobacco."

A brief outline of Matsigenka culture, followed by a sketch of the conceptual background of shamanism (soul concepts, cosmology, concepts of health and illness, and others), plus a simplified description of a shamanic séance, is necessary to define the functions and roles of the *seripi'gari* more precisely. Special emphasis is placed on the chants sung at séances by the shaman and the women accompanying him. The text of the chants sheds light on the nature of the trance affecting the séance participants, and clearly shows that the role of the attending women is greater than previously believed.

The Matsigenka (their designation for "people" or "human beings") speak an Arawak language. Linguistically and culturally, they are most closely related to the Campa, who live to the west and southwest. The

Matsigenka's territory lies between 11°20′ and 13° south latitude and 70° and 73°20′ west longitude. It includes a large region of the drainage area of the upper Urubamba, parts of the lower Urubamba, and parts of the upper Manú and the upper Madre de Dios rivers. The population has variously been estimated to be between five thousand and seven thousand, but Corry (1984, 50) has most recently indicated the group to number 11,500.

ETHNOGRAPHIC BACKGROUND

For centuries the Matsigenka have inhabited these river valleys and their hinterland, the regions of hilly and mountainous country some 300 to 1200 meters above sea level. The rivers, navigated in dugouts and balsa rafts, form their most important arterial routes, though they undertake trips on foot through the hills and forests as well.

The economy is mixed, based on horticulture, hunting, fishing, and collecting. A considerable number of Matsigenka live in local groups away from the big river valleys, near smaller rivers or streams. Structurally, the most important socioeconomic unit within the local groups is the matrilocal extended family. The Matsigenka practice polygyny (including sororal polygyny), but in most cases only a few individuals, namely chiefs and shamans, have two or more wives.

The beginnings of a class structure is noticed among the Matsigenka, for there exists a class of the unfree or "picked ups," also called "brought ups," or "slaves." Unfree people are most often orphans (having lost one or both parents), unwanted children, or children who were exchanged from one family group to another. Since the possession of a large and influential kin group means protection, security, and influence, its absence leads to the contrary: low status, insecurity, and danger. Consequently, orphans and other children who are not supported by relatives, as well as widows, are accused more often than others of bewitching people from their own settlement or neighborhood, thereby causing illness or death. In former times accusations of this kind led to the death or sale of the accused (Baer 1984, 90).

The roles of the chief (*i'tinkami, ko'raka*) and shaman (*seripi'gari*) are essential to Matsigenka society. The functions of chief and healing shaman may be united in a single person, or they may be separate.

RELIGION

Living Things

The Matsigenka distinguish different classes of "living things": man (*matsi'genka*); extrahuman beings, in other words, the various classes of spirits, which are sometimes also referred to as *matsi'genka*; culture heroes and/or deities, or named superhuman beings who transformed the primeval world to give it its present shape; and the classes of animals and plants. Animals as a group are described as "living creatures with a soul." The Matsigenka also call extrahuman persons, human beings, and peccaries (which are gregarious animals), "those who assemble." These three groups are thought to have the social trait of forming groups in common.

People and animals, especially the edible animals of the bush and the water, viewed as the good spirits' domestic animals, have a free soul or "dream ego." The dream ego may leave the body during sleep, trance, or illness, and it leaves permanently at death. Dream and trance are understood as similar, perhaps even identical, states. The experiences of the dream ego are considered real occurrences involving beings seen in dreams or trance. According to the Matsigenka, the body serves only as a cover or "dress" for the free soul. Certain trees, like the lupuna (*Chorisia speciosa*), may also have this kind of free soul.

A second soul is the "eye soul," or "the mirror of the eye," located in the pupils. After a person's death, the eye soul is believed to "go up," while the free soul (dream ego) and the bone soul (*vide infra*) "go down." The eye soul is said to reside only inside people who live mainly on divine manioc, the nonpoisonous variety that comes from Father Moon. The bones are also important components of humans and animals. When a man who has transgressed a serious taboo, such as incest, dies, his bones become a demonic "bone soul" or "one who has risen from the dead." This bone soul brings disease and death to the living. The bones of animals rot after death, and thus do not become haunting, menacing bone souls.

Finally, the center, or "heart," is an important part of men, animals, and all living things; it is occasionally identified with the dream ego.

Spirits

Spirits can be divided into two main classes: the "pure" or "invisible ones," and the "one who lets die" or "one who kills." The pure spirits are benevolent to people and are associated with continuing life. The others, on the other hand, personify death and the transformation of death-bringing demons. Like humans, they seek company among the living, but unlike humans, they change the living into beings similar to themselves, killing the living and taking them along. It can thus be said that "the dead kill." These spirits of death have occasionally been identified with bone souls or the ones risen from the dead. The religion of the Matsigenka is, among other things, an attempt to check the power of the spirits of death, allowing the individual to escape death and become a pure and invisible being.

The Cosmos and the Deities

The Matsigenka's rich cosmology can only be outlined here. Its most essential characteristic is probably the multilevel nature of the cosmos (cf. Baer 1984, 228, fig. 10; Roe 1982, 128). Basically, it is divided into three parts: the layers of sky (including the clouds), the layer of the earth, and the subterranean realms.

The underworld is where most of the dead live. Only those who have died by drowning or have been struck by lightning dwell in the layer of clouds. The underworld is also said to contain a huge body of water, which was described to the author as a kind of "sea" or immense lake named Chi'kosa. The rising mists in the morning are traced back to the waters of that lake, and it is said that the earth will come to an end if the subterranean waters of the lake rise up one day and overflow the earth.

There are invisible "closed" links between the different layers of the cosmos. These linking paths become visible to the shaman only after he has taken *ayahuasca* (or other hallucinogens). Generally, the good spirits live in hilly or mountainous country, in the depths of lakes and rivers, and in layers of the sky. They bathe in the Milky Way, imagined as a heavenly river, where they shed their skins and rejuvenate. If a human bathes in the Milky Way, he becomes immortal. The evil spirits live in the depths of the rain forest, around rock formations, or inside certain rocks, which are their "palaces." They also live in cloud regions and inside the earth with the dead. Rain and fog are the media in which these spirits like to manifest themselves.

The culture heroes and/or deities are chiefly male, and are mainly restricted to the heavenly and underworld regions. The female deities belong to the earth. For instance, 'kipatsi is the Earth. In primordial times, she was heard to speak, but now human sin has silenced her. Features in the landscape, such as rock formations near rivers, show characteristic signs interpreted as traces of the former work of certain culture heroes and/or deities. Today, the culture heroes of the earth and the underworld are immobilized or rigid. Thus, Pa'reni, Mother of Fish and of Game Animals, has taken on the shape of a salty rock. The *Pa'chakama* and other underworld spirits and deities have been "nailed." On the other hand, the deities of the heavenly spheres, namely Sun, Moon, and certain stars, have remained mobile. Apart from the sun visible to us, the Matsigenka recognize two more "suns." One of them is fixed; the other, located in the underworld, is believed to move.

ILLNESS

Causes

According to the Matsigenka's religious tradition, illness is almost always the expression and result of a previous social conflict or of the disturbance of social order. This also applies to illnesses ascribed to the aggression of extrahuman persons or powers, for the extrahuman forces are believed to cooperate with human aggressors or human witches (*ma'tsinti*) and/or bewitching shamans (*matsika'nari*).

The concept according to which a man becomes ill or dies "by himself," in other words, without the influence of a third party, is virtually unknown to the Matsigenka. When an old person dies, his vigor or vitality ("life power") might be assumed to have expired, but when younger people die, the question of cause is always discussed and the culprit sought. It has already been mentioned that widows, orphaned children, and other persons without relatives providing protection tend to fall under suspicion of sorcery or witchcraft and were, in former times, often found guilty of being human witches and, at times, were even executed.

Illness as the expression of conflict is an indication of a disturbance of the psychosocial balance of the group or the social order. The many disturbing factors include: incest; breaking of food taboos; ignoring the implications of an ominous dream or some other bad omen; and conflicts resulting from not fulfilling social obligations, such as improperly distributing food (especially game and fish), stinginess, laziness, and stealing. In one example, such a cause of illness occurred when Helena, a former shaman's wife, was having acute coughing fits. For quite some time she had been feeling weak and ill. (I had the impression that she was suffering from chronic bronchitis and tried to relieve her pain with antibiotics.) In the course of her slow recovery, Helena related the following: "When my daughter Anita was still small, she bathed in a brook. Suddenly the round flat stone next to her moved without any obvious reason. I was startled and cried out. There was a whirlpool in the brook, which was caused by a water spirit. It was he who brought the disease."

Anita's husband suggested another reason: "Maybe Helena's illness was caused by a Matsigenka called Cha'kopi ("arrow-cane"). Perhaps a witch secretly slipped into her house and entered her. Helena was probably bewitched by Cha'kopi because he could not marry Anita." (This means she was not promised to him as his future wife.)

Later a shaman blew some tobacco smoke at Helena and produced an object from her body, a leaf. Thus Helena knew she had been bewitched by Cha'kopi. The reason for her illness, according to this second version, was a social conflict: the mother's refusal to promise her little daughter to Cha'kopi and the resulting vengeance of the refused.

When a Matsigenka has broken serious taboos and thereby becomes "stained," he may be frightened; then his body opens up, and he becomes defenseless, allowing "arrows" shot by evil shamans and their demon allies to penetrate his body. This leads to illness and, under certain conditions, death. When the body is open, the dream ego can also leave the body. This constitutes a further threat of illness and death. In both cases it is the task of the healing shaman to take the "projectiles" out of the victim's body or bring back the escaped soul.

In this context it is important to note that certain patterns of face and body painting have two main tasks: First, preventing illness by "closing off" the painted person's body and protecting it like armor; and second, frightening demonic beings, like the death-bringing squirrel-cuckoo (*Piaya cayana*), so that they will release their victims and flee. A man or a woman who feels threatened and vulnerable may thus paint him/herself in order to avoid becoming ill (fig. 4.1).

The concept of "poison," *ke'pigari,* is central to illness beliefs. *Ke'pigari*

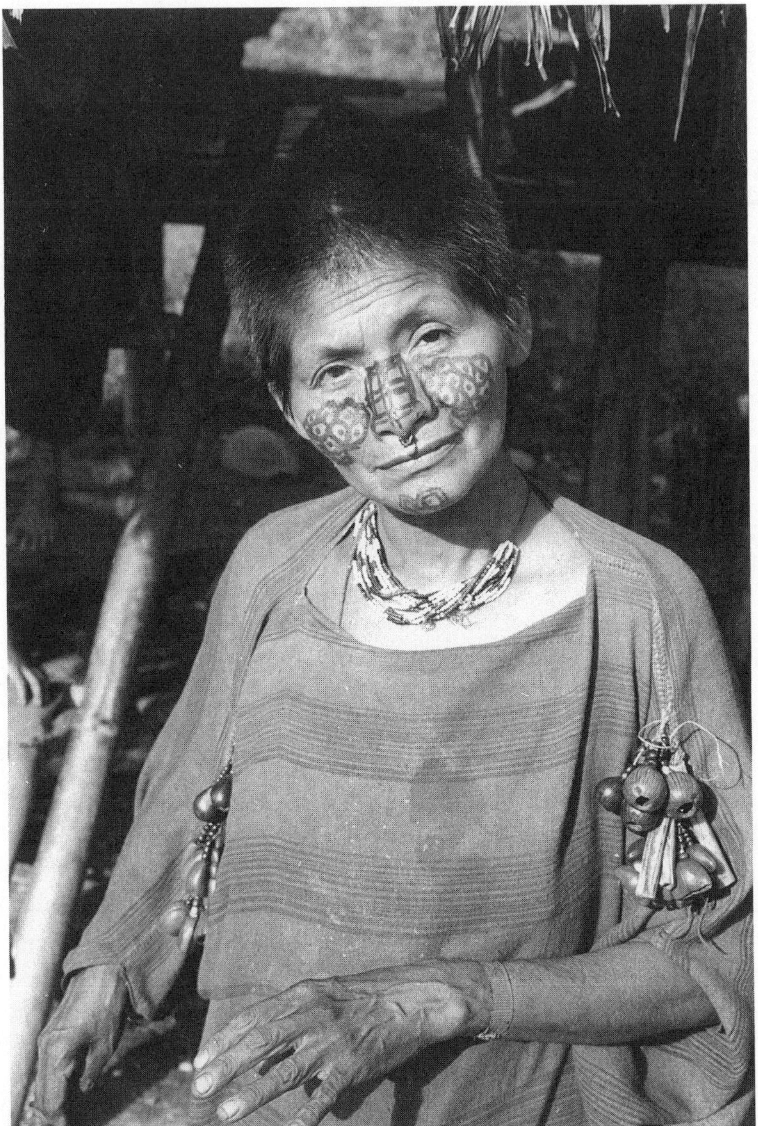

FIGURE 4.1. A Matsigenka shaman's wife with face painting, to protect against illness.

has three meanings: "poison," "medicine," and "drug." Snake venom is *ke'pigari*. For the hunter and the shaman, menstrual blood is poison too. The Kepiga'rite, or "Poison-People," are the spiritual "owners" of illnesses. Medicinal plants contain poison, which checks and frightens away the demons. Like painted body patterns, the poison of the medicinal plants seals the body of a Matsigenka, protecting him from being frightened and thereby falling ill.

Hallucinogens, like *ayahuasca* (*Banisteriopsis* sp., *kama'ranpi*), *Datura* or *Brugmansia* sp., *'saaro, ha'yapa,* are described as "sweet poisons." *Ayahuasca* is used most often; it generally contains admixtures of other hallucinogenic plants, like the leaves of *Psychotria* sp., which are supposed to make it more potent. These hallucinogenic brews render extraordinary reality visible to the drinker and enable him to communicate with the invisible ones. This applies above all to the *seripi'gari,* "the one intoxicated by tobacco." Taken in sufficient quantities, tobacco acts like a hallucinogen and is thus classified by the Matsigenka as sweet poison.

Curing

Information from many Matsigenka indicates that the sick are not cured by the shaman directly, but by his guardian spirits and auxiliary spirits. Medicinal and magic plants are also important to him. Some of them grow in gardens; some are wild. As they are put at the disposal of the shaman and his extrahuman partners, these plants are considered to be cultivated by the spirits, or to grow wild in the spirits' territory.

When treating the sick, the shaman employs various techniques: blowing, spit blowing and breathing (with tobacco smoke or simply with breath), and sucking out alien elements that have entered the sick person. The shaman sucks where it hurts. He takes out the pathogenic objects ("thorns," leaves, bones, spines, and so on), and shows them to those present. Before the sucking out, he drinks a thick tobacco juice. The blood he sucks out is said to be black. If the thorn is too big, the patient may die. Light-colored or transparent stones, especially quartz crystals, are regarded as curative. They are called *isere'pito.* Although this designation is the same as that for the auxiliary spirits, it is more correct to view them as "bodies," "residences," or material manifestations of these spirits.

The shaman acquires these stones during his initiation, or he receives them from his father or another close male relative, and carries them with him in a small bag. The Matsigenka say the shaman feeds his stones tobacco daily. If he does not do so, his auxiliary spirits, which materialize in the crystals, will leave him, and then the shaman will die.

Although the shamans of many Amazonian tribes both heal and bewitch, as far as can be concluded here, the *seripi'gari* is only a healing shaman. The wizard, who bewitches people, making them ill and killing them, is called *matsika'nari,* a term derived from the bewitching stones he uses. Although there is a myth that tells of how a *seripi'gari* was accidentally turned into a *matsika'nari,* the shaman seems to make a conscious choice: when he meets the invisible ones, a man (female shamans are reported to occur, but only rarely) decides whether he wants to heal or bewitch. The Matsigenka demonstrate ambiguous feelings of fear and hatred only with respect to the bewitching shaman. However, many stories emphasize that even the *seripi'gari* are not faultless; they boast about their real or pretended abilities and skills, and they are sometimes even arrogant.

THE SÉANCE

As a rule, a shamanistic séance takes place in the shaman's house in complete darkness. The participants include the shaman, his assistant or apprentice, his relatives (especially his wife or wives), the patient, and guests, including members of the patient's family. The patient lies on a mat in front of the shaman. The shaman and the other males in the house (apart from children) take *ayahuasca* from a pot standing next to the shaman ladder. Although women do not drink *ayahuasca,* they are vital to the séance because they sing with the shaman. In the Matsigenka's view, these ritual chants are of considerable help in inducing the appearance of the "visitor spirits" or shaman's guardian spirits. They enable the shaman to send away his dream ego or to depart entirely, body and soul, on his ecstatic journey to the invisible, pure ones (figs. 4.2–4.4). During the séance the shaman climbs the ladder several times. He sings and hums, climbs again, moves the leaf fan, and so forth. The Matsigenka say that the person climbing and descending the ladder is sometimes the shaman and sometimes one of his guardian spirits. Behind this explanation lies the belief that a drug-induced trance leads to an exchange between the benevolent invisible ones and the shaman.

Much has been written about the nature of shamanic trance and whether it is only soul flight, or whether it may also include possession.

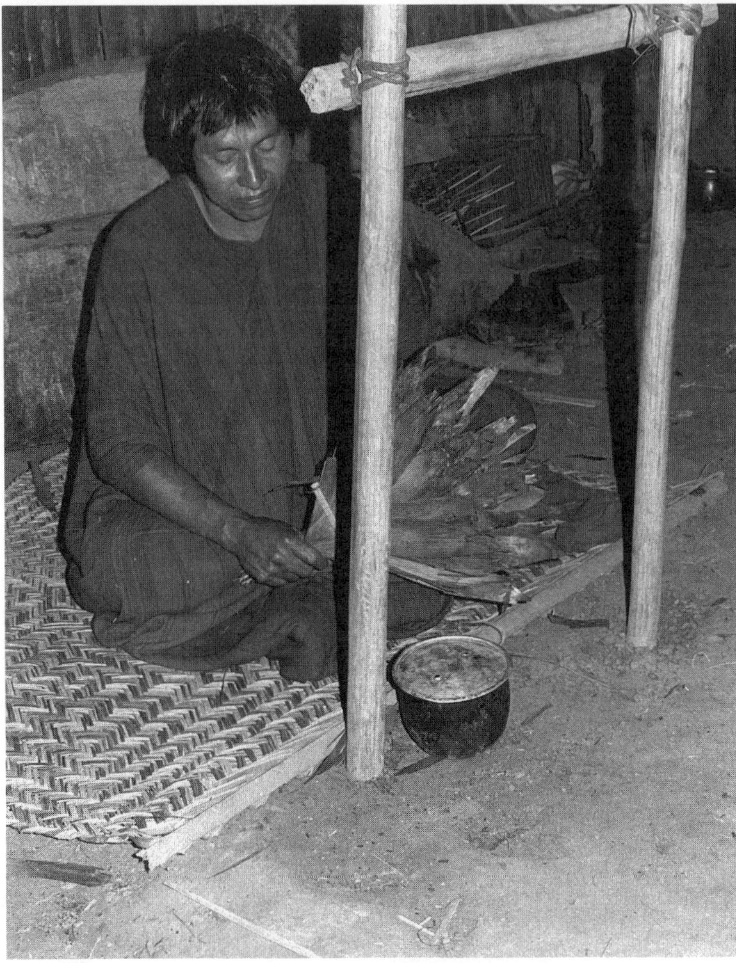

FIGURE 4.2. Matsigenka shaman chants over *ayahuasca* before drinking it. Note the shamanic ladder before him extending to the roof of the house.

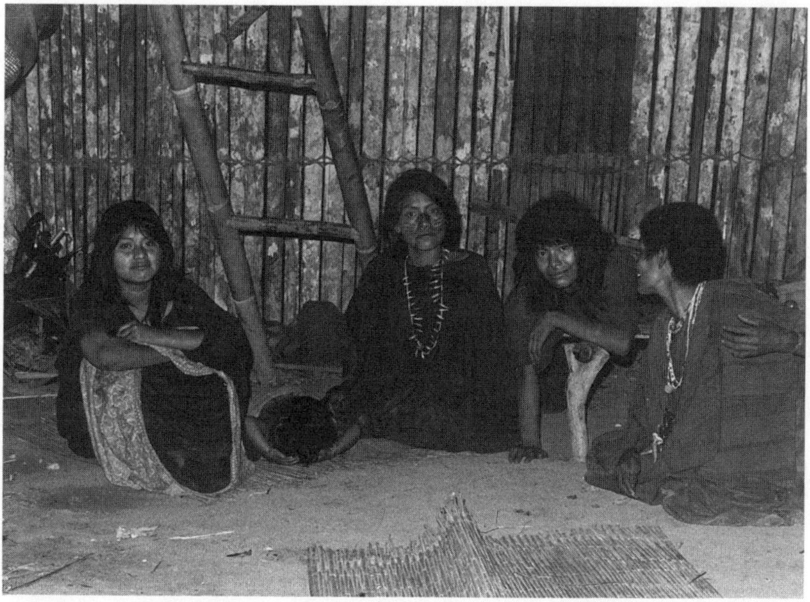

FIGURE 4.3. The Matsigenka women who will sing in the séance.

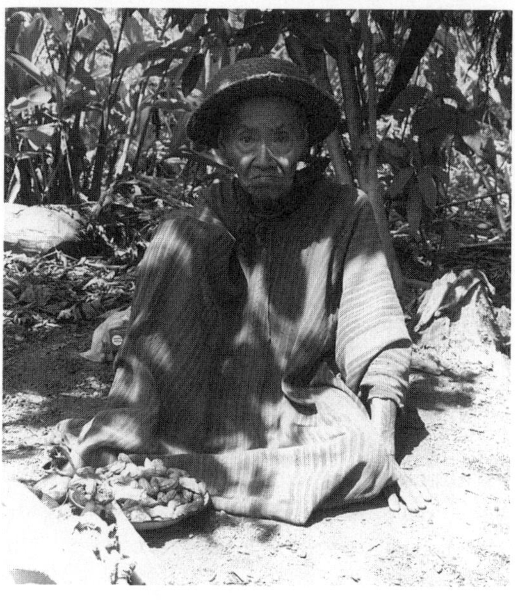

FIGURE 4.4. An old Matsigenka shaman.

The Matsigenka consider the shaman's trance to contain elements of both. They have, however, two ways of explaining what happens during a shaman's trance.

According to their first concept, after he takes the hallucinogen, the shaman's soul becomes independent and departs on an ecstatic journey to the realm of the pure spirits, it visits them, and then returns to the shaman's body. While his soul is absent, the shaman's visitor spirits or guardian spirits descend, enter his soulless ("empty") body, and appear to the participants in his shape, speaking and singing in his voice. The participants thus remark that "he is now someone else," or "he is transfigured."

According to the second concept, the shaman does not send away only his soul during trance, but he disappears "body and soul." At the moment of his disappearance, one of his guardian spirits descends and fills in for him before those present. The shaman's wife or wives receive the spirit hospitably, whereupon he sings, either by himself or with the women's accompaniment. The moment the shaman returns from his journey, the spirit that has been representing him disappears.

The light symbolism connected with the séance and the shaman's trance is highly significant. It refers to the ornaments worn (feathers), the ritual chants, and the guardian spirits that appear. An informant once said, "A shaman who really knows his business can give his guests light in the house by singing." He also said, "Some of the spirits resemble lamps. When they are alight, it is bright as day; then they sing." The light that illuminates the nocturnal darkness inside the house is an expression of the shaman's magnified, potentiated, communicative power with the pure and invisible ones. This explanation is not unlike one provided by Freud.[1]

Experiences of intense light are also produced by drinking hallucinogenic plants. A Matsigenka informant once said, "When one drinks datura, the sun becomes sad." One of the explanations of this statement was "the sun became sad because the datura [*Brugmansia* sp.] became the sun." The informant added that the "miracles of datura [the effects of the hallucinogen] caused the sun's effect." With regard to the brightness and light it produces, datura can compete with the sun; it is the sun's rival. Thus, it is no coincidence that allusions to shining light are found in many of the chants sung during shamanistic séances. For example:

We are the sons of their mothers
 [i.e., sons of the owners or spirits of the datura plants]
We
Their blossoms [of the datura plants]
Flash white
There, where they live
Their mothers
Their heads are covered with a cotton cap
Their tunics are as flaming as light
Oh, bright shining water
Where they live
Their mothers
We
Where we come from
Where they [the mothers of datura] live
Where nothing grows
The datura blossoms flash white
In the datura lake [or river?]

Most of these chants are considered to be the chants of the guardian spirits themselves (i.e., songs the respective guardian spirit sings during his appearance in the house), or chants the shaman has learned from his guardian spirits during his meetings with them. The shaman's most important guardian spirit is the *matsi'panko.* Its name probably means "charm-house." Zoologically speaking, the term refers to the swallow-tailed kite (*Elanoides forficatus*), but the birds encountered in daily life are not spirits; they are considered the "grandchildren" of the *matsi'panko* spirit. He is human in form, in other words, it/he is *matsi'genka,* as well as *i'nato,* the master spirit of the swallow-tailed kites.[2]

The following text is an excerpt from the song of the guardian spirit *matsi'panko:*

I am flying
I have come flying, over hills
Have you heard my grandchildren laughing
I hear the mortals [Matsigenka] say:
See them [my grandchildren] flying about
I turn round myself as I fly
We laugh
You have seen my grandchildren

They have brought little clouds with them
I come from the headwater region Porenkishi'ari
You call the water course Porenkishi'ari
But I say it is called Shanpavire'niari
I fly high and low, turning as I fly
Have you noticed [the master of thunder and lightning]
Who falls from above with such force
Have you seen my grandchildren
Whose caps are white
They have their caps
My grandchildren. . .

A clear distinction is made in this chant between the guardian spirit and his "grandchildren," the swallow-tailed kites who bear the same name. Although the shaman's guardian spirit is invisible and has human shape, the chant says again and again that he flies up and down, turns in the air, and so on, as if he were also a bird. The image evoked in the chant thus demonstrates a certain dualism as to the form of the guardian spirit. We find the same dualism in mythological accounts of how "vulture-people" take off their wings and appear as humans or people, and later put on their wings like garments to fly off like birds.

The complex metaphorical imagery encountered in shamanistic song is typical of the spoken or sung texts that are performed during shamanistic séances. An excerpt of text tape-recorded at a séance in 1978 serves as an example.[3] Andrés held a séance at his house, with his friend Manuel acting as his assistant. Apart from Andrés's and Manuel's wives there were several other men present. A ladder with one rung led to the roof and tied to a horizontal beam. At the bottom of the ladder a woven mat was spread out. Between the uprights stood an aluminum pot containing the *ayahuasca* drink. The men and boys present drank from it. Near the ladder there were two leaf fans used to produce rhythmical sounds. Night had fallen. The kerosene lamp inside the house was extinguished.

Andrés: What hour does the Moon show?
Manuel: The Moon has almost hidden.
Andrés: Our throat is parched.
Manuel: I am too heavy to "run" [i.e., climb the ladder, descend, climb again, etc.].

It has been a long time since I have drunk *ayahuasca.*
If one drinks and vomits, one "runs" well. My throat is getting dry. I feel like drinking.

Andrés: It is good to drink *ayahuasca,* but we are afraid to take it. We should not be afraid.
If it were like sugarcane, we would have no fear.
Ayahuasca is good for drinking, but it does not make us drunk enough.
Wild datura provides more hallucinations.

Manuel: Bush-datura can't be endured.
If I take only a little of it, my throat gets all dry. . .
You can't eat when you drink [*ayahuasca* or datura], because our throats get parched.
But if there is someone with us who takes care of us, then he gives us some lukewarm water.
When the drunkenness stops, we are healthy again.
If you can't withstand the datura, you will run into the bush. . .

Andrés: The Moon will soon hide.
[Turning to a boy] Put out the fire.
Shut the door with the mat. . .
It is dark already.
[Andrés is humming. The leaf fans sound the rhythm.]

Andrés and the women: We listen when the small bird [*ine'tsaane*] sings.
Sisters, listen when the small bird sings.
[sisters refers to sisters of the guardian spirit.]
The *ine'tsaane* is fragrant.

Andrés: ehehehehehehehehehe. The *ine'tsaane* sings powerfully. . .
I am in a serene mood.
[The singing breaks off]
I shall climb the ladder. . .
[leaf fans in motion] ehehehehehehe.
I am listening to the *ine'tsaane* [silence].

The participants offered the following explanation of this section: At the beginning of the séance, Andrés ascends, vanishing through the roof. The first *ine'tsaane,* the shaman's guardian spirit, comes down and starts singing. Then, he goes back up again and disappears. The next *ine'tsaane* does the same, and so forth.

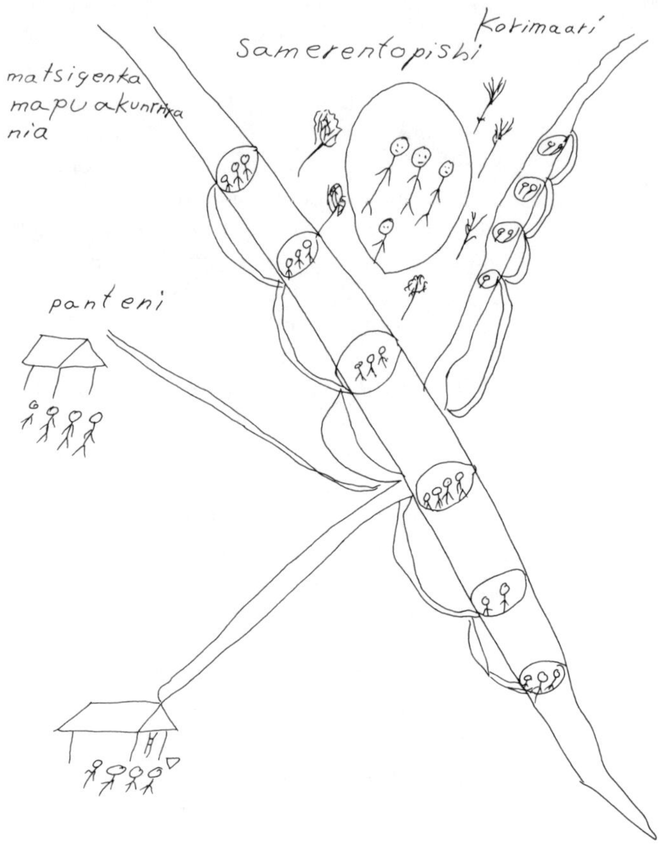

FIGURE 4.5. Matsigenka shaman's drawing of his ecstatic journey to the land of the water sources, the rivers and lakes where many spirits reside. One sees the paths that lead him, or his soul, to the water spirits (*matsi'genka mapuaku-nirirania*) living inside stones, to the reed spirits (*samerentopishi*) and to the spirits living in the "golden river" (*kori'maari*). The path leading to the house of the *panteni,* a greedy, miserable person, corresponds to a dangerous deviation from the "right path."

Andrés (above):	I have seen the yellow flowers of the Shi'mashiri tree. Those living in the flowers do not care about me [this refers to the shaman's *ine'tsaane*].
ine'tsaane (below) (guardian spirit):	Yes! Those living in the flowers cry for joy because [the shaman] has got used to them.
Andrés (above):	The orange-chinned parakeet sings *korerere'rere.*
ine'tsaane (below):	The orange-chinned parakeet is wonderfully green. [leaf fans in motion] I come from far away, from the watercourse where the yellow flowers bloom.
Andrés (below):	They are like me, those living in the flowers.
Women:	They are like us.
Andrés (above):	I whistle to my sons-in-law [*ine'tsaane*] I tenderly fondle the small birds that live by another watercourse.
Women:	So do we; we tenderly stroke our daughters [daughters refers to male *ine'tsaane*].
Andrés (above):	My sons-in-law are fragrant.
Women:	. . . The *ine'tsaane* tenderly stroke the yellow flowers of the Shi'mashiri tree. The flowers have already ceased to bloom.
Andrés (below):	But these flowers [the *ine'tsaane*] of the Ko'maro tree, do not come to an end. They are forever fragrant [i.e., the *ine'tsaane* are immortal]. Therefore, my sons-in-law are pleased with them. [feminine plural meaning the Matsigenka women are pleased with the (male) *ine'tsaane*].
Women:	The flowers do not cease to bloom. [i.e., the *ine'tsaane* are immortal]
Andrés:	I have seen the earthquakes of primordial times.
	. . .
ine'tsaane (guardian spirit):	Once I saw the earthquakes.
Women:	Once we saw the earthquakes.
	. . .
Andrés (above) *and the women:*	'Tomiri-'tomiri tree, we are very similar to you.
Andrés:	Small is the 'Tomiri-'tomiri tree.

ine'tsaane (above):	I come from the other side, where there is a countless number of 'Tomiri-'tomiri trees.
	. . .
ine'tsaane (below) *and the women:*	He has brought the fragrant herb, he who does not die [the *ine'tsaane*]. [The *ine'tsaane* goes up.] [Silence, then three knocks that indicate the arrival of a new *ine'tsaane.*]
ine'tsaane (above) *and the women:*	hmhmhmhmhmhmhmhm
	I come from the Río Manú, where the 'Tomiri-'tomiri trees stand. I come from the other side. A long time ago I saw the earthquakes and those who died through the earthquakes and who had once lived.
Women:	It is you who once saw the Matsigenka on the Río Manú?
ine'tsaane (below) *and the women:*	I said to my cross-cousin/brother-in-law: "Have pity on the Matsigenka." But he said: "No!"
ine'tsaane (above):	hmhmhmhmhmhmhmhmhmhm
ine'tsaane (below):	The Matsigenka were turning in circles. They had mixed with the demons; they died irrevocably.

An informant noted here that the Matsigenka's turning in circles refers to the earthquakes of primordial times, when darkness prevailed and there was no sun. The Matsigenka and the demons fell into the water and drowned. The earthquakes were a punishment for the Matsigenka and the demons living with them because the Matsigenka had committed incest and violated other taboos.

ine'tsaane (below):	Before the wild coca existed [*ka'sankari,* "the fragrant one"] many earthquakes occurred and there were many demons. The same will happen to you [i.e., to the Matsigenka]. When the end of the world comes, you will perish through big earthquakes.

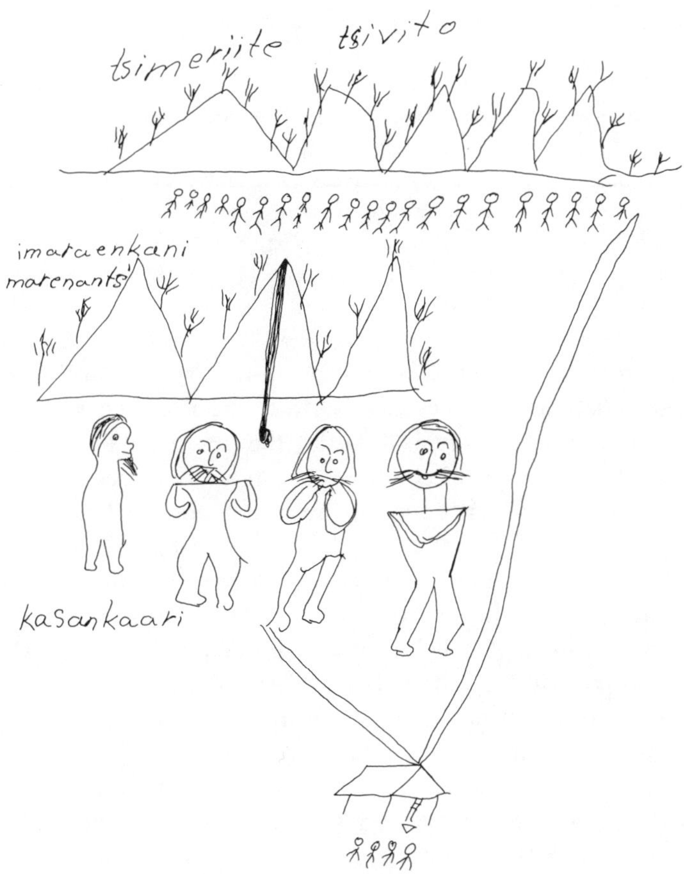

FIGURE 4.6. Matsigenka shaman's drawing of his ecstatic journey to the hill spirits, where he visits the "Bird-People" (*tsime-rite* and *tsi-vito*), and the *imaraenkani* and *marenan-tsite* spirits. These spirits only eat tobacco and keep jaguars as their dogs. They are bearded and have a fragrant smell. Thus they are also called "perfume" (*kansankaari*). At the bottom, one sees the house of the shaman and his people. The ladder (two rungs) and the recipient for the *ayahuasca* are clearly visible.

Women:	Yes, that is how it is; we shall all die when doomsday comes.
	. . .
ine'tsaane (below):	I have pity on you. Therefore, you will have a long life, and will not die. Once, the demons used to appear, but I have pity on the mortals [Matsigenka]. Once, the Sun was extinguished.
Women:	Yes, the Sun went out; but you are the one who has pity on the mortals.

What do these excerpts from a shamanistic séance tell us? Certainly they show that such séances have a ritual character. They also prove that séances are not restricted to curing the sick. They have additional functions and dimensions, because in the rite they confront the participants with primordial times and the threat of doomsday. Moreover, they demonstrate that the shaman, as a kind of mediator and go-between, stands between his family members or followers and the extrahuman persons he counts as his relatives. Hence, the shaman has human and extrahuman qualities. He is human, or, as the *ine'tsaane* say, "mortal," but he also participates in the realm of extrahuman persons and their immortality. In a way he has both "divine" and human aspects, what have been called "liminal attributes."[4]

The excerpts from the séance recording also illustrate the important role women play. The Matsigenka say the women's singing helps the shaman to induce the guardian spirits to come down into his house. Although Matsigenka women rarely become shamans, they are indispensable at séances. Further data prove that the shaman's relationship to women is ambivalent. He must abstain from sexual relations with his wife (or wives) before and during his shamanistic activities. The Matsigenka also believe that if the shaman comes into contact with menstrual blood, it adversely affects his strength.

Apart from this, many myths relate how powerful shamans were destroyed by the enmity, malice, or stupidity of women (e.g., their wives). It is striking that the shaman's life and death are dependent, among other things, on his wife's (or wives') social behavior; if she does not behave properly, he risks death. Matsigenka tradition confirms that adultery by either of the partners can lead to the guardian spirits' desertion of the shaman, and thus to the shaman's subsequent death (Baer and Snell 1974, 71–72). It is evident that the shaman not only exercises social control (e.g., deciding who is responsible for a death), but that he is also subject to the control of his group.

In summary we can say the following about the functions and roles characteristic of the healing shaman:

1. He acts as a mediator between his (family) group and the extra-human persons.

2. He protects his group from dangerous illnesses and hunger, and is able to do so because of his links with the guardian and auxiliary spirits. By the means of the ingestion of tobacco and hallucinogens, he can recognize the extraordinary, hidden reality and see future events (the gift of clairvoyance). The shaman is a seer.

3. His protective functions can be defined more precisely. The shaman protects his (family-) group from the spirits of the dead and other death-bringing demons. With the aid of his guardian and auxiliary spirits, he diagnoses and cures illnesses brought on by hostile powers (witches, demons). Thanks to his clairvoyance, he recognizes the causes of illnesses, death, and other disruptions of the social equilibrium. In times of starvation he can ask the pure spirits, and especially the master spirits of the game, to give his group meat, and may thereby avert hunger. He can foresee impending harm in dreams or trances and warn his group. On the basis of his seer-like faculties, he takes protective measures, and influences and guides his group.

4. The shaman is also a redeemer. He strives for a ritually pure life and tries to include his followers in his endeavors. If he succeeds, there is a possibility that his group will be carried off, that they will be called for by the pure ones and enter the land of the pure. Then the shaman and his people will have escaped death, for they will have become the pure, invisible ones.

NOTE ON TRANSCRIPTION

For the Matsigenka language, ' indicates stress on the following syllable. This has been adopted to follow its use by the Summer Institute of Linguistics.

Notes

1. Cf. Kakar (1978, 84): "The reassurance provided by the goddesses Sarasvati and Parvati against the terrific estrangements of infancy reminds me of Freud's account of the child who called out of a dark room, " 'Auntie, speak to me! I'm frightened because it's so dark!' His aunt answered him, 'What good would that do? You can't see me.' 'That does not matter,' replied the child. 'If anyone speaks, it gets light.' " This is a reference to Freud (1958, Vol. 16, 407).

2. The swallow-tailed kite (*Elanoides forficatus*) has been repeatedly mentioned in the literature as being of great shamanic importance (e.g., Butt Colson 1977, 55–58; Matthäi 1977, 106–7; Wilbert 1985, 1987, 161, 184, 195), but it perhaps has not received the attention it deserves as a shamanic tutelary spirit of highest rank (Matthäi 1977). Both Butt Colson and Wilbert stress the point that the swallow-tailed kite is most closely related to tobacco and the shaman's spirit experience. Among the Warao of Venezuela, the swallow-tailed kite is the supreme spirit of tobacco, and is a "bird-demiurge in the guise of the swallow-tailed kite . . . Epiphany of the God of Origin, he represents the pleni-potent sun of the zenith and acts with creative force to establish the new order of *bahana* shamanism" (Wilbert 1987, 147, 150). Among the Akawaio, Guyana, the swallow-tailed kite is the shaman's bird (*kumalak akwalu*). "First, there is the tobacco spirit; this spirit brings down the *kumalak* bird, which is the shaman's chief spirit helper" (Butt Colson 1977, 55–56). According to Nimuendajú (1914, 302), the shamans of the Apapocuva-Guarani had a close relationship to the god of the thunderstorms, Tupã, who is a son of the creator god Nanderuvuçu. Two retainers of his, called *yvyraija,* sometimes assume the form of swallow-tailed kites. Since they are closely associated with rain, and thus fertility of plants, the shamans put the tail feathers of the "thezouras" (i.e., the swallow-tailed kites) on their front diadem. Thus, the relation between the shaman and the swallow-tailed kite is widely distributed across South America, from Guiana, the Orinoco delta, and the Apapocuva-Guarani in the east, to the Tunebo, the Desana, and the Matsigenka in the west (Wilbert, personal communication).

3. The part of the text that has been translated from the tape-recording is given in Baer (1984, 274–83).

4. See Leach (1976, 71–72, especially p. 72) "The mediator, whether he is a 'real' being (e.g., a shaman or a mythological god-man) then takes on liminal attributes—he is both mortal and immortal, human and animal, tame and wild." See also van Gennep (1960); Pentikäinen (1979); and V. Turner (1974).

PART TWO

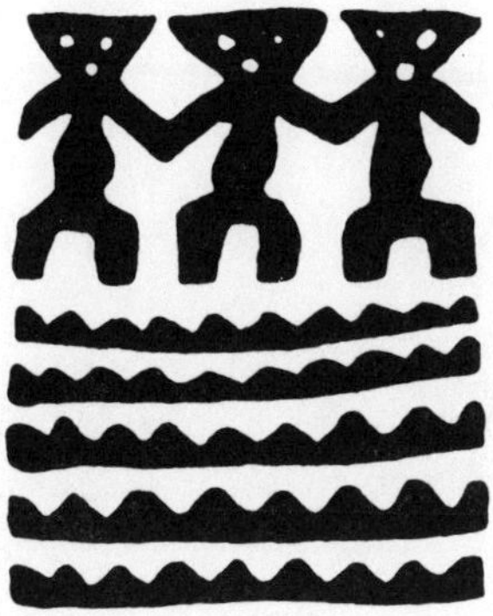

SHAMANS AND THE VISIONARY EXPERIENCE

FIVE

THE BODY OF THE GUAJIRO SHAMAN

Symptoms or Symbols?

MICHEL PERRIN

The traditional ethnological controversy over the question of "normality" or "marginality" of the shaman has clouded and limited studies on shamanism. The basic reason for this controversy, kept alive by the culturalists and ethnopsychiatrists, is a confusion between collective representations and individual behavior. I shall explore this topic through an examination of indigenous concepts and categories associated with Guajiro shamanism in Venezuela and Colombia.

Each Guajiro shaman has a specific way of recounting the events that brought her (him) to the practice of "shamanery,"[1] and that have particularly marked her (his) career (as opposed to most South American societies, eighty percent of Guajiro shamans are women). Although these autobiographical elements seem, at first, to describe intimate experiences that are highly subjective, they tend to conform to a single pattern, with a few noteworthy exceptions to be analyzed later. In fact, specific and repeated manifestations in body and dream, incorporation of tobacco, and particular patterns of behavior with regard to food and sexuality are considered traits of a distinctive relationship with the supernatural, and as true symbols of the shamanic calling and function. Moreover, these behavior patterns are expressed in vernacular language by means of words or expressions reflecting general laws of mythical thought, as well as specific cultural views and conceptions of the relations between "this world" and an "other world" on which the former depends.[2] These attitudes of the Guajiro shamans are interconnected and subject to a mode of thinking that always seeks the greatest possible degree of coherence. In other words, they form a system.

In our society, such types of significant behavior patterns and associated verbal formulations are among those regarded by psychiatrists or psychoanalysts as symptoms (in the medical meaning of the word). More precisely, they are seen as the expressions of a "body language" characteristic of hysteria: convulsive "pantomimic" crisis, food phobia, asthenias, aches, perturbed sexuality, alternation of two personalities, tendency to identification, and so on. It appears that a cultural representation of hysteria could be found in the Guajiro characterization of the "perfect shaman." Due to this "coincidence," which is also found in shamanic systems of other societies, many anthropological studies, relying on external descriptions of behavior patterns regarded as universally significant, have stressed the deviance of shamans in general, or at least questioned the shaman's normality. In fact, we are dealing with what the physicists would call a typical case of "indetermination" or "indecidability," a logical impossibility of answering yes or no.

I do not deny, of course, that the shamanic function may produce specific effects on the person who fulfills it, or that a disturbed person may be attracted to shamanism, which provides him with a "language of the body" allowing him to give appropriate expression to his mental disorders. Nor is it denied that there is a relation between shamanism and illness (see Perrin 1986a). Before drawing a conclusion, however, the ethnologist should seek to understand how shamanic manifestations form part of a logical pattern of general cultural ideas that obviously exists prior to any individual calling.[3] Once this has been firmly established, it will then become possible to perceive behavioral differences, personal motivations, social strategies, or problems involved in the adaptation "of cultural material for neurotic ends," to borrow the very terms used by Devereux (1972, 244), who emphasized the recurrence of models of hysterical behavior in traditional societies.[4]

THE SHAMANISTIC CALLING: SIGNIFICANT MANIFESTATIONS OF THE BODY

Considered essentially in its therapeutic dimension, Guajiro shamanism is associated with three classic principles. First, every human being is formed of a body and a "soul." Good health is the harmonious coexistence of the body and the soul (which, in normal circumstances, leaves the body only in dreams). The immediate cause of sickness is the alteration or departure of the soul, whatever the symptoms, whatever the ultimate causes. Death is the permanent separation of the soul from the body. For the shaman the healing of sickness initially consists of "reconstituting" the soul, or bringing it back into the patient's body.

Second, the Guajiro etiology attributes the ultimate causes of bodily disorders to powers deriving from an "other world." The shamanic diagnosis consists of identifying these supernatural agents, denoted by the Guajiro term *pülasü,* as the other world and the beings who dwell in it. (They also designate as *pülasü* phenomena or beings in "this world" that are believed to bear witness to the hidden but constant presence of "the other world." The other world and this world correspond as much to two levels of perception of "reality" as to two separate universes.)

Third, shamans are persons who may, at will, give evidence of supernatural knowledge or powers. Shamans, say the Guajiro, are *pülasü.* They can know the truth of this world by communicating with the other world, either directly, or through the intermediary of auxiliary spirits whom they can call up or request to dispatch to the *pülasü* world from which they originate. They thus discover the causes of disorders in this world—the causes of diseases and calamities. On the occasion of each cure they can confirm the relations of interdependence and complementarity between the supernatural world and the world of humans.

However, this particular faculty of the shaman is neither innate nor hereditary. For the Guajiro, acquiring shamanic power means fitting into a particular order different from the ordinary social order. It means becoming *pülasü.* This gradual insertion into the shamanistic order is reflected in specific bodily reactions. Whether desired or not, these reactions attest to a calling or a distinction conferred upon the individual by the supernatural world and recognized by the world of humans.

Almost all the shamans have suffered from phobias or allergies to certain foods.

> *Pülasü tamüin sawainrü:*
> The turtle was forbidden to me.
> If I partook thereof I began to swell. . .
> The deer too was forbidden to me, and the rabbit.
> The rabbit made me itch all over. . .
> I rejected them all because of the *wanülüü.*
> The spirit who entered my womb. . .
>
> (The shaman Reeachon Jayaliyuu, in 1973.)

> *Pülasü wanee ekülü sümüin tüü wanülüü wanainka:*
> Some foods were forbidden for me,
> because of my *wanülüü,* my spirit.
> At this time, I could not take milk, nor cheese.
> I was not able to eat beef.
> I could not even bear to smell these foods.
> If I smelled meat, I died, I fainted.
> I could only taste beef slaughtered at home. . .
> I behaved in this way in the past. . .
>
> (The shaman Maria Jayaliyuu, in 1975.)

In the Guajiro language, this intolerance to foods is expressed by the word *pülasü. Pülasü tamüin sawainrü* can be translated as "turtle was prohibited for me"; in other words, "it is dangerous for me to eat turtle," or "I am allergic to turtle." These reactions are considered implicit proof, if not of communication, of a distinctive relationship between the other world and the victim. Moreover, the intolerance in question is almost always to meat.

For the Guajiro, almost any animal can reveal itself to be a metamorphosis or the messenger of a being from the other world, more precisely of one of the Pulowi, the "mistresses" of sea and game animals, or of a *wanülüü,* their nocturnal and evil emissaries. Here, too, the language is revealing: the word *uchii,* the generic term for "savage animal," is also synonymous with *wanülüü,* as if a supernatural being could be hiding in any beast. Therefore, all animals are at least slightly *pülasü* (Perrin 1976, 1985); they can also reveal shamanic vocations. If a person does not tolerate fish, for instance, this may imply that she (he) has been singled out by Pulowi, or by one of her emissaries. The same happens for domestic animals, to a lesser extent (Perrin 1987, 1988). It is therefore not surprising that, to justify their calling, a number of shamans claim to have suffered phobias or genuine allergies to certain animal foods.

Moreover, when the person becomes a shaman, special care must be taken to avoid ingesting "wrong foods" so that the essential action of tobacco will not be neutralized. This uncommon sensitivity to food, which is the sign of a calling prior to initiation, subsequently becomes a rule for life. This is because, in relation to their bodies, shamans must live marginal lives, a fundamental requirement for them to be able to communicate with the other world.

> There is the shaman who can only blow for she does not pay enough attention to her food. She eats fried things, she eats what has spilled over onto the fire, and her spirit goes away, goes away. . . It is as though smoke were coming out of her belly and her body is swollen. . . Because of that she constantly falls sick, she dies, she faints, and her shamanery disappears.
>
> The true shaman, she who eats *yüi* tobacco, must be very careful with her food.
>
> Otherwise she will see no more than he who sees with his eyes. . .
>
> (The shaman Too'toria Püshaina, in 1977.)

To a category known as *wanülüü* (the same name as is given to the shaman's auxiliary spirit) the Guajiro assign all woes that cause great distress and are interpreted as a consequence of the departure of the soul, borne away by a *pülasü* being (see Perrin 1979, 1980, 1982a). To be a frequent victim of *wanülüü*-type sicknesses is therefore proof of a relationship with the other world and is the sign of a potential shamanic calling. This category of illness can only be recognized and cured by a shaman. Its archetypal form is the sickness known as *wanülüüsiraa,* literally, "to be the hunt victim of a *wanülüü.*" The latter word, in this case, designates a *pülasü* being who is both an emissary of Pulowi and the descendant of one who has long been dead. To kill you, he shoots an invisible arrow and takes possession of your soul. Therefore, the sickness, the supernatural being who has caused it, and the auxiliary spirit of the shaman who seeks to cure it are all designated by the same name, *wanülüü.* This homonymy, this ambiguity, is significant. To be sick, to cause to be sick, and to cure are different aspects of the relationship linking man to the *pülasü* world (Perrin 1976). It is logical that the Guajiro, in order to justify their calling, always refer to the recurrent sicknesses of their younger days, since they also attest to a certain interpenetration with the other world.

> This was already in me when I was a child, and I grew up with it. I was ill when I was young. I suffered many *wanülüü* sicknesses. It is why I became a shaman, and I feel good like this. I was ill, I fainted because of the *wanülüü* I had in me. I was very ill and I dreamed a lot in the past. . .
>
> (The shaman Maria Jayaliyuu, in 1975.)

Lapü, Dream, is also *pülasü.* Independent of man's will, he is the personified proof of the diffuse action of the supernatural world on the person experiencing the dream. For this reason dreams need to be taken seriously. They are the voice of the other world. They may reveal the source of the sickness, designate the supernatural being who is its ultimate cause, or warn against a future calamity. The Guajiro, practically, consider frequent dreaming to be an embryonic form of the auxiliary spirit, of the *wanülüü.* On the one hand, dreaming implies intercourse between the dreamer's soul and Dream who stimulates it. On the other hand, according to some shamans, Dream integrates into itself the souls of the dying.

> Dream is the one who receives our soul. . .
> There is not one soul that gets away from him:
> The souls of the foreigners, of the dogs, of the cows.
> They are all there, where Dream is.
> He is the only one who is in command of this. . .
> When we sing, we the shamans, we go up there,
> We ask to Dream, very far away. . .
>
> (The male shaman Setuuma Püshaina, in 1973.)

This continually sustained integration perpetuates the "matter" of Dream, which contributes to the emergence of the spirits of the shamans (Perrin 1986b). Thus there would appear to exist a kind of consubstantiality among soul, Dream, and auxiliary spirit. And, as asserted by some shamans, the shaman's spirit would appear to be a sort of personification or emissary of Dream.

> I have good dreams: Do it this way! I am told when I begin to sleep. I dream of dances to be organized after the treatment. We do not see with our eyes where our spirits live. We know it because of their words:
>
> I am Saamatüi, tells us this one. I come from Wapusanain, "Our Dream," he says. . . He comes out of the dream, and we dream with him. . .
>
> (The shaman Aana Püshaina, in 1979.)

To remove "shamanery" when it becomes harmful has the consequence of erasing the dream while taking away the spirit (Perrin 1986a):

> When it [shamanery] came to me, I had good dreams. But I did not want to suffer because of this.
> Take it away from me, I do not want to suffer, I said. A shaman removed it. Then I was ill for a year, and I did not dream anymore. Nothing, not a single dream. Before, my dreams were very good. . .
>
> (Aura Jayaliyuu, in 1979.)

Perhaps the shaman is a kind of dreamer-to-order, a waking dreamer who is not subject to the haphazard qualities of dreams, but, on the contrary, can establish at will a communication with the supernatural.

Mention should also be made of another implicit connection between dreams and shamanism. Dreams are considered to be neutral intermediaries that can, without risk, formulate an accusation in a system partially based on the projection and delegation of responsibility. Similarly, in his dealings with a sick person or the community, the performing shaman is "other." He is reputed not to be the master of what he says, does, or requests. He is a mouthpiece, a mediator, a third party consulted for the purpose of obtaining a diagnosis. He himself obtains this diagnosis from another third party, his auxiliary spirit or spirits, who themselves consult Dream of other beings of the *pülasü* world. At the end of this series of links "words are spoken" from the shaman's mouth.

> We the shamans, we eat tobacco and we chant.
> We keep our eyes closed and we see. . .
> It is as though someone were in front of us.
> It is our auxiliary spirit, our *wanülüü.*
> His words pass through our mouth,
> But they are different from the words of ordinary people.

It is like a telephone that comes into our head. . .
We go where Dream is.
Our spirit travels continually, very far away, and he comes back immediately.
He is as swift as our gaze. . .

(The shaman Too'toria Püshaina, in 1977.)

Hence it is not surprising that those who have become shamans claim to have been "good dreamers." In earlier times they had therapeutic dreams that attracted attention and demonstrated their shamanic vocations. Generally these dreams revealed the proper diagnosis and treatment of childhood illnesses. The "good dreams" were proof of an interrelationship with the "other world."

Thus a coherent network of "significant symptoms" and signs may gradually be woven around a person, demonstrating her (his) permeability to the *pülasü* world. This calling, or "penchant for shamanery" (*outseewa*), is confirmed on the occasion of a further *wanülüü*-type sickness. The shaman consulted reveals the true nature of the pain.

This is not a bad sickness, a fierce *wanülüü*.
It is a good *wanülüü*.
It is her (his) desire to be a shaman: *outseesü*(*shi*).

Then the dreams become more precise, frequent, and premonitory, revealing sometimes the nature of the ready-to-come auxiliary spirits: male or female, Indian or foreigner, young or old. But this communication with the other world is still uncertain, not at will. Finally comes the "crisis," the fainting fit, the "near death" (*ouktapünaa*), and the summoned shaman will make it clear:

It is ready now, it is ripe *jakütüsü, keerain*. . .

A "reversal" occurs (see Perrin 1986a). The pathogenic spirit is now regarded as a "good *wanülüü*," in other words, a future auxiliary spirit. Signs previously interpreted as significant symptoms will shortly be interpreted as shamanic symbols, provided that this reversal is confirmed by "the tobacco proof."

SHAMANISM, TOBACCO, FERTILIZATION, AND SEXUALITY

Tobacco is essential in the symbolic systems of a large number of Amerindian societies, smoked or chewed as the case may be. All Guajiros smoke tobacco, industrial made cigarettes or local cigars, but only shamans drink tobacco juice, known as *yüi makuira.* I have shown elsewhere that tobacco is indirectly linked to the jaguar, which is clearly associated with the extraordinary power of nature (Perrin 1986b, 220–23, 1992). By ingesting tobacco the shaman incorporates a symbolic object of *pülasü* power, and the effects become its tangible expression.[5] These *pülasü* effects enable the shaman to see by other means than the eyes, to perceive the true nature of beings, to recognize the various manifestations of the other world, and even to dominate it. It therefore follows quite naturally that one cannot drink tobacco juice without precautions, without restrictions, and without consequences.

This is why tobacco juice is a test substance at the time of the fainting fit, the state of near death that always marks the culmination of this slow process, a culmination announced by the shaman who is urgently summoned. Chewing tobacco, this "initiating" shaman introduces some into the mouth of the person who has fainted and then, blowing, sprays some on her (his) face and body. The "dead person" regains consciousness. The shaman again makes her (him) drink tobacco juice. If the "patient" does not tolerate it, if she (he) vomits, it indicates that she (he) will experience difficulties as a shaman, that her (his) spirits are bad. If, on the contrary, she (he) tolerates it, she (he) may become a true shaman: a relationship now exists between the other world and that person who has "opened himself up." Afterward, when a sick person consults her (him), she (he) takes tobacco and again, in the actual words of the Guajiro, will "open herself (himself) up all through her (his) body." She (he) will open herself (himself) up to the *pülasü* world; she (he) will communicate with the supernatural world through the agency of her (his) spirits. She (he) will go elsewhere during a journey triggered by powerful shamanic tobacco (*pülasü yüi makuira*). She (he) will know the truth directly, assisted by the spirits who will reveal it to her (him):

> Those who die go toward the east, toward the roots of the sky. I see them because of my good *wanülüü,* my spirit. It is he who takes me over

> yonder and then I speak to those who are dead. . . I saw the wife of Huya with her enormous vagina.
>
> Take it easy, don't touch that! I was told by my father Maleiwa, the Culture Hero. I hid and looked through a hole. . . Thus is Maleiwa, he is very nice to me.
>
> (The shaman Maria Jayaliyuu, in 1975.)

Tobacco is at once a "vehicle" and a "catalyst" acting upon the shaman's body (Perrin 1982b). It is also the symbol of this "meeting" between the shaman and her (his) spirits on the occasion of each cure. By means of tobacco, the new shaman clearly perceives her (his) auxiliary spirits, who until then had been but diffuse and remote presences, never revealing themselves directly. With it, the spirit "takes bodily shape," he "descends" on the shaman who sees him or feels him above: *tajuunakai,* "he who is over me," is the other generic name for the shaman's spirit, synonymous with *wanülüü.*

Tobacco is a substance that is ingested by shamans to give concrete form to their power. This is perhaps the origin of the correlations established between sexuality, fertilization, and shamanism. The question is, over and above the general remarks just made, how do the Guajiro view the action of tobacco on the body of the shaman?

Sometimes the role assigned to tobacco the first time it is taken is one that facilitates a dilation comparable to the experience of the body of a woman in childbirth. It is the "bringing into sight" of something that, until then, was hidden in the abdomen of the new shaman, but that originally comes from somewhere else, from the other world. The person who takes tobacco "opens himself up," "is split open," as though a communication is established between the inside of the shaman's body, where the tobacco is—hence, "shamanery"—and the *pülasü* world, accessible only to those for whom this communication is established:

> He who is going to be a shaman faints.
> A shaman blows on him.
> He prepares *yüi* tobacco and puts it in his mouth.
> He makes him swallow it.
> Then his voice comes out of his belly.
> For it was taking shape there,

> It was swelling out in his belly. . .
> There it is, he is a shaman now. . .
>
> (The male shaman Setuuma Püshaina, in 1973.)

More commonly, the action of the tobacco juice on the body is indirectly associated with fertilization through the mouth, comparable to the impregnation of a woman during the sexual act: the tobacco juice, ingested by the novice, literally causes "shamanery" to become "ripe" or to "grow" in the belly of the shaman to be. Moreover, the Guajiro are quick to stress "the first time" for tobacco juice, just as they emphasize the first time for the sexual act, which "pierces" women. Both occasions are linked with fear, danger, and desire, and both are strictly subject to social conventions.

> At the time, it was as if I had no legs. I was the victim of a snake, I was like a snake. In my dream, it coiled up all around me. . . He said to me, showing tobacco, here is your food! Are you going to accept this tobacco for us? The *wanülüü* arrived then.
>
> Hold it, we bring that for you, take it now! he said to me about a green piece of tobacco, still fresh. It was inside a little crocheted bag. . . I took the soul of that, its image, and I ate it. I was afraid, but I had a longing for tobacco, because my *aa'in,* my soul, my heart was asking for it. I ate some to settle that, and something happened. I was as if I was dead. When the sun set, I had not regained consciousness. That's the way it happened when my spirit arrived. . . Then, I still had my grandmother, who was a shaman.
>
> There is no remedy for that, she said. It is here, in her belly, one day she will eat tobacco, the song of my grandmother told me. . .
>
> (The shaman Maria Jayaliyuu, in 1975.)

To be socially useful—not only to society in general, but also to the family of the woman concerned—to be safe, both the use of tobacco and the sexuality of the maidens have to be controlled. All the more so, because both are associated with economic interests. In Guajiro society, the virginity of the girls is highly valued, and female adultery severely punished, in particular by economic sanctions. In the same way, the access to the shamanic function can be a way to relative wealth (Perrin 1986b, chapter 10, and 1992).

There are additional connections between shamanism and sexuality that contribute to a coherent system, or a shamanic model of sexuality that can induce a shaman to observe certain characteristic attitudes. Each time such attitudes are expressed, they become confirmations of shamanic qualities.

> This shaman was very powerful, very *pülashi.* He asked for horse races and shooting games. For the *yonna* dance, he wanted only the maidens.
>
> Those who already "did the thing" with men cannot come, he said; If one claimed to be a maiden and was not, he knew it.
>
> You, you will not dance, he said; he was very clear sighted. . . It was dangerous for people to couple in his presence. If they did so, the heart of that shaman filled up. *Pülasü nümüin:* it was dangerous for him, it was taboo. There was something like froth in his mouth, because of what comes out of men, sperm. . . This is what happened once, because of that:
>
> Why did you let them enter? This had to happen! Why did you let them dance? His spirits told him about two young persons who had made love.
>
> We'll see if this *pülashi* will die, they had said to themselves. But straight away he had felt a bad taste and nausea. Already he knew: his spirits had protested and told him.
>
> Sit down, we do not want to die, they had also said. Because of that, this shaman fainted away. Then, he drank a lot of tobacco, and he sang again. But, after that, he fell sick. He stayed inside for a month, eating only tobacco juice. . .
>
> (The shaman Aura Jayaliyuu, in 1979.)

While this, in a way, confirms the links between virginity and shamanism, this story also reveals a relationship between sperm and tobacco juice. The sperm finds its way metaphorically into the mouth of the shaman and chokes him. The mouth of the shaman is likened to the sexual organs of a woman absorbing a bad product and being blocked up by it. Only a good product, tobacco juice, can neutralize this pathogenic effect. Hence sperm and tobacco juice are incompatible. The fact that they hold the same paradigmatic position makes them exclusive of one another, since they occupy a concurrent position in relation to the other world. Like the tobacco juice, human sperm is supposed to get its power from the *pülasü* world (Perrin 1985, 118–19).

This is expressed somewhat differently in the following tale. Here, it is the guilty parties, more than the shaman, who suffer from the consequences of their misplaced sexual act. But again, the shaman's breath, full of tobacco juice, neutralizes the pathogenic effect.

> We are going to have a *yonna* dance, said the shaman. But if the dancers do what they shouldn't, they'll swell up. . . Soon, however, a woman was there, recumbent, and the man too.
>
> Help them, don't let them die, people said to the shaman.
>
> Help them fast for they are already huge! The shaman went and had a look at them. . . He blew on them with tobacco juice: Pshuuuu! Then they woke up, they were saved. Thus are the shamans who are very *pülasü,* very powerful. . .
>
> (Sepaana Epieyuu, in 1977.)

Is it this image of a female sexuality associated with shamanism that causes Guajiro who are not shamans to say that all women shamans are man-eaters and men shamans homosexuals (a "theoretical" position that does not prevent the circulation of many stories demonstrating the heterosexuality of many male shamans)? In any case, this sexualized image associated with the shaman's tobacco accords with the fantasy descriptions of shamanic sexuality expressed by others. Note the following conversation between two men.

> What's best to become a shaman, to be a man or a woman?
>
> If you're a man, you're said to be a fag, but if you're a woman, you're said to be a whore and to change men all the time. . . The male shaman is fucked by his spirit who copulates with him. But the female shaman too is the wife of her spirit. And the spirit hates the husband of the married female shaman; he won't let him get near her. . . That's true, all the Guajiro say so.
>
> (Makantre Uliana and Moono Jinnu, in 1979.)

Moreover, this image of a female sexuality associated with shamanism is compatible with the masculine status of tobacco juice in Guajiro thought. The shaman's tobacco is associated with Jaguar, who, as a great seducer of maidens, symbolizes masculine power and is opposed to the cultural hero Maleiwa, just as untamed nature is opposed to the humanized world. Here too a considerable degree of coherence is apparent.

The shamanistic function is considered to be incompatible with normal sexuality, tending instead toward sexual excess, as some Guajiros say, or toward continence, as most shamans claim.

> This was a very good shaman. Her husband could not sleep with her. They could not lie one beside the other, because her spirit became angry at once. To be able to sing, she could not have a man for a year. . .
>
> (The shaman Too'toria Püshaina, in 1979.)

> The shamans who have husbands are liars, and the male shaman who is *pülashi* has no wife. . . If the very *pülasü* shaman tries to copulate, her spirits say to her:
>
> If you go on, we will kill you. We will fasten your head down if you don't stop. After that, she falls ill, she suffers headaches. Those who have men are only lying. They are like the white doctor who is married to the money he gets. . .
>
> (The shaman Setuuma Püshaina, in 1973.)

> For the female shamans, men are *pülashi:* forbidden and dangerous. They die because of them. It is forbidden to copulate: these things are *pülasü.* Likewise with my husband:
>
> You will not do that with me, you will be like a son. Then you will stay alive, and I will stay alive. It is what we say when we are together. . .
>
> (The shaman Reeachon Jayaliyuu, in 1973.)

Jealous spirits, so it is said, may even prevent procreation in women shamans.

> My little baby dies in my womb.
> One of my spirits ate him. . .
>
> (The shaman Ouusilia Jayaliyuu, in 1977.)

The Guajiro shamans find chastity imposed by "the other world." They then advocate abstinence and make of it, as they say, a way of life. The shaman's death is considered to be the effect of a sexual act, refused until then, between him and one of his spirits. It is asserted by the shamans themselves that formerly they lived close to one another, the life of a couple, but without union. Nothing can neutralize the effects of this fatal joining, this coupling with the supernatural. Tobacco juice itself is of no avail.

> A shaman dies when her spirit has copulated with her. She dies pissing blood.
>
> My spirit took me, she says before dying. He made love to her and took her over yonder that she may be his wife. . .
>
> (The male shaman Setuuma Püshaina, in 1973.)

Tobacco, however, will be used one last time.

> When a shaman dies, his mouth is opened wide, liquor is poured into it and then a piece of tobacco is placed in it. Then his jaws are shut tight. . . Later two pieces of tobacco are placed in his hands. In this way his soul will not reappear. Otherwise it would keep coming back to ask for tobacco. . .
>
> (The shaman Too'toria Püshaina, in 1977.)

Here tobacco is no more than the commonplace sign of the shamanic function. It is no longer the powerful substance that has acted continually upon the shaman's body. The shaman here is portrayed as no more than a drug addict craving his drug. We have left the strict Guajiro shamanic logic and entered into the Guajiro logic of death.

THE PENCHANT FOR SHAMANERY

Apart from the cures they effect, the Guajiro shamans lead a life outwardly similar to that of the other people. They are occupied by domestic tasks and kinship roles, and are not full-time specialists. They adopt the position of shaman at the request, for instance, of a sick person and his or her group, of a family wishing to be sure of the non-evil, non-*pülasü* nature of the land they are intending to settle, or, in earlier days, at the request of a "chief" who wanted to know the outcome of a war before continuing with it. Thus they are called according to circumstances (Perrin 1986b, chapter 10, and 1992). A shaman does not normally take tobacco except when effecting a cure; therefore, his use of it is socially regulated. The shaman is not normally an addict or a being subject against his will to "shamanic crises." If he behaves differently, there is a disorder, and this disorder is expressed by a category of Guajiro etiology: *ira'iraiwaa,* literally "to be taken by the spirit *ira'irai,* the spirit who causes trembling" (Perrin 1982a, 53–54).

> She falls down in a faint; her teeth clamped together. Tobacco must be put into her mouth, or else she'll die. She chews it and at once she feels better. She seizes her rattle; she shakes it vigorously. She trembles with the rattle in her hand. And soon it stops, because of the tobacco. . .
>
> (Isho Jayaliyuu, in 1975.)

> The *ira'rai* is a *wanülüü,* a shaman's spirit. If we have it, we faint away incessantly. Then, when we sing or when we take tobacco juice, we are shaking all over, our wrists are stiff. We spit out a lot, we stay half dead. . . The one who has the *ira'irai* is frightened of everything. The barking of a dog, etc. I am not afraid of this, because my spirit is good. I feel like this only if the feast was not organized well, the feast I asked in order to help the sick person. . .
>
> (The shaman Maria Jayaliyuu, in 1975.)

The victims of these passing crises (somatic crises with a hysteria-type symptomatology, according to a psychiatric description) are, to some extent, tobacco dependent. According to them, only tobacco can bring relief. But such shamans very soon lose their clientele and their function, assuming they held one before. These spectacular crises are regarded by the Guajiro as abnormal (*mujusü*).

This is not true of the comparable crises that the shaman may undergo if his patient's family does not pay in full what he has asked them. Then on the occasion of each cure, the Guajiro shaman, by means of his body, may express his displeasure and goad or blame those who have consulted him. This bodily behavior is also linked to the consumption of tobacco, which alone can bring back his normal state.

> If I'm underpaid I get cramps in my hands, my feet swell up and I may faint. Then I quickly swallow some tobacco juice and that makes me feel better. . .
>
> (The shaman Aana Püshaina, in 1979.)

These shamanic upsets are based on the logic of a series of linked debts, the operation of which is described in the following tale.

> All that was missing was a cow the color of a squirrel with straight horns. No one could find one. So I died in my hammock, I fainted.
>
> They don't pay attention to you, my spirit had said to me. He escaped at the moment that I died, for his words and his requests had

> not been respected, and he did not see how he was going to be paid.
> I stayed twenty days without moving. . . My spirit had been caught by ghosts of the dead there with the soul of the person I was tending. . . It was when he came back that I came to my senses again. I started to breathe, because of the smell of the tobacco.
>
> (The shaman Reeachon Jayaliyuu, in 1973.)

The auxiliary spirits who take on the responsibility of bringing the patient's soul back from the supernatural world make the shaman pay whoever summoned them. This payment is calculated in jewels and cattle with clearly specified qualities whose "souls" will be kept by the spirits and whose "bodies" will be kept by the shaman. The shaman consequently informs his client's family of the demands of his spirits. If they are not satisfied, a crisis occurs. The patient will not be able to be cured, which becomes the responsibility of his family. Also the shaman may fall sick, victim of one of his dissatisfied spirits, himself a victim of the supernatural being who holds the sick person's soul. Hence there are four intermediaries, three of whom are in the position of debtors one to the other.

In Guajiro logic the crisis just described is justified. But this is the outer limit of the system. This crisis, which is a source of blame for the patient and his group, is a sword with a double edge. Excessive use of it may well give rise to a change of attitude toward the shaman. Instead of being the accuser, he may become the accused. Crises that occur too systematically would be interpreted as the symptom of an *ira'irai* sickness or simply as a false pretext for "eating money."

Some Guajiro also evoke other manifestations in their biographies that do not conform to the usual pattern but that leads them, nevertheless, to "shamanery," or to a broken career. Here are two examples. The first one is that of a shaman whose vocation, she says, emerged after an emotional shock due to the death of one of her adult children.

> This is the way I have been made: long ago, I suffered a lot, but this is somewhat new. It was after my son's death, around six years ago. . . He died in a brawl. Before that, another child had died of diarrhea, very young. I used to cry every day, every day. I would cry for years before I

> found shamanery. . . Before I would never dream. Then, because of my son's death, I found it:
>
> If you want to be *pülasü,* to have supernatural powers, if you want something to come from your son's death, something will come out one day, the dream told. Then, much later, a person came out. She told me things about minor diseases. From this moment onwards, I have cured children. I am not a shaman who has eaten tobacco. . .
>
> (The shaman Kataliina Aapüshana, in 1973.)

The next example is more dramatic. It shows how a woman, also distressed by the death of a child, was willingly dispossessed of symptoms interpreted to signify a shamanic vocation. In this narration, troubles of personality and shamanism are closely linked. This near-fictive connection helps to clear up a temporarily difficult psychological situation.

> I used to have very good dreams. It [shamanery] was there, but they removed it. They snatched it from me. . . One day, one of my children fell ill and died. Then I was crying all the time. At this very moment I started feeling bad. Then, one of my youngest brother's children died. I went to his burial. I was crying and the same thing happened as before. I fainted, and I was taken to the Lower Guajira.
>
> I would like to die very soon to stop suffering. I would say to myself.
>
> You're going to be well, you'll get cured, I heard then in my head. Nothing will happen. Just as you are, you're close to it [shamanery]. I had pains, I didn't feel well. Everything seemed to be dark on my way.
>
> Accept it, my parents were saying. But I did not want to suffer because of shamanery. I went to see a *pülasü,* a shaman.
>
> Take it out of me. I don't want to suffer, that's what I told her. So, the shaman took it out, and it made a lot of noise. I got rid of it, but I was sick for a whole year. . .
>
> (Aura Jayaliyuu, in 1979.)

Let us reconsider the Guajiro notion *outseewa,* translated as "wish to be shaman," or "penchant for shamanery" (Perrin 1986a). This real nosological category is a syndrome on which are projected all kinds of personal problems, associated mainly with the consequences of acculturation and the exodus to urban areas, a process that particularly modifies the feminine condition (Perrin 1986b, 1992). In fact, at the present time, many women claim to have a vocation of shaman. But a seventeen-year retrospective enables us to assert that very few of these vocations come to be realized. The proportion of "fully recognized" shamans did not increase during these years. On the contrary, it seems that it decreased somewhat, if we believe the Guajiro themselves.

What conclusion can be drawn? We can accept that among the Guajiro "collective or individual neurosis" has developed—a phenomenon that can be observed in societies subject to acculturation. Devereux speaks of "acculturation neuroses," which are expressed in a particular form (Devereux 1970, 72). Why do we find specifically this type of "ethnic disorder" associated with shamanism among the Guajiro? To put forth a hypothesis taking into account Devereux's suggestions: if the members of traditional societies tend to express their personal confusion first in the form of hysteria, and, among the Guajiro, if the model of the shamanic vocation corresponds to a cultural representation of hysteria, as suggested above, there is nothing surprising in the fact that women, completely troubled by the present changes, express their confusion by evoking a "desire for shamanery," a language of the body particularly appropriate.[6] This could be all the more desirable because they can expect secondary benefits from this type of attitude.

However, if we observe the facts of who actually becomes a shaman, we are led to a conclusion that contradicts some of Devereux's arguments. Very few women who feel called to shamanery actually become shamans. The shamans who are called on to confirm shamanic calling make strict selections from all the implicit requests they receive, even if they tend not to refuse them openly. They may readily agree that a *wanülüü* spirit upsets their patient, but they don't easily declare that she is "mature" for shamanery. In the name of an idealized definition of the conditions required for access to shamanism, they firmly control the social reproduction of the shamanic system. And it could be supposed that because of this present excess of requests, the selection, increasingly rigorous, requires greater conformity.[7] Thus, none of the five cases fully observed during twelve years led to anything conclusive regarding the women's capacities as shamans. Two of the women concerned still sometimes "have good dreams" and are subject to fainting spells and pains that they consider consequences of the aleatory visitations of their spirits. The three others no longer feel any sign of shamanery, since the shamans consulted did not meet their expectations or did not respond to the expression of the women's pathological states.

SHAMANISM AND HYSTERIA

At the end of this analysis, one question arises. Why is there this cultural model of hysteria? Two hypotheses can be suggested. From a genetic point of view, one could suppose a connection, at the origin, between a universal human desire to relieve others' suffering bodies and a structure of hysterical type, associated with deep-seated mental processes and expressed by a specific "language of the body." Now, the human body and its essential functions are, in preliterate societies with only simple technology, a fundamental source of thoughts, metaphors, and images underpinning representations. In other words, the first shamans would have been "real hysterics" before the system they have slowly created was accepted fully as a logical and formal representation, made up of elements of hysterical nature but now semi-independent of its psychological origins.

It is also possible to consider the problem from a more general angle and to adopt the paradoxical standpoint formulated by Lévi-Strauss when he stressed the difference between magic and science from the point of view of determinism.

> One can go further and think of the rigorous precision of magical thought and ritual practices as an expression of the unconscious apprehension of the *truth of determinism,* the mode in which scientific phenomena exist. In this view, the operations of determinism are divined and made use of in an all-embracing fashion before being known and properly applied, and magical rites and beliefs appear as so many expressions of an act of faith in a science yet to be born (Lévi-Strauss 1966, 11).

It might be said of shamanism that it is the expression of an unconscious perception of the relations between man, his body, and the world, which the psychological and psychoanalytical sciences are endeavoring at the present time to understand scientifically. This does not mean, to paraphrase what Lévi-Strauss says further on, that it is necessary to go back to the "crude view" of shamanism as "a hesitant tentative form" of psychoanalysis.

> Magical thought is not to be regarded as a beginning, a rudiment, a sketch, a part of a whole which has not yet materialized. It forms a well-

> articulated system, and is in this respect independent of that other system which constitutes science, . . . (Lévi-Strauss 1966, 13).

It is, indeed, a particular conception of the relations of the world to man and to his body expressed by shamanism in a "tightly knit system." In this system, intolerances or phobias of certain foods, dreams, somatizations, hallucinogens, and a "third sexuality" serve as both symptoms and symbols. Similarly, psychoanalysis builds up a tightly knit system with the same terms but according to different arrangements and with different emphases. It bears witness to a very different outlook on the world and a very different relationship between man and the world.

However that may be, to consider the shamanic calling as no more than the manifestation of mental deviance would be to associate in our own cultures the functions of the priest, doctor, or psychoanalyst with particular types of "madness," or to judge medical and psychoanalytical theories, or principles of the Church, by the yardstick of those madnesses. It would be to deprive oneself of the possibility of discerning possible forms of deviance in relation to a dominant cultural model. Conversely, as this study shows, care should also be taken not to gloss over the cultural representations of the body in the shamanic system by seeking to disregard, in reaction, all but the intellectual and spiritual aspects of the shaman's calling or function.

NOTE ON TRANSCRIPTION (GUAJIRO)

The transcription of the Guajiro language used here is a simplified system taking account as far as possible of the spelling and pronunciation of local Spanish. For an English reader, the major drawback to this system is the use of the letter *j* to convey the sound *h.* The sign *ü* signifies a central closed vowel situated between *i* and *u,* as in *mürülü* (domestic animal), and ' a mute occlusive glottal consonant, as in *ka'i* (sun). Long or geminated sounds are not shown.

Notes

1. I venture this neologism to translate Guajiro expressions conveying the idea of "shamanic function," or the idea of an "alteration of behavior char-

acteristic of a shaman." It has the advantage of underscoring an implicit parallelism between an inclination toward sickness and an inclination toward shamanism (see Perrin 1986a, 119–20). In this, specific meanings can be distinguished from the far too general sense given by anthropologists to the word "shamanism." We will also use the verb "to shamanize" as a literal translation of the Guajiro word *outajaa,* from which derive *outsü* (feminine) and *outshi* (masculine): "shaman."

2. Even though, for instance, in his work on the Mojave shamans of North America, G. Devereux constantly alluded to a "process of cultural fashioning," to a "social prestructuring," or to "culturally structured experiences," he never fully explained these concepts. He suggested them merely in order to go on to emphasize the importance of "emotional behavior" or "neurotic reasons," and, subsequently, this attitude becomes more pronounced (see for instance Devereux 1970 and 1972).

3. Ethnographic data on this subject are rare. A. Métraux, for instance (1967), to mention only the best known, does not seem to have suspected it in his studies of Amerindian shamanism. Devereux, already mentioned, never did a thorough analysis of what he calls the "Mohave surnaturalism." A vast field of comparative research still has to be explored.

4. See, for example, in Devereaux (1970, 67–68) translated from "Normal and Abnormal: The Key Problem of Psychiatric Anthropology." In *Some Uses of Anthropology: Theoretical and Applied,* Washington, D.C., The Anthropological Society of Washington, 1956, pp. 23–48; and especially Chapter 9 in Devereux (1972), translated from "Dream Learning and Individual Ritual Differences in Mohave Shamanism," *American Anthropologist* 59:103–45, 1957.

5. Usually, nicotine is not classified as a hallucinogen by botanists or pharmacologists. But it is recognized that tobacco juice (here *Nicotiana tabacum*) in large quantities produces hallucinatory effects (see Wilbert 1987). In any case, tobacco, in Guajiro shamanism and in other Amerindian shamanic systems, occupies a place comparable to that of "recognized" hallucinogens in other shamanistic societies.

6. Devereux would certainly label "ethnic disorders" or "typical disorders" the Guajiro food phobias, characteristic dreams, and *wanülüü* sicknesses (three elements surely associated in some other shamanic systems), i.e., "psychological sicknesses proper to the type of society that produces them" (1970, 62). But, let us again lay stress on that point, the similarity of many shamans' biographies is so striking, the correlations between the "symptomatologies" they present and the Guajiro world representations (what Devereux calls "surnaturalism") are so great that they almost coincide. Moreover, Devereux implicitly admits this difficulty; it is only afterward when people manifest other symptoms (then qualified as "atypical") that it would be possible to recognize "hidden" or "covered" forms, i.e., pathology (see Perrin 1986b, 721–35).

7. In fact, the reality is more complex: it is a dynamic system in a complete upheaval. Some people are making individual decisions and are finding themselves in new contexts, on the edge of traditional society and of Western society. This way, completely abnormal people can hold therapeutic positions temporarily, and even claim to be new shamans on arrival in a new sphere, at the end of a migration, with the help of privileged contacts with the whites, supposedly to reinforce their powers. Considering the distress of Guajiro populations recently arrived, they can be sure, at least for a while, to have some success.

S I X

HE WHO DREAMS

The Nocturnal Source of Transforming Power in Kagwahiv Shamanism

WAUD H. KRACKE

The concept of "shamanism," like many basic concepts in anthropology, is a generalization of a concept from one culture as a tag for similar phenomena in others. It is true that the institution of a healer who goes into trance as part of a curing ceremony is one that recurs in different cultures throughout the world with some remarkable similarities. But there are also striking differences from culture to culture, both in the practices of such healers and in the way of conceptualizing the process of the cure and the healer's part in it. These tend to be masked by the use of a single term. Even in the current literature, in otherwise excellent discussions, one encounters debates over whether the "true shaman" uses possession or magical flight (e.g., Peters 1982, 22), or whether "the shaman" is invariably schizophrenic, is typical for his culture, or is exceptionally well-adjusted (a discussion that ignores not only differences between cultures, but also between individuals in a culture).

Such assertions give an illusory sense of uniformity in curing institutions that can be highly misleading. Yet if true shamans are only those who use magical flight, then others who depend on possession must be something else. I would not go as far as Lévi-Strauss did with totemism and assert here that the concept of shamanism is an illusion corresponding to no real phenomenon. We would be better served to examine cases with an eye to identifying dimensions of contrast between shamanism in different cultures, both on a regional level and between individual cultures within a region. A more specific focus of this sort may not only bring out different configurations of shamanism, but may also bring to attention new features central to certain shamanic systems that have not been noted or regarded as important in shamanic systems hitherto studied.

One such distinct configuration of shamanism, which occurs in several South American cultures, is a system of beliefs in which the shaman's power is expressed predominantly through dreaming. For example, the Parintintin Indians of the Madeira River in Brazil hold that many of a shaman's most important effects on the world are executed through dreams. The Parintintin are a Tupi-speaking, tropical rain forest culture of the western Amazon region of Brazil. Traditionally they lived in small settlements consisting of a single longhouse each, two at most, scattered along the banks of tributaries to the Madeira River. They made their living by hunting, fishing, and growing corn and manioc in slash-and-burn gardens cut from the tropical forest. They still practice these subsistence activities (though they hunt with guns and have lost their traditional varieties of corn), but they have been in contact now for nearly seventy years, and much has changed. Brought into permanent contact in 1923, the Kagwahiv are now highly integrated into Brazilian interior society. They are dependent on a monetary economy for goods from sugar to shotgun shells, and they are locked into selling Brazil nuts and the other jungle products they gather to pay for them. While they still speak their language and observe moiety exogamy and many other traditional practices, other aspects of their ceremonial and religious life have fallen into abeyance—including the rites of curing, and the specialists who conducted them. Thus most of what I have to report on Kagwahiv curing is a retrospective reconstruction, based on the memories of older informants, of something that has not been practiced for some years.

The shaman, or *ipají,* is one casualty of the process of contact. None are left, and some of the reasons for this will become clear in the following discussion. The information on shamans presented here comes from the more elderly Parintintin, who have seen them in action and in some cases been cured by them.

The Kagwahiv curer and principal religious practitioner—*ipají,* "one possessed of power"—performed cures in a ceremony in which he (or his spiritual emanation), in a trance, contacted the Sky People and other spiritual beings and beseeched their help. In this "magical flight," the Kagwahiv *ipají* resembles the image Eliade (1964) and others have built up of the "shaman." But in some other ways, the Kagwahiv individuals with such powers were quite different from the Tungus shaman who is the source of the concept (Shirokogoroff 1935). In particular, for the *ipají,* being healed from an illness caused by spirits had no part in the acquisition of power. Rather, the central image for being empowered in Kagwahiv shamanism was dreaming. Dreaming was not only a mode of gaining knowledge of the supernatural world and communicating with higher beings (as it still is for some nonshamans), but was the vehicle through which the shaman *exercised* his power to change or influence conditions or events in the world: through his dreams a shaman could make a particular kind of game available for a hunter; he could assure vengeance against an enemy in warfare; he could send illness; or he could cause a woman to conceive a child who would later become another shaman, his successor.

THE NATURE OF SHAMANIC POWER

The question of terminology brings us to the heart of the question of what the Kagwahiv curer was—the Kagwahiv conception of his nature. There is no noun to refer to the curers. Rather, they are designated by a verb, *ipají,* meaning "possessed of power"—one of a class of verbs I call "attributive." (Helen Pease in her [1968] S.I.L. grammar calls them "descriptives.") They are verbs that tend to assign qualities to their subjects, and they are like predicate adjectives in English (e.g., *ipohýi* means "it is heavy"). As they are ergative in form, that is, the subject of an intransitive attributive verb has the same form as the object of a transitive one, there is a certain implication of passivity or recipience, so *ipají* might best be translated "is empowered." Thus, the Kagwahiv do not think of *ipají* as a named role, like chief or headman (*ñanderuviháv*), but as a quality that inheres in certain individuals: one is empowered as one is generous or tall, angry or beautiful.

Nonetheless, the curers with such powers did occupy an important role in Kagwahiv society, and it is useful to have a noun to designate them as such. If one were to describe them by their activity, one might call them "singers" (as the Navajo do when referring to their medicine men), for they are described as having spent much of the day pacing back and forth on the plaza singing, and it was through song that they communicated with the spirits of the upper realms. But, they are not denoted with such a term in Kagwahiv. In Portuguese, such practitioners are designated by the Tupi-derived term *pajé.* This is the term with which the Kagwahiv refer to the empowered ones when speaking Portuguese, so it will be used here to designate their role.

The powers that are attributed to such empowered individuals are varied but mostly involve the power to transform or to bring something into being. Besides curing (or causing) illness or death, one who is *ipají* can cause game animals to be available for another man to hunt successfully—or the reverse. One bisexual *pajé* was described as turning his male genitals into female ones for a tryst then changing them back. In myth, when a character transforms himself or someone else into an animal, or effects a change in the environment, it is often added as in explanation: *ipajiheté ga,* or *ipajiheté hẽ*—"he/she was very powerful." The little insects that hover around manioc when it is being toasted into manioc flour, during which it pops up rather like popcorn, are, as one informant told me, "*muito ipají*"; they make the flour expand as it toasts.

Such power is not exercised these days; or at least, no Kagwahiv *pajé* now survives. The last two real *pajés, ipajiheté,* Capitão and Igwaká, died several years before my first fieldwork with the Kagwahiv and before the *pajés* could train their successors. Hence, my understanding of this power is limited.

THE TOKÁIA AND THE PAJÉ'S COSMIC JOURNEY

Several informants have described the curing ceremony that was the focal ritual for these practitioners. The term for the curing ritual, *tokáia,* refers to a small shelter built of palm fronds (*pindóv*) in the center of the clearing, in front of the rectangular longhouse that constituted a traditional Kagwahiv settlement. (The same term, *tokáia,* refers to a small shelter built as a hunter's blind, or to a chicken coop.) Within the shelter prepared for the occasion of the ceremony, out of sight of the audience, a *pajé* would go into trance and communicate with the various spirits he successively approached for help in curing his patient, while another *pajé* would wait outside and question each spirit as it arrived in the *tokáia*.

The ceremonies described by Paulino and Catarina, who had seen at least four of them, involved two *pajés,* one inside the *tokáia* communicating with the spirits who spoke through his voice, the other outside with the people, questioning the spirits as they arrived. The last ceremony they remembered was conducted by Capitão and Igwaká, two *pajés* of Pãi'ĩ extraction who were the last true *pajés* to practice among the Parintintin. They took turns, night by night, being in the *tokáia.* Igwaká, who took the first night, had a red band (presumably of urucú) across his chest, and something red "like cloth" over his head. Preparations for the invocation of spirits included making a pair of pictures on a tree in the plaza before the ceremony of each spirit to be invoked.[1]

The first spirits to visit the *tokáia,* by most accounts, are *añang*—ghosts or forest spirits who live under the ground—in this case named ghost-spirits with distinct individual personalities: Namiremi'ga (who looks like a dog, doesn't eat fruit, and kills people, and who comes out of the cemetery and hides against tree trunks); Nambikwara (literally, "Pierced-ear," who is encountered in overgrown fields, bedecked with macaw feathers hanging from his ears and limbs, with a pet tinamou on one shoulder, and a jacamim—*gwɨrajehe'ó,* "weeping bird," a trumpeter—on the other); Añanga-hapukai ("Screaming *añang,*" a pregnant *añang* who appears upside down); and others.

Next come the spirits of animals, whose order varies somewhat from description to description. Paulino once said that first the small birds (*gwɨra'í*) came, then large birds (*gwɨrahú*), but most of the lists of appearances start with fish and aquatic animals. Singing the songs he remembered from a *tokáia,* Paulino began with the song of the small fish (*jijuhú*), then sang the land turtle's (*jabuti'í*) song, then that of a wood duck, then another fish, the *acarí* (mailed catfish). Following these come the songs of other assorted animals: a large caterpillar, *jatɨtá;* the small frog, *juitarág,* which lives around houses, and, Diré said, urinates; and the squirrel, *quatipurú* (*kutivúruhu*). Peccary and jaguar are animals that one or another informant also recalled coming down into the *tokáia.*

Aruká gave me a song of *mbɨrɨtí* (buriti palm, used for flooring)—commenting, "also a *santo.*"

If the presiding *pajé* is merely *ipajitĩuhũ,* a lesser "white" *pajé,* the parade of spirits stops with the animals. But if he is *ipajiheté,* a "real *pajé,*" then the performance climaxes around daybreak with the appearance (invisibly, in the *tokáia*) of the Ɨvaga'nga, the Sky People themselves, including their chief, Pindova'úmi'ga, and his sons, Arukakatúi'ga (with his son Shashámi'ga), Kwatijakatú'i, Mboave'ɨm, and Pɨrahamarána'ga. The culminating appearance is that of the *ipají* of the Sky People, whose name, Mohãng, means "medicine"—"because he knows," commented Paulino. "Mohãng is a great *ipají,* therefore his song is the highest medicine."

Each spirit, as it comes into the *tokáia,* engages in a formulaic exchange with the shaman-interlocutor outside. The spirit introduces itself:

Frog spirit:	*Juitará-ramo ji rúri*	I come, the house-frog.
Capitão [outside]:	*Gará-ramo nde rúri?*	What have you come for?
Frog spirit:	*Momé ji kwaitáv?*	Where is my task?
Capitão [indicating the locus of the illness in the patient]:	*Ki-kotɨ nde kwaitáv.*	Over here is your task.

Then the spirit sings its characteristic song, and, invisible to the audience, blows on the patient. The song the spirit sings generally dramatizes, poetically, a quality of the species it represents, especially the habitat it frequents, or the kind of food it eats. An *añang,* for example, sings:

Ha, haha, haha.	
Kavavetĩ óguhu, ore 'gwɨramó	The big settlement Kavavetĩ is our place
Ɨvɨ'am ingwánguhũ ore moka'ñɨ	In the red clay [ground] we hide

Here is the song of the *acarí,* "mailed catfish" (fam. Loricariidae), a bone-plated (*cascudo*) fish, which tends to hide in holes in the banks of small streams, as sung by Aruká:

Toré, toré,		toré, toré
Ɨvɨ'am ingwánguhũ ji rúvi.	*Toré, toré*	In a red clay bank I live
Iporová ko ji rúvi	*Toré, toré*	A tough fighter I live

The little *jijuhú* fish:

Jireruapɨ-apɨ parana'já. é-í	Dancing like a river, *é-í.*

A duck:

Ñimbɨ-, ñimbɨape ji hoi	Downriver, downriver I go
ɨreru'já	As if dancing

Some songs involve metaphors, sometimes mediated by a myth. The jaguar, for instance:

Kwari aho-uhu Marité-ve	By day I go indeed to Marité
Ipinĩmongɨuhu ji rupáva ra'e	All dabbed with spots was my hammock
Ñuhũeteuhu reháva ji rupáva ra'é.	In the big savannah a turning-around place was my hammock.

This song refers to the analogy of the reticular pattern of a hammock, with the pattern of spots on the jaguar's hide, which is also manifested in traditional dream interpretation: to dream of a hammock predicts an encounter with a jaguar, because of the analogy of the patterns. This association between jaguar and hammock may be reinforced by the myth in which the jaguar encounters and is bested in a game of bravado by Tupã, the Master of Thunder, who frightened the jaguar nearly to death with thunderbolts while lying in his hammock in the sky.

On the other hand, the songs of the Ɨvága'nga, the Sky People, who appear at the climax of the ceremony, refer primarily to their curative powers. Thus, Pindova'úmi'ga's song, as sung by Aruká:

Ore orotĩa-pɨpe ore rekoi	We are within our binding [?]
Ko ji ore, ore pohã'gí, wẽ	I have our, our little medicine
Ko ti pehepíahete	You [pl.] will see indeed
Ore rovɨtéripe okóvo	Sitting in the middle of our sky
Arɨrɨ, arɨrɨingwãnguhũa	A large, red moth

The red moth, Aruká explained, refers to illness.

The final and climactic song is that of Mohãng, the *pajé* of the Sky People, whose power is presumably the greatest possible. (Here as sung by Diré):

Nde repíaga ji ruri mbogwerápa	I come to see you and restore you
Mbogwerávamo ji ruri nde repíaga	In order to restore you I come
Mohãngamo ji ruri nde repíaga	As medicine [or: I, Mohãng]
	I come to see you

The word, *mbogwerá,* means, literally, "bring back to life" (*mbo-,* causative prefix, + *-kwerá,* "come back to life"). *"Opɨ. Ipají ga,"* concluded Diré. "He blows (curatively on the patient); he is powerful."

The *pajé's* successive trance encounters with spirits are conceived in various ways by different informants. Most frequently they are spoken of as a kind of spiritual journey—"visionary magical flight," in Eliade's phrase quoted by Larry Peters (1982, 22). Others speak of the spirits coming into the *tokáia* to visit the *pajé* there, or the *pajé* going up and bringing the spirits back to the *tokáia.* In a third account that reconciles these two, and seems to be the most precise, Paulino (my principal informant on ritual matters) spoke of the *pajé's rupigwára* going to the sky and bringing the spirits back to the *tokáia* for their negotiations with the *pajé.*

Rupigwára is a key concept for understanding the relation of the *pajés* to the spirits of the universe; but it is at the same time a complex, shadowy, and multifaceted concept. The spirits of the animals that come into the *tokáia* are referred to as the *rupigwára* of the officiating *pajé* in the *tokáia.* His power is judged by the range of *rupigwára* he can call on: a truly powerful *pajé,* one who is *ipajiheté,* can summon the Sky People, as well as the spirits (*ra'uv*) of animals. *Rupigwára* are invisible to non-shamans (*"ñande ndohepiagi nga-ndupigwara"*), and in the *tokáia* it is they who actually cure, who blow on the patient and "administer the medicine" (*opohãnong*). In other contexts, if a shaman can cause death by snakebite or by the attack of a jaguar, the snake or the jaguar is spoken of as his *rupigwára.* In this usage, it seems to refer to any spirit over which the *pajé* has a degree of control, or with which he has a reciprocal relationship, such that he can summon them into the *tokáia,* or send them to perform a task for him—including even the Sky People themselves. Paulino spoke of Mbirova'umi, chief of the Sky People, as being Igwaká's *rupigwára.*

The term seems to be applied in a more restricted sense to a single animal spirit that has a more intimate relationship with a particular *pajé,* which "goes away" when the *pajé* dies. Paulino mentioned the *ɨhoguhú,* a large stinging caterpillar, as Igwaká's *rupigwára*. Another *pajé*, Jahɨra'ga, had a *tajahú* (white-lipped peccary) for his *rupigwára*, through which he could provide hunters with peccary.[2] A third, the Apeiran'di *pajé*, Kwã-rãntã, had a bat (*andɨra'i*) for his *rupigwára*, which he had tattooed on his chest. Kwãrãntã also had the piranha and a small caterpillar (*ɨho'gi*) as other *rupigwára*. A *pajé* of a different tribe[3] had an unspecified monkey, which enabled him to feel no pain when he was shot full of arrows. In these examples, *rupigwára* seems close to the idea of a "familiar spirit," except that they are even more closely identified with the *pajé* himself than that term usually implies. They are probably the same as the spirit who is incarnated in the *pajé* at his birth, in the dream-birth phenomenon discussed later.

In some instances, the *rupigwára* seems to have an even closer identification with the *pajé*'s self, as in the beliefs just described about his cosmic journey. In this context it seems to be a kind of alter ego, a spiritual part of the *pajé* himself. It is neither his *ra'úv* (the spirit that is associated with dreaming, and which leaves the body at death), nor is it his *'ang* (shadow, associated with the ghost, *añang*). It is the *pajé*'s *rupigwára* that is spoken of as being active in his dreams while the *pajé* himself sleeps.

The *rupigwára* is a complex topic that needs more clarification; but further elucidation would require discussions with an actual Kagwahiv shaman, something no longer possible among the Parintintin. New, closely related cultures now coming into contact, which were not known at the time I began work with the Parintintin—such as the Uru-eu-wau-wau, and the Cawahib of the Madeirinha—may provide further opportunities for investigation.

The cosmological underpinning for the *pajé*'s journey to the sky (or his *rupigwára*'s) is the origin myth of the Sky People, the story of Pindova'úmi'ga. This cosmographic myth depicts the outlines of the Kagwahiv universe. As Paulino recounts it:

> Pindova'úmi'ga [or Mbirova'úmi'ga, as some storytellers insist he is called] was angered by his children fighting in the woods, and told them: "Now I am going to take you far off, to the sky, and leave you! I don't like the people here." ("He was talking to us," inserts the storyteller.) He went to investigate the sky, but there were vultures all around. He came back and said, "There are vultures there." He went into the

> ground next and saw *añang* [ghosts, evil spirits]. So he came back up and told about them. Then he dove into the water, and there were fish there. He returned to his wife and said, "It won't do, because there are a lot of fish." So then he went into a tree, but there was honey in the tree. Finally, he went once more up to the sky—there are two skys, and he went up to the second level. There were no more vultures up there. He came back and said, "We're going there. The forest is no good here, and there it is beautiful."
>
> In response to his children's sadness about leaving their playthings, he said, "I'll take it all." He took his wife and sons, Kwatijakatú'i, Arukakatúi'ga, and Pɨrahamarána'ga, and gathered them on the roof of the house. As it went up, he tossed out a beam, which turned into an electric eel. He threw out a piece of firewood, and it turned into a cayman. He threw out a firefan which turned into a stingray. He left us here, and he left us the earth here. We never saw him again. He is *ipají—nhanderuviháv* [our chief].

The soul journey of the *pajé* (or his *rupigwára*) in the *tokáia* ceremony closely follows the path pursued by Pindova'úmi'ga in his myth, as the *pajé* successively visits *añang,* the spirits of the fish and other animals, and finally the Sky People themselves. The teller of the story stresses the identification of himself and his listeners with those abandoned below. The *pajé* is the only link with this lost father. In a sense, the *pajé is* Pindova'úmi'ga, and/or the other Sky People, his sons. Not only does the *pajé* represent each of the Sky People in the *tokáia* as he successively sings each of their distinctive songs, but he may also be a reincarnated child of one of them, mediated by the dream of another *pajé.*

If *pajés* are metonymically related to Pindova'úmi'ga and the Sky People, however, they are metaphorically related to Mbahíra, the trickster/culture hero who brought fire from the vultures, made mosquitoes from the smoke of a campfire, and brought many other amenities to mankind along with his pranks. For it was Mbahíra who most consistently used his magical powers not only to create, but also to heal. It was he who repeatedly brought his companion, Itariáno, back to life when he had come to grief trying to imitate Mbahíra's inimitable feats. These cures were accomplished by the universal method of Tupi *pajés*, blowing on the injured part, or successively on various parts of a dead body to bring it to life.

Cosmologically, these two mythic sources of the *pajé*'s craft draw together two geographically opposed poles. Pindova'úmi'ga is of the sky, and associated with raptors: his pet is a harpy eagle (*kwandú*), linking the Sky People conceptually with the Kwandú moiety. But Mbahíra is distinctly terrestrial. Mbahíra and his people live in a large rock on the earth's surface, and his adventures take place on the ground—or, frequently, in the water: he fished his daughter from the river as a catfish, and obtained arrows by swimming past a settlement disguised as a large fish, tempting the men to shoot all their arrows at him. His pet is the ground-nesting game bird, the mutum (curassow), eponymous bird of the Mɨtúm moiety. The *pajé* is man's link with the Sky People, but his domain includes the cosmos here below.

DREAMING AND THE SHAMAN'S POWER

These are the mythic models for the *pajé*'s practice, providing the dimensions of the universe within which he operates. An equally central metaphor for *ipají*—and one that links the *pajé* to his mythical/celestial source of power—is the act of dreaming. "Anyone who dreams," I was told more than once, "has a little bit of *pajé*."

When I first heard this phrase, I took it to refer to the predictive value of dreams. As in many cultures, Kagwahiv dreams are held to be interpretable as symbolic portents of future events—especially death, illness, or success in the hunt (see Kracke 1979, 130–32). (On arriving at a settlement I had never visited, I was sometimes greeted with the announcement that my host had dreamed I was coming.) Alternatively, vivid dreams may be interpreted as direct spiritual communications or perceptions. A nightmare may be taken as a direct sensing of the presence of an *añang* close to the dreamer, or an erotic dream might be a direct perception of the feelings of the person dreamed about. At a relative's death, his or her ghost will appear in one's dream to announce the departure.

These beliefs are only part of the elaborate Kagwahiv system of dream beliefs (discussed more fully in Kracke 1979); but they imply that dreams are an important mode of perceiving not only the future, but the spiritual state of the immediate surroundings as well: the presence of evil spirits, the health of one's kin, the disposition of others toward one. Hence, dreams are taken quite seriously, and their meanings may be earnestly discussed when they are recounted in the morning. For ambiguous or obscure dreams, the opinions of knowledgeable old people are sought and weighed carefully. (Naturally, the *pajé*'s knowledge of the meaning of dreams would have been especially valued, and special attention paid to his dreams.)

Furthermore, dreams are another mode of access to spiritual beings in various levels of the sky—the only mode of access to them, perhaps, other than the *pajé*'s trance journey in the *tokáia.* Once when a child was ill, Mohã'gí—an old man who evidently would have loved to be a *pajé* had the calling been open to him—dreamed of going up to the sky to implore the help of the *ikã'nã* ("the crippled ones"), benign spirits who live on nectar and have curative powers. (On another occasion he wrestled with my cold, personified, in a dream.) In both these instances, he was able through a dream to take on some of the *pajé*'s ability to interact with the spirit world.

As I learned more about *ipají,* I found that dreaming played an even more direct role in a *pajé*'s actions; for dreams are one medium through which a *pajé* exercises his power to affect the world. In particular, the *pajé* has a crucial part in the conception of a child; and this, too, is carried out in a dream.

When a *pajé* wants to cause a particular man to have good hunting, he dreams it, either literally or symbolically. (In the example my informant gave, to dream up game he dreams of making love with a woman.) The term to describe this action is the verb *-hãmongó,* "bring good hunting through a dream."[4]

Such dreams by a *pajé* would seem to contrast with ordinary people's dreams in being actually causative of future events, rather than just predicting them. Yet these causative, or agentic, dreams are not unrelated to the premonitory, or mantic, dreams that ordinary people can have. For one thing, the outcome of such an agentic dream may be mediated by the same symbols that mediate the predictions of ordinary mantic dreams; a dream of making love with a woman is one of the *portents* of good hunting.

In addition, I argued in my earlier article on Kagwahiv dream beliefs, there is some ambiguity in this limitation for ordinary people as well (Kracke 1979, 166). Dream predictions can be canceled out by certain ritual acts: telling the dream by a fire, or, more elaborately, performing the ritual of "breaking medicine" (*opohãmondók*), which consists of tearing a palha palm leaf (the type used in thatch) to pieces, bit by bit, reciting with each bit torn off a phrase denying causative intent for the dream (*ahayhú-tehe ko ji rẽ—ndopo'rúí-ate ko ji rẽ,* "I dreamed at random/for no purpose—he will not suffer [the outcome I dreamed of]"). This imparts to the dreamer a degree of control over the outcome of his or her predictive dreams, which gives the dreams themselves a kind of causative quality.

In any case, dreamers seem to experience their predictive dreams in this way, for some of those who reported such dreams in their depth interviews spoke as though they felt some responsibility for the event foreshadowed by the dream. (One old man who dreamed of a fire in my sleeping quarters, a dream predicting that I would suffer fever, seemed guilty about the dream and hastily reassured me that he had averted my death by performing the ritual of breaking medicine.) And a woman spoke disparagingly of her son who had not gone hunting when she dreamed up the game for him.

These examples suggest that ordinary people may sometimes have dreams that go beyond the mantic to take on an agentic quality; but these dreams are likely to be spontaneous and inadvertent. (The old man who dreamed of my fever was angry at me at the time, but had not intended to express his anger, of which he may not have been aware, in quite so drastic a fashion.) Perhaps the difference between a *pajé's* *ohãmongó* and an ordinary person's predictive dream of game is not so much that one is causative and the other predictive, as that the *pajé* is able to gain conscious control over the agentic dreams that he produces. This may give a fuller sense of what is meant by saying, "Anyone who dreams has a little bit of *pajé.*"

A *pajé's* dreams have an even more crucial part in the lives of at least some Kagwahiv, for a *pajé* can bring about the conception of a child through a dream. A *pajé* will have a dream in which a child comes to him wishing to be born (*jihuvotár*), and the *pajé* directs him to enter a certain woman. The "child" who comes in the dream is a spirit, in some cases one of the Sky People, in others an animal spirit. The next baby born to the woman to whom the *pajé* referred the child would then be considered to have been engendered by the *pajé,* and is spoken of as the *jihúv* ("offspring") of the *pajé* who dreamed him, as well as of his natural father. The *pajé* is also said to have "caused the child to go into" the mother, or to have "given him" to her (*omondó,* "causes to go" or "gives"). The child may also be said to be the *jihúv* ambiguously either of the spirit that announced itself to the *pajé* in his dream, or, if it was a Sky Person who came in the dream, then of that Sky Person's father.

The case described in most detail was that of Carlo, the eldest son of Jovenil and Aluza, who was "dreamed" by the *pajé* Igwaká. The Sky Person Shashámi'ga (the son of Pindova'úmi'ga's son Arukakatúi'ga) came to Igwaká in a dream asking to be born to a woman, and Igwaká told him to enter Aluza. When Julio was born, he was given two infancy-names (*mbotagwahav,* literally, "play thing"), one of which was Shashámi'ga, in recognition of his being a reincarnation of that Sky Person. Igwaká was said to have "given Julio to Jovenil as his child" (*omondó ga-pe pi'a-ro*). Julio is now Jovenil's offspring (*jihúva'ga*), but also the *jihúva'ga* of Igwaká—and, in a third sense, of Arukakatúi'ga.

Multiple paternity is a familiar concept to the Kagwahiv, who share the widespread Amazonian belief that the child is a product of repeated intercourse, and is "fed" by every man who sleeps with the mother during the child's gestation. The *pajé* adds one more "father" to the list; but whether, like a child's cogenitors, he was treated as a father (expected to obey the food taboos during the pregnancy and after birth, for example) is not clear.

The children "dreamed" by a *pajé* were specifically destined to be apprenticed to him and become a future *ipají.*

Much yet needs to be learned about the exact mechanisms of the power of those who are *ipají,* and about the full part that dreaming plays in exercising that power. It is evident, however, that dreaming plays a vital part in Kagwahiv shamanism.

DISCUSSION

The Kagwahiv *pajé* had two principal sources or vehicles for his power: trance and dreaming. To these may be added the ritual acts of singing, blowing, and spells, although these seem to have functioned primarily as adjuncts to one of the principal ones (e.g., singing in the *tokáia* ritual), or by themselves in less important or negatively valued tasks such as warding off rain, or sending illness.

Between these two principal sources of a *pajé*'s power there seems to have been a kind of division of labor. Trance was reserved for the crisis ceremony of curing. The *pajé*'s trance journey in the *tokáia,* with its mythical precedent in Pindova'úmi'ga's journey, drew on all the spiritual power of the cosmos, bringing it to bear on the cure of the patient for whom the ceremony was performed. The *pajé*'s dreaming, on the other hand, influenced less critical, but equally important, everyday life processes, birth and sustenance (hunting). Yet as Mohã'gi's *ikã'nã* dreams indicate, supernatural contact for curing can also be initiated in a dream. This particular instance may be an artifact of necessity, an adaptation of the loss of shamanic contact with the Sky People, but it raises the question whether there is a real hard and fast functional distinction between trance and dreaming, or whether trance may not be (as Guss [1980, 305] termed the Makiritáre drug-induced hallucinations) "a simulated dream."

Another way of dividing it may be a more real distinction (in Kagwahiv terms). In affairs to do with the preservation and creation of human life—curing and birth—whether that be through dream or through trance in the *tokáia,* the *ipají* serves primarily as a conduit for spiritual intervention in human lives. In the *tokáia* ceremony, it is clear that the spirits who come down are called on to put *their* curative powers to work for the patient on behalf of the *pajé* (*"Momé nde kwaitáv?"* asks each spirit as it arrives—"Where is your job to be done?"), although one informant asserted that it is the *pajé*'s *rupigwára* that treats (*opohãnong*). In less crucial matters, the *pajé* uses his own powers more directly, through dreaming in a matter as important as hunting or divining the outcome of a war expedition, and through spells in such things as warding off a rainstorm. These last may be thought of, too, as matters of primarily individual concern, while sicknesses and the birth of children are things that affect the welfare of the whole community. Still, there is one major distinction between the services performed in trance and in dream: dreaming a child and *ohãmongó* are done privately for an individual mother or hunter, trance curing is done in a public ceremony.

Are the powers that the *pajé* channels asocial in origin? Insofar as they are the powers of *añang,* who are in origin ghosts and of animal spirits, we can certainly say so; these are domesticated in the context of the *tokáia.* Yet, the Sky People also come; and while they can be said to be *extra*social in having renounced (or abandoned) the society of this earth, they constitute an ideal society—one without social strife or economic hardship—and so, in some sense, are consummately social. If the *pajé*'s own powers have their origin in Pindova'úmi'ga's, the same conclusion applies to them. Yet, insofar as they are modeled on the powers of Mbahíra, who (though the civilizing culture hero) always stood at the borders of society—acquiring fire, but also making mosquitoes, creating the daughter who concocted *cauĩ* (corn beer), but also tricking men out of their arrows—its origins are more ambiguous.

In the *pajé*'s trance journey to the sky in the *tokáia,* both space and time are condensed. Cosmic space is condensed into the ritual space of the *tokáia,* where the *pajé* is simultaneously present within the hearing of his audience, and (according to some accounts of the journey) in the sky talking with the Sky People and other spirits.[5] Mythic time is condensed into the ritual time, inasmuch as the *pajé*'s journey might be regarded as a reenactment of Pindova'úmi'ga's cosmic peregrinations. Geographic space, too, is condensed, for the various spirits contacted represent all regions of the cosmos visited by Pindova'úmi'ga, the rivers (*jatuarana*), the jungle (*añang* and jungle animals), and the sky. Moreover, since earthbound Mbahíra has as much claim as Pindova'úmi'ga to prefigure the *pajé*'s healing power (especially, perhaps, the power of blowing in the cure, which comparative evidence from other Tupi tribes with extant shamanistic traditions [Jangoux 1977] suggests may have greater importance in curing than my retrospective accounts of the *tokáia* indicate), wider mythic and social polarities may be condensed into the symbolic meaning of the *tokáia.* Pindova'úmi'ga, with his pet harpy eagle, is associated with the Kwandú (harpy eagle) moiety, and Mbahíra, with his pet curassow, with the Mɨtúm (curassow) moiety. (To stretch a point, one might also argue that the *pajé,* identified with both Pindova'úmi'ga-hawk and Mbahíra-curassow, is simultaneously predator and prey. Animals that serve as *rupigwára* include both eagle and turtle.)

Dreaming, unlike the spirit journey in the *tokáia,* appears to have no mythic precedent (although one could argue that Pindova'úmi'ga's taking the best game with him to the sky places the control of game within the mythically sanctioned domain of shamanic activities); but the dreaming of children does seem to involve contacting about the same range of spirits and Sky People who are contacted in the *tokáia* trance journey. Hence, these dreams, as well as curing dreams like Mohã'gi's, also bring spiritual energies from all parts of the cosmos to bear on the perpetuation of human life.

Since trance and dream play such similar roles as expressions of the *pajé*'s power—trance in a public ritual, dream in a more private context—the question naturally arises, what is the conceptual relationship between these two states of consciousness? I do not have the data for a definitive answer to this question, and probably a full answer would require the study of an active shamanic tradition with living *pajés,* who could give fully informed instruction on the subject; but I suspect that a clue to the answer might lie in a deeper understanding of the concept of *rupigwára,* and of its relation to the concept of *ra'úv,* "dream image," or "soul," a key concept in the understanding of their dream theory (Kracke 1979, 127).[6] Whatever the exact conceptual connection, since trance and dreaming are both regarded as modes of contact with the spiritual world, and, in particular, with the celestial spirits and the Sky People, it seems likely that they are regarded as closely allied states of consciousness. A *pajé*'s dreams and trance states of mind are set off from those of ordinary people by the *pajé*'s ability to direct them—to willfully dream a dream of successful (or unsuccessful) hunting, or to call on a particular healing spirit in trance or dream. Yet insofar as everyone dreams, everyone participates to some degree in the *pajé*'s power: "everyone who dreams has a little bit of *pajé.*"

COMPARISONS

The Kagwahiv, of course, are not the only culture in which dreams have an important place in the shamanistic complex of beliefs. What distinguishes them, and places them in a small group of those cultures whose shamanic curing practices have been described in the literature, is that a major part of the manipulation of reality by shamans is carried out in dreams.

Dreams play a variety of roles in shamanistic beliefs. Most commonly—or at least most centrally a part of the established concept of shamanism—they are a medium for the initial contact with a suprahuman being: the "call" to shamanism by a spirit (Eliade 1964, 33–66; in South America, Butt Colson 1977, 46; Gregor 1977, 335; Sharon 1978, 15). Or dreams may be a mode of attaining special knowledge, with shamans being either specialists in interpreting them (Siskind 1973b, 155, 163; cf. Tedlock 1981), or especially attuned to receiving messages in dreams from spirits or other shamans (Sharon 1978, 56). The idea that shamans have a special bent for attaining knowledge through dreams may edge over into the idea that dreams are an actual source of power for the shaman, and is perforce a part of the shaman's dream powers in cultures where a shaman exercises his power through his dreams (Bartolomé 1977; Crocker 1985, 224–25, 234, 245; Faron 1964, 143; Guss 1980, 300–301; Métraux 1948, 90, 92; Wagley 1943, 66, Wagley 1977, 194).

In lowland South America, several cultures have been described in which dreaming is a prime source and vehicle of the shaman's powers. Those I am familiar with are Wagley's descriptions of Tapirapé shamans (1943; 1977, 181–212) and David Guss's recent (1980) discussion of the part of dreams in Makiritáre shamanism. (I have not had the opportunity to consult Bartolomé's treatise on Guaraní shamanism for this writing [Bartolomé 1977].)

Wagley's classic description of Tapirapé shamans contains practically all of the major dream elements that appear in the Kagwahiv *pajé*'s armamentarium, although the emphasis is somewhat different. According to Wagley, "knowledge of the supernatural world is gained chiefly through the dream experiences of shamans or *panché.* For among the Tapirapé shamanistic power derives from dreams and from powers revealed in them. . . Obviously anyone may dream, but frequent dreaming is evidence of shamanistic power" (Wagley 1943, 66; 1977, 181). "Sorcery . . . is believed to be the action of shamans in dreams" (Wagley 1943, 70), and *panché* engage in epic dream battles with ghosts (*anchúnga*) and with one another (Wagley 1943, 65–70; 1977, 182–83, 185–86), and meet and befriend other spirits in their dreams, recruiting them as familiars (Wagley 1977, 183–85). *Panché* also dream to bring children to mothers for them to conceive, stealing them from Thunder or from animal spirits; and *panché* are responsible for the maintenance of a good supply of game—although they do this last on behalf of the community rather than for individuals, and by rather different methods from Kagwahiv *ipají:* in dreams they visit the hill that is the "home of wild peccary" and have intercourse with the females for the increase of their offspring (Wagley 1977, 194).

Tapirapé shamans do not use trance in healing, but cure by blowing smoke over the patient, or by sucking out witchcraft objects amidst vomiting, induced by swallowing tobacco smoke (Wagley 1943, 73–74; 1977, 191). Trance is part of a very different ceremony, however: the Thunder Ceremony that takes place during the season of violent thunderstorms in December and January. During the four days of this ceremony, all the shamans of a village, dancing in the plaza, go into trance, aided by swallowing tobacco smoke, and do battle with Thunder (Kanawána) and his minions, the *tupi* (Thunder's "pets" or children) and the *panché iúnwera,* "deceased *panché*" (Wagley 1943, 84–91; 1977, 199–211). They are invariably vanquished, collapsing in spasms, though the more powerful *panché* persist longer and get closer to Thunder himself. In many ways, this is an exact inversion of the Kagwahiv *tokáia* rite. Rather than beseech curative spirits for help in curing the patient, the *panché* do battle with hostile spirits. Rather than one *pajé* confined privately in a *tokáia,* screened from the audience, many *panché* dance publicly in the open plaza. Pindova'úmi'ga is an idealized culture hero living in the sky, governing his immortal children; Kanawána is a wrathful nature deity living on a mountain across the Araguaia River and presiding over a host of strange spirits and ghosts of *panché.* This reversal, in a sense, typifies the difference in emphasis between the Kagwahiv *ipají* (as portrayed retrospectively by people who were not themselves *ipají*), in a cooperative relationship with spirits, and the Tapirapé *panché* constantly at war with them.

Contrasting though they are, both ceremonies are unique (or nearly unique) occasions in which the shamans go into trance rather than exercise their power through dreams. For the Tapirapé, there is one other occasion, which might be regarded as intermediate: novices who do not dream may be put into trance (again with the help of smoke) by their *panché* mentors, in order to induce dreams (Wagley 1943, 82; Wagley 1977, 198). This also suggests a close conceptual relationship between dream and trance among the Tapirapé.

Although I am not familiar enough with Tapirapé mythology to identify a foundation myth for the practices of *panché* like those of Pindova'úmi'ga and Mbahíra's cures, and Wagley does not cite one, he does summarize in full a myth featuring a legendary *panché* as its protagonist (1977, 181–84). Again, in contrast to the Kagwahiv situation, the myth does not provide a prototype either for curing or for the trance ceremony, but for shamanic struggles with spirits in dreams: Waré's exploits consisted largely of tricking and killing *anchúnga* in his dream travels.

David Guss (1980) describes a somewhat similar set of beliefs among the Cariban Makiritáre (Ye'cuana). The power of the Makiritáre *karainto* (shaman) is also conceived in terms of dreaming, but in a somewhat different sense. An ordinary person's dream is believed to be an account by his or her spirit double (*akato*) of the spirit voyage (*adekato*) it took while the dreamer was asleep. During these voyages the *akato* is in danger of capture by spirits. If this happens, the shaman may free the captured *akato* by locating it in a "simulated dream" using hallucinogens (apparently the smoke or powder of *ebenê* inhaled through the nose: Schuster 1976, 94) in which he retraces the steps of the *akato,* and, having found it, restores its memory of the world it left. The shaman is able to free this spirit double because his own *akato* is transformed into a *damodede,* a dream-double that, unlike most people's *akato,* responds to his conscious control: he is able to take his *damodede* out of himself (whereas an *akato* wanders off on its own during sleep), and is able to *direct* the course of his dreams. (The *damodede* is evidently to some degree parallel to the Kagwahiv *rupigwára,* though with significant differences.) The dreams of the shaman, and his hallucinatory "simulated dreams," thus differ from ordinary people's in that he is able to control them and consciously direct them, enabling him to carry out intentional action in the spirit world through them.

It is not clear from Guss's article, or other sources on Makiritáre shamanism I have consulted, whether shamans can act through their dreams proper—during sleep—or whether the spiritual action of the *damodede* is limited to the "simulated dreams" of hallucinatory trance; but clearly the hallucinations in trance are conceptualized as a kind of dream, so the power of the shamans is conceived as operating through his dreams. In any case, the mythic precedent is clear; it was through dreams that the culture hero Wanadi battled the demonic enemy of mankind, Odo'sha.

In each of these cultures, dreaming is conceptually the core of the shaman's power. There are indications in each one that trance is conceptualized as either a public form of dreaming—a "simulated dream" in Guss's (1980, 305) phrase—or a mode of facilitating dreaming (Wagley 1977, 198). Yet in none of these cultures does dreaming stand alone as the sole mechanism for the operation of the *pajé*'s power, or the only medium for its expression. In each case, it stands in contrast to another altered state of consciousness—autohypnotic trance, trance induced by tobacco, or a drug-induced hallucinatory state—as a marker of some opposition, albeit perhaps a different opposition in each culture: public ceremony versus private arrangement, communal benefit versus individual, and (perhaps in Makiritáre) the controlled "dream" of the shaman versus the erratic and perilous dream of the ordinary person.

It is not surprising that dreams are regarded as vehicles for shamanic power in some cultures, for they are the most vivid and frequent experience we can have of a reality that transcends the physical and social limitations of the waking world. The limitations of dreaming as a model for shamanic power are twofold: dreaming is essentially a private experience, unsuited for public ceremonial display; and dreaming is accessible to all, making it difficult to distinguish the shaman from the ordinary person (though with the termination of the Kagwahiv shamanic succession, this has become a saving grace). A third problem is that dreams are unconsciously constructed, not usually subject to conscious direction.

Each of the cultures discussed here solves the first problem by combining dreaming with some other form of expression of supernatural power on the shaman's part, but an expression that can be regarded as a form of dreaming. The second limitation of dreaming can partly be canceled out by the third, however. For in each of these cultures, it proves to be important that the shaman or *pajé* acquire an ability to control his dream. Both Guss (1980, 306) and, further afield, Larry G. Peters in an account of shamanism among the Tamang of Nepal (1982, 35–37), compare this ability to direct the dream or hallucination while within it with Tart's (1969, 170) concept of "lucid dream," in which "you feel as rational and as in control of your mental state as you do in your ordinary state of consciousness, but you are still experientially located in the dreamworld" (Tart 1977, 176, quoted in Peters 1982, 35). This control is what distinguishes the shaman from other dreamers, and enables him to direct the power in his dreams to its intended ends. To fulfill this requirement—a demand in accord with the shaman's need to be receptive to the emotional communications of those he treats—the shaman needs to be someone in touch with his own unconscious processes.

NOTE ON TRANSCRIPTION (KAGWAHIV)

The transcription of Kagwahiv words generally follows the Betts-Pease orthography: *v* is a bilabial fricative (as in Spanish) but in final position is pronounced as a bilabial stop, *p; j* is pronounced *dzh,* and *ch* is *tsh,* as in English; *ɨ* represents a high back unrounded vowel (Russian *yerih, ee* pronounced with the mouth wide open as in gargling); *ñ* is a palatalized *n* (like Spanish *ñ*). Other vowels and consonants follow Portuguese transcription. The stress in a word varies and is indicated by an acute accent. ' represents a glottal stop.

Notes

1. Paulino, 1967 (Field notes I 181, Feb. 11). In 1989 Paulino made examples of such pictures, including one of Añanga-hapukai.

2. If peccary were scarce, he would cut a hoof from a peccary foot he kept on hand, plant it, and a peccary would emerge, grunting, from the soil. If occasion demanded, he could also turn the peccary into a tapir: one hunter saw an animal emerge from the ground that appeared to be a peccary, but he followed it, and it turned out to be a tapir.

3. Named Kupehava'ga.

4. Third person form, *ohãmongó.* The derivation is somewhat ambiguous. -*mo-ngo* (*-mbo* + *-ko*) means "cause _____ to exist," but the first syllable could either be from *hang,* "strong," "perduring," or *'ang,* "shadow." The latter reading, "cause a shadow to exist," might refer (since *'ang* has otherwordly connotations: cf. *añang,* "ghost") to the supernatural mode of action of such dreams, and seems more likely.

5. Thus, Kagwahiv *pajés* combine the supposedly opposed categories of soul journey (or "visionary magical flight") and spirit possession (cf. Peters 1982, 22).

6. In Kagwahiv dream discourse, the image of a person or thing appearing in a dream is spoken of as his/her/its *ra'úv* (whence the "dream-tense" marker *ra'u* used when narrating a dream). This includes the self: the dreamer's own appearance in a dream is *ji ra'úva,* "my dream image." But the term *ra'úv* has an ambiguous meaning. In some cases it means an iconic representation: when a stone is used in play to represent a cooking fire, it is spoken of as *"tata ra'úva,"* "play representation of fire."

SEVEN

DREAM, SHAMANISM, AND POWER AMONG THE TOBA OF FORMOSA PROVINCE

PABLO G. WRIGHT

Research regarding the conception and the role of dreams in non-Western societies has demonstrated that dreams occupy an important place in native systems of collective representations, and also that they are embedded in social mechanisms and cosmology (Eggan 1949, 1964; Eliade 1961; von Grunebaum 1964; Guss 1980; Hallowell 1964; Spencer and Gillen 1927; Wallace 1958; P. Wright 1981b). The link between dreams and society is absent in our evaluation of dreams. We consider them as individual psychological phenomena, integrated neither into the collective set of ideas nor into social life (Freud 1948). Our category of reality coincides with the experiences of wakeful life, while the oneiroid ones lack that ontological basis and are understood as fantasies of the individual psyche, the contents of which cannot influence the course of social life.

In aboriginal societies, the dream experience is integrated as an important factor in the course of history (Bastide 1976, 59). It operates as a threshold to spheres of reality not accessible in daily life. The beyond, the words of the dead and of the gods are clearly explained.

The unknown future is revealed and turned immutable (Caillois 1964, 43). In the oneiroid worlds we find the symbols, images, figures, and happenings that constitute the mythologies; dream and myth dynamically relate to each other, acting as channels that feed back knowledge and proof about the nature of the world (Eliade 1961; Ullman 1960).

For the Toba, dreams, along with visions and "apparitions," have an important role in connecting them to the levels of nonhuman reality, whose contact and communication play a fundamental role in the operation of their sociocultural system.[1] Nonhuman alludes to an ontological condition radically different from that of humans. Because of their peculiar nature, nonhuman beings have power and knowledge that the Toba wish to possess and that nonhumans wish to give. This articulation of gifts determines the circulation of power in the Toba cosmos. Dreams offer the possibility of communicating with these beings, who, in one way or another, govern the totality of what exists.

Presented here is a discussion of the importance and uses of dreams in Toba culture and society. In addition to establishing contact with other levels of the universe, they allow the Toba to interpret the events of daily life and also have an important healing function. Although the Toba have undergone acculturation, and many are members of Pentecostal cults, dreams have continued to maintain their important role. Using Toba narratives of dreams, we shall compare the symbolic contents and uses of dreams between the traditional Toba and the Pentecostal converts.

HISTORICAL AND ETHNOGRAPHIC BACKGROUND

The Toba, who call themselves *qom* (people), belong to the Guaycurú linguistic family and live in the Chaco plain in northeastern Argentina. Traditionally they were organized into bilateral nomad bands of extended families. They migrated throughout a defined hunting territory, gathering together at certain times of the year to conduct trade, marriage agreements, and ritual activities. Living together during these periods permitted the circulation of news and a sharing that created a sense of belonging to the regionally located unit (Braunstein 1983; Miller 1979; Reyburn 1954).

The basic social unit was the extended family, a group of relatives who cooperated and shared resources without a mechanism of centralized authority. Redistribution prevented individuals from accumulating goods, and labor was divided by sex. Men were responsible for hunting, gathering, and fishing, while women gathered, cooked, wove fibers and wool, and cared for the children (Miller 1979; Reyburn 1954).

The shamans acted as mediators between men and nonhuman beings. They mediated the conflicts believed to be due to the transgressions of humans of the norms imposed by the nonhumans, such as the breaking of hunting taboos, or menstrual proscriptions. Poor hunting and, in some cases, illnesses were considered punishment for such offenses, and the shaman was required to return the situation to normal. When the ecological habitat used by the nomad band was exhausted, the shamans directed the group to a new territory based on their knowledge of nature and guidance from nonhuman beings (Miller 1979; Reyburn 1954).

Traditional leadership was drawn from the heads of the large families. The position was inherited, but the *cacique* (leader) had to confirm it as well, demonstrating a strong personality, exceptional skill and courage in hunting, and shamanic powers, such as the curing of illness. The leader's reputation was based on the use of knowledge and power for the group's benefit. At times of famine or war, powerful leaders sometimes arose who directed several bands as regional authorities (Miller 1979; Reyburn 1954).

The arrival of the Spanish in the sixteenth century modified the life of the native settlements of the Chaco. There was an increase of illnesses and Indian mortality. Horses were incorporated into their culture, and tribal life was redefined starting from this element (Miller 1979; Reyburn 1954).

The next century was characterized by the Spanish punitive expeditions against the natives, while a small number of white settlers established themselves in the proximities of military posts. During the wars of independence in the nineteenth century, the Chaco was nearly abandoned. The colonization process accelerated at the end of the century, with the organization of the national government, who sent the army to the Pilcomayo region.

The economic basis of the Chaco colonization was agriculture and cattle rearing. This led to conflicts with the natives, who resented the intruders in their hunting grounds. Lumbermills were established for the exploitation of red quebracho tannin, as were sugarcane plantations, which induced the Toba to work in them. Conflicts with the settlers increased to armed encounters. These were violently subdued by the Argentine army at the beginning of the 1920s.

Today the Toba live in dispersed agricultural and sedentary communities generally on state-owned lands. Here a certain number of extended families group together, work individually and communally, and consider themselves as a distinct social and political entity (Reyburn 1954). The extended family, consisting of three to four generations, is the basic economic unit. It owns the land in common, which is managed by the family head (Miller 1966). The traditional circuits of redistribution of goods continue to follow the lines of kinship.

Agricultural activities combine the cultivation of maize, sunflowers, manioc, sweet potatoes, and squash. Hunting, fishing, and gathering, although these activities are greatly reduced, complement the agricultural foodstuffs and purchased goods. The Toba serve as wage laborers in order to increase the family group's income; at times it is the only resource, which results in the migration of an individual or group to other locations, such as to the sugarcane plantations, lumbermills, or urban centers.

Participation in the labor market and the changing socioeconomic structure has resulted in a progressive cultural disintegration involving changes in patterns of subsistence and worldview. Little by little they have adapted to new and adverse exterior conditions, and with these changes their set of spiritual assumptions about the world and man's relations with it have changed. The rising of Pentecostalism among the Toba, as we shall see later, seems to be intimately connected with this gradual process of cultural loss (Miller 1967, 1979; Reyburn 1954).

Leadership, although it has suffered the consequences of contact, still maintains its usefulness. Today it is important that the *cacique* knows Spanish, since he represents the community to outsiders and travels frequently to raise money or job opportunities. Leadership, as before, is based on family heads who possess strong personalities. Decisions involving the entire group continue to be based on consensus.

In the 1940s, Pentecostal presence in the Chaco influenced Toba culture intensely. Toba migrants in the coastal towns heard the missionaries. The Pentecostal emphasis on song, dance, ecstasy, and glossolalia impressed these natives, who, on their return to their homes, began to spread the Christian message, reinterpreted according to their own Toba religious vision (Cordeu and Siffredi 1971; Miller, 1967, 1979; Reyburn 1954; P. Wright 1983a).

The Toba Pentecostal religious movement spread to such an extent that by the end of the 1950s an entirely Toba congregation was organized. The members of the church hierarchy are native with an organization modeled after the white Pentecostal church. Currently almost every Toba community has at least one church, and generally whites are absent in its organization. Other missionary groups have also found great acceptance by the native population. In most cases they are of foreign origin and financed by international organizations.

Present-day community leadership coincides with the religious one, such as occurred in the past. A good pastor, in order to be a good leader, must have a strong personality, as well as curative abilities due to his contact with the Christian divinity. Church fellowship frequently coincides with the interfamilial social groups where people recognize consanguineal bonds or affinity, and among which tensions or rivalries may spring up for prestige, political power, or even therapeutic efficacy (Reyburn 1954).

Traditional shamans continue to cure the sick. Many of them attend Pentecostal cults, participating as any other "brother in the faith." The more powerful shamans still preserve part of their political prestige due to the continual success of their therapeutic achievements.

Many aspects of traditional Toba ritual are synthesized in the Pentecostal cults: healing, dance, ecstasy, as well as expressions of Toba social life—such as speeches of the headman, communal interpretation of dreams, explanation of witchcraft cases, solutions to problems of subsistence, and so on. The interpretation of the Bible and the apocalyptic preaching is supported by traditional mythology that stresses cosmic cataclysms by water, fire, or darkness. For the Toba, there is the omnipresent possibility of a "change of the world" identical to that which occurred in mythical times (P. Wright 1981b). The Bible is used as a sacred object with curing power in therapeutic rites during religious services, and it is also conceived as an impersonal authority for leadership purposes (Reyburn 1954).[2]

The traditional Toba conception of the universe consists of various domains organized in three overlapping levels. The earth is in the middle level and is conceived as a more or less rounded flat surface of dry earth. The Toba live in the center, at a location shown to them by the mythic heroes *ašien* and *taanki'* (P. Wright 1989). On the earth they recognize different parts, such as the village, the low grasslands, the forest, the water, the swamp, and the palm grove (the latter two closely connected with the water).

On the inferior level, known as the "other earth" or "inside the earth" dwell strange beings who live in a rhythm opposite to that of humans, though their landscape is quite similar (Cordeu 1969–70). Underneath the "other earth" there is water that completely surrounds the universe and that also feeds the earth's marshes, rivers, and lakes. The course of the sun during the day on earth continues during the night in this subterranean world, a fact that explains why the sun sets in the west and rises in the east. West is considered the end or boundary of the earth where the ground ends and water begins. This cardinal point is also called "sky," because it is here where sky and earth meet.

The sky is above the surface of the earth. The clouds, winds, sun, moon, storms, and rain are found in this sky. Higher still, there is another sky that is the habitat of the stars and of other celestial beings, such as the Pleiades (Cordeu 1969–70; Miller 1967, 1977).

The night is considered a different domain in the same way as the forest or the grasslands. It exists within the interval between sunset and sunrise, landmarks that are determined by the song of specific birds. It is the time during which the beings of the "other earth" wake up and roam through the world of men.

As mentioned, the Toba distinguish between human and nonhuman entities. Among the latter there are a series of beings associated with the diverse phenomena of the empirical world who are endowed with power and intention toward human beings. The native term that designates the nonhumans is *jaqa'a* (other, strange, unknown); the rain or the wind, for instance, are *jaqa'a* beings. In other contexts this word indicates that something is distant from the whole, for instance a river branch that has separated from the main course of the river. *Jaqa'a* is semantically opposed to *jaqaja* (brother), which refers to a family relationship and which in other contexts defines everything that is known and familiar.

Toba cosmic geography is structured in such a way that each part with its subdivisions possesses a nonhuman entity that governs it. Thus, there is the "owner" of the water who dominates, directs, and protects all the animal and plant species living there. In many cases, each species has its "father" and its "mother" who act as specific or subordinate "owners" of the "owner" of the band (Cordeu 1969–70; L. Vuoto 1981; P. Vuoto 1981). In the same way, the "owner" of the night directs the beings of the "other earth" and the night species. In addition, there are also "owners" of activities such as dancing and chanting, as well as of different instruments, and so forth (figs. 7.1, 7.2).

This principle of domains and hierarchies is reproduced in all parts of the Toba universe, including the community, where the headman acts as "owner" of that space.

As mentioned, the term *jaqa'a* designates the ontologic "otherness" of the nonhuman beings, who are defined as different and possessing power. The denomination *no'wet* in its most general sense coincides with the meaning of *jaqa'a,* while in its particular meaning it refers to these specific entities who contact men in order to give them their power. We might say that, in the Toba cosmos, *no'wet* assumes the role of receptacle and measure of the numinous, including the generality of what is powerful, of "das Andere," as well as the specific nature of the nonhuman beings (Cordeu 1969–70, 84; Otto 1925).[3] We shall use the words *jaqa'a* and *no'wet* (the latter in its particular meaning) as synonyms when we refer to nonhuman beings.

The relationship between man and *no'wet* is vital for humans' physical and social well-being, and the shamans are primarily, but not exclusively, in charge of these connections. To be a hunter and a shaman ultimately requires the revelation of a *no'wet*'s will, who gives that person his power and the knowledge to carry out his tasks efficiently. This power expresses itself concretely in the *no'wet*'s cession of auxiliary spirits (*ltawa* "his auxiliary"), who facilitate the performance of specific tasks.

The benefit of the *no'wet* for humans expresses itself in power (*halojk, napiišek, l'añağak*) and knowledge (*jawan*). *Halojk* implies an ampler notion of power, while *napiišek* is restricted to shamanic power. *L'añağak* is associated in certain contexts with this type of power, though its most frequent use makes reference to an individual's physical strength or strength of character. "Knowledge" (*jawan*) differs from normal knowledge (*jajaten*) connected with the learning of educative patterns or of everyday tasks where there is no revelation by a nonhuman being.

Among the Toba the term "power" refers not only to political processes that imply decision making and exercising authority, but also to

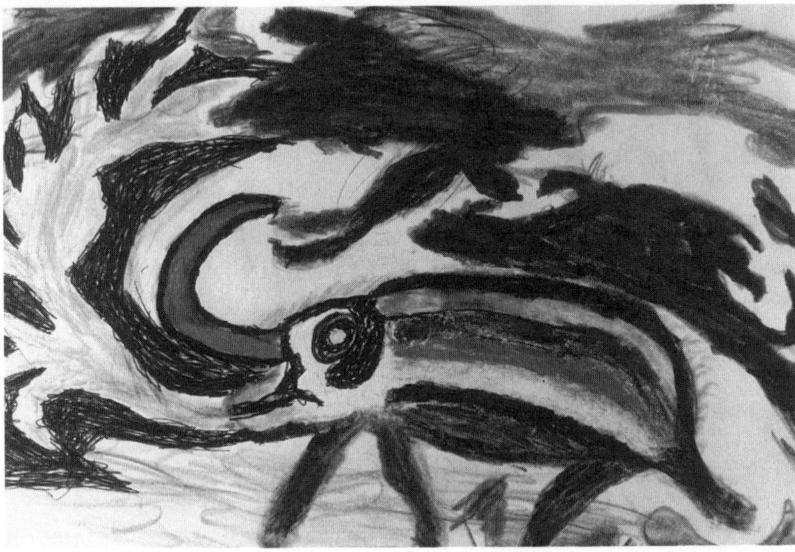

FIGURE 7.1. Gasogonaga, Owner of the Storm, in her celestial world throwing out lightning from her mouth. The Toba informants all agreed that her elephant shape and her multicolored body are related to the rainbow and rain. © Angel Achilai.

a control of the forces in the universe that permit good health and well-being (Miller 1977, 306). The usual ways in which humans gain this power and knowledge are through dreams, visions, and through "meetings" or "apparitions" in person.

Dreams are distinguished from visions because they always occur when the individual is sleeping, while visions occur when the person is awake. The same happens in "meetings." According to the informants, they are characterized by the sudden presence of a nonhuman entity that appears or blocks their way.

Although any individual may have contact with these nonhumans through the experience of dreams or "meetings," the status of shaman *pi'oǧonaq* is marked by a greater amount of power due to his special relation with nonhumans, which enables him to cure. Unlike ordinary

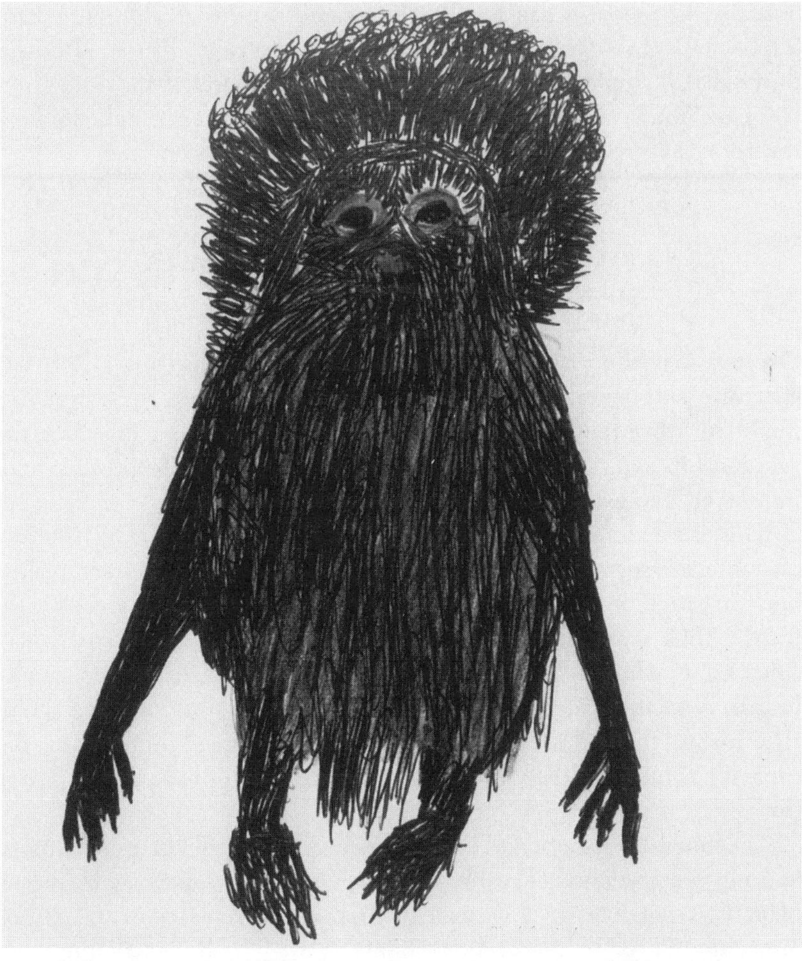

FIGURE 7.2. Here Angel Achilai has drawn the fearsome Pel'ek, Owner of the Night. His ugly form is similar to that of humans, but his profuse hair and colored eyes, general traits of all night beings, characterize him as a *jaga'a* being. © Angel Achilai.

humans, the shaman can handle visions and dreams at will. He enters into ecstasy through song, rhythm, and, in some cases, dance. Although they do not employ hallucinogens, and it is not clear if they did so in the past, Buckwalter (1980, 209) affirms that they once did, smoking the root called *pa'a,* which contains hallucinogenic properties.

DREAMS AND THE ACQUISITION OF POWER AND KNOWLEDGE

Dreams, as well as visions, operate among the Toba as levels of experience that are ontologically qualified compared to daily life. In a way, we might say that they are a real cosmological environment in which the relationship and communication with the nonhumans are possible and, moreover, necessary.

This is rendered clear in the traditional narratives in which heroic characters resort to dreams in order to get to know a distant reality, be it in space or time. This usage becomes exemplary and archetypical for the Toba, who personally prove the virtues of this kind of experience. The beings who appear in mythical accounts demonstrate their superhuman capacities, such as changing their morphology at will—an action that makes them deserve the name of "transformer"—or having the capacity to control their dreams at will. Both are proof of the power they possess.

The oneiroid experience confers on the individual the possibility of getting to know areas of reality inaccessible to daily existence. By means of it, it is possible for a shaman to reach strange places in the sky or in the depths, or to approach the limits of the world, contributing later with his personal experiences to the traditional knowledge about the nature and conformation of the universe. In these cases, myth and the oneiroid experiences operate in a vital interdependence favoring the perpetuation of the Toba worldview (P. Wright 1981b).

Not all dreams have a revelation of a nonhuman entity or provide the possibility of entering sacred areas. Those that do are classed as "true" dreams and are conceived as "given," that is, not ascribed to individual psychological phenomena. Because they are given, they possess a teaching that should be interpreted in a personal way, and, if considered suitable, communicated to others later. A dreamer who does not reveal an oneiric experience important for the community is thus responsible for the dangers that may occur.

For the Toba, the dream is the exit of a psychic component of the individual, which they call "image-soul," and which roams outside the body of the sleeper (Ducci 1904; Karsten 1932; Loewen et al. 1965; Métraux 1937; P. Wright 1981b). The image-soul differs from another psychic element of the Toba individual, the "shadow-soul," which is the shadow cast by the body (Cordeu 1969–70, 110). This shadow-soul seems to be associated with the destiny after death in the subterranean world, a destiny that transforms it into an entity whose sight frightens living men.

If the individual has the power of a *no'wet,* it is said that his image-soul can walk and see at night as if it were day. The initial contact with the *no'wet* may originate in a "meeting," in a dream, or in a series of dreams where the nonhuman entity expresses his teaching.

Every Toba who becomes related to a *no'wet* through dreams is considered to gain power and knowledge. They then have a status similar to that of the shaman's since they have contact with the *jaqa'a* entities empowering them to undertake a determined activity, such as hunting, seduction, or knowing the future. Successful activities are attributed to the action of auxiliary spirits, the ultimate sources of whatever talent a Toba may have.

The following informants' narratives will illustrate this point.

> A young man said that he had no girlfriend nor could he get one, that he wasn't lucky. Then one night the Trickster Fox appeared in a dream and told him, "Look here, my son, I'll show you a way in which you can have a woman." The young man asked how, and Trickster Fox replied, "You must get an herb called *kadjalom.* That herb is in the midst of the lakes, on the edge of the lakes. It is an herb of a very red color and has the shape of a climbing plant. You must look for it and bring it. Also look for *wolčenalom.* Pull out the roots and save them, keeping them well dry. You must also look for *joqwi lawoǧo,* a small herb with a yellow flower and keep it.

In this oneiroid revelation, the *no'wet* teaches the manufacturing of a love-magic packet. The Trickster Fox of mythical tales is connected with seduction, lying, and deceit. He transmits his knowledge to the youth, and operates in this dream as an auxiliary spirit, presenting the characteristic attributes of the paradigmatic figure of numerous Toba traditional narratives.

Another informant claimed to know how to prepare many of these magic bundles, making them for many people. After asking their wishes, he waited at night for his *no'wet* to reveal through dreams the ingredients necessary for each desire.

The following statement comes from an informant who gained power from the "owner" of the entertainment activities while dreaming.

> Šigitağajk teaches me so that I may become skillful in singing and beating the drums. Father of the Drum and Father of the Dance also appear to me. He indicates that I must play hard during the whole night. I must sing and beat the drum. When I dream with Dance Father, I have to jump in the dance like a toad.

These *no'wet* are closely related to seduction and sexual excitement. The Fathers of the Drum and Dance have the power necessary to beat the drum skillfully, to know its songs, and to dance well without tiring. They are subordinate to the "owner" of the entertainment practices, Šigitağajk, who is higher in the hierarchy of powerful beings.

The owner of the countryside establishes contact with men to enable them to hunt successfully.

> An old man went to hunt without knowing how this was done, and he found an ostrich, but he was in a great hurry, so he left some meat thrown about. Then a *no'wet* arrived at night. The hunter dreamed about a person dressed for hunting, such as when one is going to shoot an ostrich. Then that man appeared at night with very long palm leaves like the clothing of a dress of long leaves. He saw the hunter and spoke to him, "And how were you hunting yesterday and left some pieces of meat lying about, of an ostrich?" "Yes, because I was in a great hurry; therefore I left a bit behind." The other told him, "Well, let it be the last time, for only once will I give you four ostriches. Tomorrow I'll come this way." When the man dreamed about the man of the countryside, he was dressed as a man, but with palm leaves. This man said he would prepare a heap of grass and also said, "I shall burn this tomorrow. There you will find the four ostriches." Early in the morning the hunter got up and went according to the sign the man of the countryside had pointed out. Then he saw the grass. There seemed to be smoke, but it didn't burn.

When the *no'wet* present themselves in human form, they possess certain symbolic traits characteristic of their conditions as "owners" of this or the other respective species or area (Cordeu and Siffredi 1971; Pagés Larraya 1982). The "country man's" instruction includes a sermon about the behavior of the hunter toward his booty, a common trait in these nonhumans' teachings. This relationship with the *no'wet* is vital for the hunter, because it enables him to secure a more or less regular provision of food.

The Water Owner imparts the rules of behavior for fishermen and indicates the locations by having plenty of fish sent by him.

> A man dreamed that the Water Owner had made him a dream so that he would know, and he went to the water. He had confidence, for he already knew, because Werajk had given him a dream for his people to go search at night. Then he got up very early and called his companions and they went to fish in the place the water owner had indicated to him.

Visits to the world of the dead, the "other earth," are quite common in dreams when a person is very ill or feels threatened by an impending illness. The abode of the dead is imagined to be in the west, although, according to witnesses, what exists there is the threshold of the subterranean domain inhabited by the deceased.

SHAMANIC POWER AND DREAMS

The volition of the *no'wet* is decisive for access to the shamanic condition, although an individual may wish to seek the revelation of such beings, that wish being summed up in the expression "I seek a grace or a gift." The various ways of gaining power include: transmission of power by a shaman relative, by "meeting" the *no'wet* in person, through dream apprenticeship, and through self-healing.

Transmission of Power by a Shaman Relative

This practice involves a relative, such as father, uncle, or grandfather, placing his saliva into the child's mouth. As the child grows, his power (*halojk*) will develop until he can begin to cure the ill. With the saliva, "power objects" are passed on and conceived as illnesses that he will later be able to heal, and whose nature is nonhuman (Cordeu 1969–70; Loewen et al. 1965; Miller 1977, 314; 1979). These objects find a place inside the child's body, especially in his heart.

Meeting the No'wet in Person

This occurs in the forest or in any of the different habitats, and may be unintended or sought for by the individual in the loneliness of the forest (Reyburn 1954). The *no'wet* appears humanlike with certain animal or plant features indicating the species or place he governs. He usually introduces himself and explains what power he can offer (Miller 1977, 315). He asks the person what he wants of the gifts he has at his disposal and suggests that the person choose at will. It is customary to select only part of the power offered, since possession of too much *halojk* can be dangerous, for it may drive the individual crazy or kill him. Once accepting power, it is best not to withdraw for the same reasons.

On some occasions, *no'wet* takes the person to his dwelling and reveals to him the quantity and quality of the power he wishes to offer. The "owner" of the animals usually takes men to his dwelling place in the forest and shows them the species he rules, so they may choose those from which they want power.

Dream Apprenticeship

Through dreams or visions a man can initiate contact with a *no'wet* who, in a series of experiences, communicates his volition of giving power. Gradually the *no'wet* imparts knowledge. As the dreams continue, the bond between the two becomes stronger with the consequent transmission of power and knowledge. This dream apprenticeship implies the occurrence of dreams taken as revelations of great importance that are treated, directed, and interpreted according to their culture (Heredia 1978; Miller 1970; P. Wright 1981b).

Self-Healing

When a person heals himself without any external help, it is considered to be evidence that he has some kind of power. From this point, the disease from which he suffered will be part of his personal power and he will subsequently be able to cure others suffering from the same disease.

In all these cases, the power transmitted by nonhumans to the future shamans entails the giving of auxiliary spirits that help them to heal and/or produce disease. According to the informants, the shaman's power implies that he has diseases inside his body that are nonhuman entities called *lawanek,* which are located primarily in the shaman's heart. These entities function to protect shamans from other shamans' spiritual aggressions. They also heal, or they may cause harm.[4] The hierarchy of vigilants seems to be inferior to that of the companion spirits, which in this case would behave similarly to the "owners."

During the initiatory experiences, the person undergoes a metamorphosis in his character. He will hide his condition until his power has developed completely and his healing skill is mature. He must not seek patients, but must wait until they come to him because they believe or they have been informed that he has shaman's *halojk.* Once he has gained their confidence, he is able to display his shamanic status openly, which will be strengthened if his cures are successful.

The Toba identify "classes" of shamans according to their power and the aims of their actions. Thus, there are shamans who cure or harm (Loewen et al. 1965; Miller 1979). The most powerful shamans are those who are associated with the spirits of the dead. These shamans are called *oikjağajk* ("powerful," "those that show their power"). During therapeutic sessions, they demonstrate their contact with the spirits of the dead by "dialogues" that all attending can hear but not see. The great Toba leaders, such as the *cacique* Moreno, were powerful shamans and authentic *oikjağajk* because of their exceptional qualities that distinguished them from the other political and religious leaders.

The acquisition of auxiliary spirits and vigilants determines the shaman's degree of power. It can be said that the more auxiliary spirits a shaman has the more quantity of power he will have. As mentioned, the *jaqa'a* are hierarchically organized regarding the extent of their power. The power quality inherent in them is linked to their place of origin, the greatest degree being the "above" (sky) and decreasing toward "below" (earth) (Cordeu 1969–70; Miller 1967, 1977, 1979).[5] Shamans thus make efforts to contact the more powerful entities, although they are often more dangerous and demanding. These *jaqa'a* entities determine the differences between the shaman and other men and function as entities of his own soul constitution.

The possession of *jaqa'a* guarantees the shaman's capacity for healing or harming, as well as guaranteeing his own personal health. The latter is closely related with the shamanic power struggles, in which they compete to prove who possesses more *halojk*. The power circulates among the winning shamans, who accumulate the power of the defeated (Cordeu 1969–70; Miller 1979). The struggles begin during the dreams when the image-souls leave the sleeping shamans and meet those of other shamans. Then, with the help of the auxiliary spirits and the vigilants, they take part in fierce fights, which result in the accumulation of power by the winner and loss of power by the defeated. Such a loss is conceived as the escape of the shaman's soul entities, thus leaving him without protection against other shamanic attacks that will make him ill. A sick shaman is, almost certainly, equivalent to a dead shaman (Loewen et al. 1965; Miller 1979).

Obviously, the Toba shamans have an agitated night life as their image-souls travel to other domains of the universe, talk with nonhumans and other shamans, and struggle for power. Due to their faculties of penetrating the nonhuman universe through dreams, they are considered the most qualified to interpret important dreams, whether their own or of others, and to prescribe necessary actions to be taken. Dreams also have their role in the shamans' therapeutic practices.

Toba etiology attributes the causes of illnesses to be from shamans who send nonhumans to enter the victim, from "witches," and from the transgression of taboos generally sent by entities that are "owners" of the species or substance the taboo involves. The shaman must identify the cause in order to cure the individual.

The healing ceremony starts when he uses his gourd rattle, a power instrument, to call his auxiliary spirit.[6] A dialogue begins through singing, in which the shaman asks his "companion" about the patient's illness. Sometimes the shaman goes into ecstasy, a state considered optimum to contact the auxiliaries. If the spirit identifies the illness, he tells the shaman how to cure it; otherwise, he tells him to instruct his patient to consult another shaman.

Once the cause is identified, the Toba shaman passes his hands over the patient's body, and proceeds to suck, blow, or sing, according to instructions given by the spirit. The therapeutic singing is revealed to the shaman by the auxiliary and is regarded to be the "same voice" of the *no'wet*. After locating the illness, the shaman tries to persuade the harmful agent to leave the patient's body. Once he has achieved that, he usually shows the "object" that caused the illness to those present or to the patient. Little stones and sticks, worms, and other elements of poorly defined morphology can be seen on his palms. He may then throw them far away or put them into his mouth in order to increase his own power.

However, on some occasions the shaman must wait until his auxiliary spirit tells him through dreams how to cure the harm.

> A shaman didn't know what was the matter with a boy; then one night a *no'wet* appeared in his dreams and told him, "Your son has an illness called 'sore.' In order to cure it you must look for *čajk, kokalja* and *čjela,* those plants." So he looked for them, boiled them and gave them to the boy on that same day.

In another case, the shaman's auxiliary was unable to locate the cause of a child's illness resulting from his parents' transgression of a food taboo. Ideally, during the ritual the spirit should have aided in locating what taboo was broken and then directed the dialogue with the offended "owner" in order to reach an "agreement" favorable for all. In the following case, the shaman had to wait for a dream.

> At night he had a vision from a *no'wet* as in a dream. He dreamed that the parents had eaten ostrich. The raven gave him the revelation. He said, "Your patient will soon be cured of the 'infection.'"

The shaman's auxiliary spirit, the raven, told him that the patient's family had eaten ostrich, whose meat had been thrown away in the forest and the "owner" of the ostriches had sent the "infection" as a punishment.[7]

As noted by Perrin (this volume) payment by the patient is an important concluding element in the curing process. Once cured, the patient must pay the shaman in the form of goods of various kinds. If this payment is not made, the shaman is in danger, since his auxiliary spirits could get angry and interrupt their association with him. Like the sick shaman, he is left unprotected and without powers to cure.

DREAMS AND THE PROBLEM OF WITCHES

The Toba have a category of individuals who cause harm and are not shamans, the *qonağanağae* or "seizer." Generally, they are considered to be women, although men occasionally are also accused. Like shamans, they are associated with nonhumans that have revealed their power to them, but their techniques are always directed to produce harm. Their procedures are also different from the shaman's, for they operate using contagious or sympathetic magic and not object intrusion, as do the shamans. Their name describes their techniques, because they "seize" some personal object of the victim (clothing, utensil, hair, etc.) to cook or elaborate a packet that is then introduced into a reptile's mouth. The power of the packet is made effective by means of prayer, and the victim is condemned to a certain death (Miller 1979).

The witches keep their actions secret and do not have a public recognition of their status. The traditional way to discover a witch is through dreams, when the victim meets the witch responsible for his suffering.

> Before his death, a man summoned his family and told them, "Well, I shall die, so I shall tell you everything that happened. That woman [the witch] said I earned too much, and she didn't like that." The woman had said, "It is better to kill this man." The man heard that in his dream. When the man was about to die, he already knew everything that had happened to him.

As is common elsewhere, witchcraft accusations are related to interpersonal and intercommunal tensions.

Sometimes not only the witch is revealed through a dream, but also the procedures used that allow the victim to be cured. The following narrative describes such a case.

> While I remained like a dead man, there was a place, the palm grove where there was a palm trunk. They said they had put my photograph there. There was also a bird head. Then they killed a snake, opened its mouth. *Empayenar* is what they did to me.[8]

This victim, through dream, was able to identify the causes of his illness in time. Then, praying to God, he saved his life from certain destruction.

Such cases of self-healing are rare, and this individual began to be regarded by the community as having power from a *jaqa'a* being. Others suspected that he was a secret witch.

We still do not know the exact nature of the nonhumans with which the witches associate. The Toba say that they are known through revelation, the contact occurring in dreams, or in "meetings" in person in a desolate place. Some have said that it is possible to inherit some relative's harmful power.

DREAMS AND PENTECOSTAL CULTS

The importance and functions of dreams for the Toba continues among those converted to Pentecostal cults. In general, dreams are used and interpreted in the traditional way, though reflecting Christian symbology. It is one way to establish contact with God and to receive power from Him.

Frequently, joining a church is preceded by an illness, the healing of which is attributed to God. In these cases, revelations are usually received that indicate God's role as healer. The sick person often dreams of beings sent by God, who give out a shining light, or whose words calm down the sleeper's uneasy spirit and cause a therapeutic effect.

> When I was ill, someone seemed to speak to me whom I couldn't see. I only heard the words. "The cross is very difficult to follow, but if you do, you will succeed. The word of God is heavy," he said to me. After going several times to the religious services, I got well and joined the Gospel.

Conversion to the Gospel is a gradual process in which the believer is progressively convinced of the goodness of God's power. Such goodness is proven by the acquisition of health, material prosperity, the experience of glossolalia, and reception of the Holy Spirit. During the religious services, singing, dancing, and prayers offer a favorable framework for the participants to enter into a state of ecstasy or to have visions that permit communication with the divine world, as does the shaman in his rituals. The Holy Spirit takes the role of shamanic auxiliaries.[9] He protects the believer from dangers and illnesses, usually appearing in dreams to communicate to the believer.

> I was in bed, sleeping alone, and feverish. Then a man dressed in white appeared. My eyes were closed, but I could feel the sound of a person praying for me at the bedside. Then I said, "Who is praying for me? I left the door well closed and someone is praying for me by my bed." Then I looked closely at the man. He was fair haired, but the hair was all like curls on his head. He was very young. Then I watched him and thought, "Ah! He is not from here as the other brothers; he is dressed in white." And in that moment I could hear very well the words he said to me as he sang in Spanish, "God is love, God is love, God is love." I had never heard that before, and as he was singing that, he was ascending. He was already ascending. Then I woke up and I felt fine. I had a bath and was cured. Later I told my husband about it. It happened that the man who had sung was coming from Heaven and I was already feeling joy.

The apparent transformation of the dream to Christian conceptions is clear. This being of heavenly nature from above, dressed in white, young and non-Indian, says a prayer for her cure. The message is that of the Church. After waking up, the dreamer made the traditional purification from illness, the bath, thus ending her therapy. The joy that she feels is an internal happiness similar to a "fire," one of the basic manifestations among the believers of their relationship with God. Note that she told her husband of the significant dream.

In the same way that dreams can reveal the shaman's contact with the spiritual world and indicate his calling, dreams for the Christian Toba occur as revelations coming from God.

> I saw a big hole and that hole was sinking. I was inside the hole and stones fell into it. Everything loosened and then a voice told me, "Now look at the sky. Look up. Put your eyes in the sky." I did so and the voice told me, "Call the God of Israel." Meanwhile, I remained in the hole. "Look at the Holy God of Israel." That's what the voice told me in my dream. And so I looked at all the stars. All of them looked like at nighttime in my dream. But what he pointed at were the Pleiades, and I said to myself, "Ah! The Pleiades show me that it is the Holy God of Israel, *dapiči.* There it ended and I awoke and kneeled to pray to God, and I thanked him for showing me that.

Here there is a confluence of traditional mythical elements, the hole and the constellation of the Pleiades, and the Pentecostal Holy God of

Israel. In ancient times, the Pleiades were especially venerated as an important celestial deity (Tomasini 1976; P. Wright 1981a). Their annual cycle marked the seasonal cycle of animals, and the Toba prayed to them as a deity for power and for securing food. Here the role of the Christian God coincides with the one previously played by that constellation.

As in traditional times, dreams considered to be relevant must be retold to the community during their cult ceremonies. Each of the faithful testifies to his "brothers" these experiences of contact. He demonstrates his power by his dreams, describing the voices, gleaming beings, or speaking Bibles, and the "messages" that God desires to give to his "children." The faithful then interpret the dreams according to a personal reading of the Bible, adapted to the multiple circumstances of the oneiric discourse.

The following narrative illustrates the continuing belief in witches and the role of the Church in protecting its followers:

> A witch who was preparing remedies to kill people appeared to him. He said that the witch showed him that they were preparing a snake and the beak of a pool bird. He also saw that they had two little bones and then they threw everything away in the forest. He saw it as in a dream, and he sent P. S. to take everything out, but P. S. trembled; he was afraid of digging the hole. P. S. took out the bones and carried them together with the beak and the snake to church.

Here, as in the previous narratives, the sick person saw in his dreams the characteristics and location of the packet that had been made to cause him harm. Without doubting, he sent a friend to the place he had dreamed about, and, as expected, the frightened P. S. found the packet and removed it from the hole. Rather than being taken to a shaman, it was taken to the church, where they fought against the harm by means of collective prayer.

The first Catholic missionaries in the Chaco identified the *no'wet* figure with the Christian devil, and his actions were considered evil (Cordeu 1969–70). Nowadays, the Pentecostal preaching, reinterpreted by the Toba with the orientation of a few missionary translations in Toba, follows the same course. *No'wet,* in its different manifestations, has diabolic characteristics typical of the Biblical "world devils" that imply sin, illness, and the ruin of man. Shamans are often considered to be related to these diabolic powers and for that reason the cult preaching tends to deprive them of authority.

> When I was at home, he always came at night. He was like a devil. He always came, but I don't know for what purpose. Before I joined the Gospel, he used to step on me. I suffered a lot. He who came at night was that *pombero.* They also call him *pel'ek.* He is short, but he has a lot of hair and no clothes. Once, at night, he came into my body; I was like possessed by the devil. The *pombero* enters those men without faith. Sometimes he tells me, "I am the *pombero.* You, son of God, are good for nothing." He has a great strength and the person possessed jumps a lot and hits, and when he leaves him, the body remains limp.

The figures of these "beings of the night" and their behavior with respect to men is characteristic of the Toba tradition. They journey on the earth during the night and return to the underground world during the day. Their behavior toward men is ambiguous, and they generally tend to frighten them, at times causing a physical discomfort. Meetings with the *pel'ek* may also occur in person. The Toba *pel'ek* is associated with the Spanish *pombero* and the devils of the Bible that possess men of little faith. In the dreams he makes the traditional form of appearance, introducing himself and showing hostility toward the believer's faith.

In spite of the large number of converts and the Pentecostal opposition between God and the shaman, there are many shamans who are believers and many believers who seek shamanic cures. In reality this opposition is not a deeply held doctrine. The Toba, including the believers, still consider these "devils" to have a power that is vital, according to their vision of the world, for the well-being of the individual and the community.

NOTE ON TRANSCRIPTION (TOBA)

The native terms have been transcribed according to the phonological notation established by Braunstein (1981, 11). Such an alphabet is distinguished from the Spanish one as follows:

1. All Toba words are stressed on the last syllable, so intensity is not marked.
2. The labiovelar semiconsonant or semivowel or in contexts followed by the vowel *i,* the voiced fricative bilabial consonant is represented by *w.*
3. Semiconsonant or palatal semivowel is represented by *j.*

4. Voiceless postvelar occlusive *q*.
5. Voiced postvelar fricative *ǧ*.
6. Voiceless glottal fricative *h*.
7. Glottal stop ’.
8. Voiceless velar stop *k*.
9. When the following consonants, voiceless apicodental stop *t*, voiced apicodental fricative *d*, voiceless fricative (grooved or flat) *s*, and apicoalvelar nasal *n* appear in contexts followed by the vowel *i*, they represent the voiceless affricative prepalatals (it may alternatively appear as *č*), the voiced affricative *y*, the voiceless fricative *š*, and the nasal *ñ*, respectively.
10. Regarding the vowels, the same Spanish signs are used, though the high back *u* and medium *o* appear in a free fluctuation, a fact that makes the presence of one or the other irrelevant; however, the closed high front *i* must be differentiated from the other open one, somewhat lower, that appears together with the closed or open front medium *e*.

Notes

1. Data are based on fieldwork carried out in the Toba colonies of Misión Tacaaglé and La Primavera during 1979, 1981, 1982, and 1983. The last three sessions were conducted as Fellow of the Consejo Nacional de Investigaciones Científicas y Técnicas (CONICET) in the Centro Argentino de Etnología Americana, Buenos Aires, Argentina. These Toba from the eastern Formosa Province are linguistically and culturally different from the other Toba of the Chaco region. I would like to thank Inés Terradas, Carlota Romero, and Jorge Wright for their translation of this article from Spanish to English, and Jean Langdon for her final revisions of the translation.

2. Miller (1970, 1977) asserts that Pentecostalism caused a secularization of the Toba culture. We disagree, since the cognitive and cosmovisional structures were not substantially modified.

3. Consult P. Wright (1981a) about the term *no'wet*. According to Miller (1967, 1977, 1979), and Loewen et al. (1965), *no'ouet* is the owner of an area, a powerful figure of the forest. Buckwalter (1980) says they are guardian spirits of nature. Tomasini and Braunstein (1975, 108) are in closer agreement to us and to Cordeu (1969–70), “*No'wet* is an ambivalent theophany that may act positively or negatively. It is positive in the shaman’s initiation. It is negative when it brings about illness and death. Certain mythical characters, as for

example the owners of the animal species, are or possess *no'wet* as long as they share their kind of power." Tomasini (1974) should be consulted for the western Toba's idea of *pajak,* which is similar to that of *no'wet.*

4. This notion of vigilants as nonhuman entities is not completely clear because the Toba notion of person is not totally clarified. For the moment, our explanation is based on our current understanding of the theme. Miller (1977) uses the word *ltaxaỹaxaua* ("the companion who speaks to him or to her") for auxiliary spirits (*ltawa*). He also mentions *ñinaigaxaua* ("my companion") and *lỹa* ("his other one"); pointing out for all terms the relation of companionship established with the shaman.

5. This point has not yet been proven by our own field data. Cordeu (1969–70, 88) states the existence of tense opposition among the three levels of space: the sending of dangerous beings and calamities of heavenly origin would be restored by the earth level through the control over the heaven level by sacred entities of earthly origin. In the same way similar relations with the subterranean level can be detected.

6. The gourd rattle is a hollow receptacle the contains power elements, little stones of different shapes. There possibly exists a symbolic identification of the shaman's heart, where his "vigilants" or "illnesses" are said to be, with the rattle that contains power objects. In Toba mythology it appears that the gourd rattle is the heart of the mythical fox (P. Wright 1989).

7. It is usual among the Toba that the curing of "infection" coincides with the giving of a name to the child. Generally, the "owner" of the offended species suggests the name, which may be connected with the characteristics of that species or with the particular circumstances of the transgression, saying that he will be cured if the name is given to him. We find that almost all Toba adults have at least one vernacular name originating from a situation of "infection" during childhood (L. Vuoto 1981; P. Vuoto 1981; P. Wright 1981a, 1981b, 1984b). This kind of naming action is related to the idea that the individual gradually incorporates soul entities during his life that give him "power." The name is conceived as one more of these entities.

8. *Empayenar* means to make a *payé,* a word of Guaraní origin that the Toba use to refer to the magic packets, which may be used for multiple purposes.

9. Our data differ from Miller's (1977) when he describes the differences between the shamanic auxiliary spirits and the Holy Spirit. He states that, while the latter are not always with the shaman and therefore must be summoned, they always accompany the believer. Our information indicates that the auxiliaries and *lawanek* are always with the shamans, the latter inside their bodies. Otherwise, the shaman could get ill at any time. These entities are soul components of the shaman, although their possession is temporary because of the shamanic struggles for power.

PART THREE

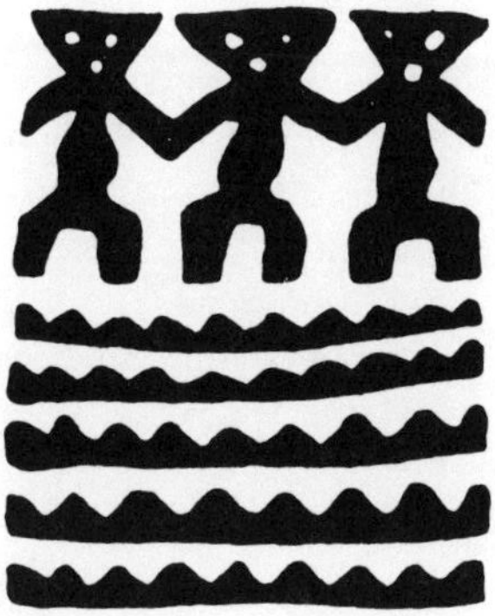

EXPRESSIVE CULTURE AND SHAMANISM

EIGHT

A MUSICAL AESTHETIC OF RITUAL CURING IN THE NORTHWEST AMAZON

JONATHAN D. HILL

In a recent survey of the literature on shamanism, Noll (1983) argued against the misleading view of shamans and other ritual healers as marginal individuals whose curing practices arise from a predisposition to alienation and mental pathology. Western observers of shamanism, including some anthropologists, have fallen into the trap of the "cognicentrist preoccupation of pigeonholing unusual behaviors as psychopathological" (Noll 1983, 450). Experiences with indigenous curers of the upper Rio Negro basin of Venezuela lead this author to strongly support Noll's contention that shamans are exceptional individuals whose mastery and control over altered states of consciousness contrast starkly with the loss of control and psychological coherence that characterize the victims of mental illness. Among other things, the description of indigenous Amazonian curing rituals that follows will demonstrate that ritual healers are central to, rather than alienated from, the ongoing concerns of everyday social life. Moreover, their ritual curing powers are a creatively practical process of musical naming that is used to "tune," or situationally adjust relations within individual human bodies, the social order, and the macrocosmos of nature that surrounds and supports human social life (Moore 1976; V. Turner 1977).

Anthropological studies of shamanism have been limited by the assumptions of structuralist rationalism and other language-centered models for describing, translating, and interpreting shamanistic performances. For example, Lévi-Strauss (1963) began his famous analysis of a Kuna curing ritual with the assumption that shamanistic curing supplies meaningful order and content to otherwise emotional, but meaningless, bodily experiences of pain. The primary means by which shamans effect cures is the semantic meaning of the texts of songs and chants. "The cure would consist, therefore, in making explicit a situation originally existing on the emotional level and in rendering acceptable to the mind pains which the body refuses to tolerate" (Lévi-Strauss 1963, 197). Lévi-Strauss never considered that semantic meaning alone cannot possibly account for the shamanistic abreaction and its generalization to a social group consisting of the patient and her family. Shamanic language of the Kuna is characterized by densely metaphorical, poetic, and esoteric nuances of mythic meaning that are, at best, partially intelligible to nonspecialists (Sherzer 1983). Semantic meaning, naming, and allusion to mythic beings and episodes are all highly significant to the effectiveness of shamanistic and other ritual performances (Munn 1969). However, by reducing shamanistic performance to a sort of "language," the more fundamental means of expressing shamanistic power through gestures, musical sounds, and other nonverbal media are excluded from the interpretive framework or treated as epiphenomena that reflect a primary linguistic ordering.

Lévi-Strauss's model of shamanistic performance makes an a priori distinction between reason (or meaning as a linguistic function) and emotion (or experiences of bodily pain as a physiological function). For Lévi-Strauss, shamanism is a sort of balancing act, or "see-saw," that serves to "cool out" overwhelmingly "hot" emotions of fear, anger, grief, and so on by restoring a balance of meaning and emotion. This approach to shamanistic ritual reifies "meaning" to a level of reality existing independently of the actors who produce meanings through practical, creative, intentional actions. For Lévi-Strauss, semantic (or tropic) meaning is conceptually and spatially distanced from emotion and the practical motivations for doing shamanism (or for being shamanized). We are left with the impression that people perform shamanistic rituals primarily to satisfy their intellectual need for balancing structures of meaning.

In contrast to Lévi-Strauss's intellectualist approach, the following analysis of shamanistic curing in the upper Rio Negro region of Venezuela is based on the notion that shamanism is, first and foremost, to be understood as a practical, sociophysiological activity of curing and recovering. Although shamanism does work through collectively shared modes of social consciousness, it does not do so in the way that Lévi-Strauss imagined. Nor is the alignment of collective ideologies the primary motivating force that generates shamanistic ritual activity. By treating shamanism as a process of practical creativity or practical signification, this analysis aims to restore the sensible as an integral part of the intelligible (Dougherty and Keller 1985; Keller 1985). As Ulmer pointed out, Western social scientists in the modernist period tended to view the world through the lens of logocentrism, or the cultural predisposition to place "the purely intelligible prior to the merely sensible" (1983, 87). A corollary of the logocentrist predisposition is the view that meaning is an abstract, mental concept that can be understood apart from the genres of activity through which it is produced. By isolating an abstract level of meaning, ritual action is stripped of social context and emotion, making it impossible to understand ritual efficacy except as an arbitrary, emotionless imposition of reified concepts (T. Turner 1985).

All of these dichotomies—meaning versus emotion, intelligibility versus sensibility, and practical versus expressive—are manifestations of a Western, rationalist tradition of the radical splitting apart of subject and object and the reification of rationalist categories into "objective" (or extrasocial) entities. In small-scale, technologically simple societies that lack a written historical record, logocentrist and other rationalist dichotomies severely distort the organization of artistic activity. Consider, for example, Brown's conclusion about magical hunting songs of the Aguaruna, a Jivaroan people of the Peruvian Amazon, ". . . the songs are part of a general ordering process that encompasses the strategic use of thoughts, speech, objects, and acts to achieve practical ends" (1984, 545).

Like the Amazonian curing songs to be discussed below, Aguaruna hunting songs bring into play evocative imagery which is far too richly textured to be reduced to the practical goals of the performer, yet their performance aims at effecting highly practical changes in the performer's environment. Aesthetic and practical thinking are masterfully integrated in native Amazonian musical performance. In empirical terms, curing rituals in the upper Rio Negro of Venezuela are based on a musical aesthetic of ritual efficacy, which is simultaneously concerned with an artistic conception of the world and a practical logic of curing.

ETHNOGRAPHIC SKETCH OF THE WAKUÉNAI

The Wakuénai, or "People of Our Language," are a Northern Arawakan society whose ancestral lands center around the Isana and Guainía rivers and their tributaries in Venezuela, Colombia, and Brazil.[1] Like the more well-documented Eastern Tukanoan societies of the neighboring Vaupés basin, the Wakuénai organize themselves into several exogamous phratries, each consisting of a number of named patrilineal sibs ranked in a hierarchical order (Goldman 1983; Hill 1983; C. Hugh-Jones 1979; S. Hugh-Jones 1979; Jackson 1983; Oliveira and Galvão 1973; Reichel-Dolmatoff 1971; R. Wright 1981). Social ranking among Wakuénai sibs is reckoned by order of emergence from the mythical center of the world at Hípana, a village on the Aiary River in Brazil. Within sibs, hierarchy is primarily a reflection of differential control over ritual powers to effect orderly transformations of individual sib members' identities in rites of passage and restorations of orderly growth and development of sick individuals in curing rituals.

Despite the great importance of rank and hierarchy in Wakuénai society, everyday social and economic relations are thoroughly egalitarian in character, and even the most powerful ritual specialists are active manioc gardeners, fishermen, and, less frequently, hunters. Similarly, relations between exogamous phratries are horizontal ties of alliance between competing affinal groups of equal status. The dual tendency toward equality and hierarchy in Wakuénai society frames a process of dynamic interaction between symmetrical, homogenous relations and more specialized, unequal relations. Over time, this process favors the cumulative development of a structured hierarchy of ritual specialists whose leadership can be called on in difficult times as a power resource for restoring order to individuals, or groups of individuals (Hill 1983, 1984b; Wright and Hill 1986).

MYTHOLOGY AND COSMOLOGY

Wakuénai mythology outlines a complex cosmic history that continues into the present through the mediating activities of ritual specialists, known as shamans (*malírri*), chant owners (*málikai limínali*), and master shamans (*dzáwináitairi*). In Wakuénai myths, the world began in the distant past at Hípana with the origin of the trickster and culture hero, Iñápirríkuli. A cycle of myths about the distant, miniature past at Hípana describes a world inhabited by presexual, precultural animals whose social division into kin and affines was the source of unceasing violence and warfare. The myths of Iñápirríkuli are hard-working social narratives that focus on basic rules and axioms that organize everyday social experience. Bride service, patrilocal residence, exogamy, and other social norms that shape relations of kinship and marriage are portrayed as emergent qualities of an ongoing process of competition between Iñápirríkuli and his animal affines. These social animals, and Iñápirríkuli in particular, provide insight into how the Wakuénai conceive of their social order as part of the precultural, natural environment. The myths explore an analogy between, on the one hand, conflicting interests of social groups of kin and affines, or phratries, and, on the other hand, the adaptive behavior of natural species that protect their own interests at the expense of other species. Through the cycle of myths about Iñápirríkuli and the precultural, miniature world of the mythical Beginning, the Wakuénai reach a sociological understanding of their own society.

The space-time of mythic beginnings is an undifferentiated, presymbolic ordering of reality that surrounds and infuses the later, verbally and sexually differentiated worlds of human society and history. The Wakuénai concept of mythic beginnings is a specific example of the more general idea of the mythic primordium, or the belief that human society and history resulted from the fragmentation of an original oneness of humanity and nature (Sullivan 1988). Language and other differentiating symbolic orders came into being as part of a fiery cosmic transformation that divided humanness from other, nonhuman (or semihuman) presymbolic modes of existence. These transformations are evoked in ritual and in ceremonial evocations of the cosmic fire as an ongoing process of constructing individual humanness and collective human sociality by controlling the passage of foods and other "substances" (including sacred names and sounds) through bodily orifices and across collective social boundaries. However, the movements of individuals and society through the differentiating, fragmenting process of language acquisition, socialization, and ritual power always remain in a constant, irreducible tension with the presymbolic mythic primordium. Control over the dynamic interrelations between the human social world and the mythic primordium is accomplished through producing musical and other nonverbal (or semiverbal) sounds that evoke imagery of a cosmic flooding of the world. Sound production, and especially poetic manipulations of the musical dimensions of spoken, chanted, and sung speech, are the primary means of regenerating symbolically structured humanness and social life (Basso 1985; Hill 1983, 1985, 1987, in press; Seeger 1986; Sherzer and Urban 1986; Sullivan 1988). "Music, rather than language, is the 'primary modeling system' organizing human bodies," and sound symbolism serves as the ultimate reality on which temporal orders are founded (Sullivan 1988, 282, 223). Sound is also the source of shamanistic power (ibid., 483).

Wakuénai cosmology and shamanistic rituals concretely exemplify these generalizations about the importance of musical and other sound symbolism in the indigenous poetics of lowland South American peoples. Through applying context-sensitive sociolinguistic and ethnomusicological methods in various lowland South American societies, researchers have begun to rethink native aesthetic and religious practices along totally new lines. Language-centered approaches, such as structuralism or ethnoscience, are being profoundly revised toward a view of language as a process of socialization and differentiation that is, in turn, subsumed by more dynamic, powerful processes of transformation, regeneration, and creativity that are rooted in musical performance, dance, spatial relations, and other nonverbal or semiverbal ways of creating social meaning. The Lévi-Straussian view of a simple dichotomy between nature and culture has given way to far more sophisticated understandings of a spectrum of a more-to-less socialized (or naturalized) being that unfolds in the dynamic interplay between primordial formlessness and contemporary meaning construction (Graham 1986; Seeger 1986). Sullivan (1988) has correctly identified the mythic primordium as the source of cultural innovation and creativity throughout South America. Although care must be taken not to assume equivalence of the meaning of the mythic primordium in different social and historical contexts, it is probable that the concept of mythic primordium is as widespread and significant for indigenous South American peoples as is the concept of Dreamtime among aboriginal Australian peoples (Hill 1988).

In a second cycle of myths the Wakuénai explain how the distant, miniature past of the mythical Beginning is transformed into a more recent, life-sized, and dynamic past of the primordial human beings. The central characters of this cycle are Iñápirríkuli, Amáru, the first woman, and Kuwái, their son. Kuwái is an extraordinary being whose body consists of all worldly elements and whose humming and singing form a "powerful sound that opens up the world" (*kémakáni hliméetaka hekwápi*) and brings into being all species of forest animals, fish, and birds. The birth of Kuwái sets in motion a rapid process of expansion in which the miniature world of Iñápirríkuli opens up into the life-sized world of forests and rivers inhabited by human beings and the various species of animals and plants. Kuwái teaches the sacred songs and chants (*málikai*) of initiation to Dzúli, the first chant owner (*málikai limínali*). Then Iñápirríkuli kills Kuwái by pushing him into a Great Fire, and the world contracts back to its miniature dimensions of the mythical Beginning. Out of Kuwái's ashes grow the plant materials for making the sacred flutes and trumpets played in initiation rituals and sacred ceremonies. Amáru and the women steal these instruments from Iñápirríkuli, setting off a long chase in which the world opens up for a second time as the women play Kuwái's instruments throughout the world. Eventually, the men regain the flutes, and the primordial father, mother, and son leave this world to stay in celestial regions of the cosmos.

The Kuwái myth cycle introduces human physiological processes of conception and birth, and all the ensuing processes of growth, development, and decay that form the basis of cultural differentiation in human society: male/female, parent/child, newborn infant/child, child/adolescent, adolescent/adult, mythical ancestor/living descendant, and living descendant/recently deceased person. The myths about Amáru and Kuwái describe the transition from a precultural past of undifferentiated social animals to a more recent time in which human individuals each came to have a unique personal and sexual identity, or *likáriwa,* as well as an animal-shaped and collective identity, or *líwarúna,* shared with other members of the same patrilineal sib. In the myths, human physiological processes are not viewed as passive forces on which cultural forms are grafted, but as transitions from one state to another that impel "the mind to formulate symbols and thereby bring into being a conceptual order that did not previously exist" (Drummond 1981, 646). The bodily processes of growth and development take on enormous, cosmic proportions in the Kuwái myth cycle and are equated with the expansion of the entire natural, physical world to its present size.

These physiological, or cosmic, forces must be controlled, or they will simply devour the social animals instead of leading to an orderly, controlled system of processes in which the social animal is not destroyed but transformed into a fully cultural human being. The myth cycle represents this transformation in terms of a strict dichotomy between control over hunger and its opposite. Control over hunger through ritual fasting allows the individual to participate in the creative and transformative powers of Kuwái and his music, whereas failure to control hunger leads to premature death. At one point in the myth cycle, Kuwái transforms himself into a rock cavern and devours three young boys who had broken their ritual fasting during initiation. One boy, however, was spared from death and became the first initiate because he withstood the pain of hunger. Ritual fasting is a form of voluntary suffering to which individuals must submit if they are to demonstrate that they are fully cultural beings capable of controlling their own destinies, rather than social animals caught up in a perpetual cycle of violence and revenge.

Accordingly, food and eating are central objects of symbolic thought and action in Wakuénai rites of passage at childbirth and puberty. Ritual specialists control the period of fasting and set up a number of densely interwoven symbolic equations between the events and characters of the Kuwái myth cycle, on the one hand, and the actions and participants of rites of passage, on the other. The end of ritual fasting is marked by performances of sacred songs and chants (*málikai*) that, together with tobacco smoke, are used to blow the world-opening power of Kuwái into a pot of sacred food (*káridzámai*) and, through eating, into the individuals undergoing ritual passages.

A third cycle of myths explores the processes of alienation and decomposition that lead to illness and death. Some illnesses are seen as a result of failing to observe ritual fasting and other restrictions on everyday diet and activity. Eating raw foods or foods that have not been properly named in *málikai* by the chanter owner can lead to a sickness called "raw" (*fiókali*). The other causes of serious illness are sorcerers, or poison owners (*máhnetímnali*), witches, or master shamans (*dzáwin-áitairi*, "Jaguar People"), and evil omens (*hínimai*).[2] In cases of serious, life-threatening illness, both the patient and the patient's kinsmen must fast on manioc drinks over which the chant owner has blown tobacco smoke and sung a special genre of *málikai* for counteracting witchcraft. Regardless of its cause, serious illness among the Wakuénai is seen as a process of disintegration in which the individual, human body–shaped soul (*likáriwa*) becomes separated from the collective, animal-shaped one (*líwarúna*). A complex cycle of myths centers around the processes of separation that lead to illness and death. At basis, these myths portray the lethal consequences of unsolicited, unmediated contacts between individuals in this world (*hekwápiríko*), the spirits of the dead (*lidánam*) in *íyarudáti,* and the bee spirits (Kuwáinyai, or "Kuwái People") who control access to the celestial paradise of Iñápirríkuli.

Chant owners and shamans seek to restore the connection between the two parts of their patients' souls by using their extraordinary ritual powers to travel to the two worlds of the afterlife: the chant owner journeys in his *málikai* songs to the celestial home of the Kuwáinyai, whereas the shaman travels in *málirríkairi* songs to the dark netherworld (*íyarudáti*) of recently deceased persons. The musical journeying of ritual curers acts as a means for symbolically controlling relations between living human beings in this world, mythical ancestors in paradise (*likáremi*), and recently deceased persons in the netherworld (*íyarudáti*). Through fasting and ritual music, the two souls of sick individuals are reintegrated, and proper relations between the living, the ancestors, and the dead are renewed.

Spiritual transformation and renewal in the world of living people has its counterpart in the belief that the souls of recently deceased persons transmigrate to rejoin their respective sib ancestral souls in celestial paradise after a period of painful separation in *íyarudáti.* The Wakuénai concept of immortality arises from a juxtaposition of two opposing views of human mortality: the continuous, vertical journey of collective *líwarúna* souls to paradise, and the discontinuous, horizontal transformation of individual *likáriwa* souls in this world into *lidánam* souls in the shadowy world of *íyarudáti.*[3] The period of time during which individuals must remain in a limbo status as recently deceased souls depends on the manner of death rather than behavior during life in this world (Hill 1983, 209; Matos Arvelo 1912, 95).

Once the *lidánam* souls have been purified in fire and have transmigrated to the celestial paradise of Iñápirríkuli, they enter into a state of eternal bliss where all souls are brilliantly white, live in beautiful houses, eat only the purest food (honey in great quantities), and bask in the eternal sunlight (Hill 1983; R. Wright 1981).[4] Like the Kuwái myth cycle and the rites of passage through which it is enacted in the human life cycle, the soul's journey after death is a twofold process of cumulative, irreversible transformation from which there is no turning back. Once the *lidánam* souls have transmigrated to paradise, they never return to the world of living people (Hill 1983, 201). Thus, Wakuénai cosmology explores the dichotomy between individual death and collective continuity in order to construct a belief in individual immortality and salvation rather than attempt to short-circuit this paradox through beliefs in the reincarnation of individuals as living members of this world.

RITUAL HEALERS: OWNERS OF MÁLIKAI AND SHAMANS

The ritual healers whose music forms the topic of inquiry in this chapter are the senior men living in a village on the lower Guainía River in Venezuela. The two are members of a highly ranked sib of the Dzáwinai ("Jaguar People") phratry, and their wives belong to the top-ranked sib of the Waríperídakéna ("Pleiades' Grandchildren") phratry. The younger of the two brothers is both a chant owner (*málikai limínali*) and village headman, and his fame as a ritual curer is augmented by a reputation for being a powerful diviner who can detect the presence of sorcerers, locate missing persons and objects, and predict future events.[5] The chant owner's older brother is a shaman (*malírri*) who uses hallucinogenic snuff made from the bark of a tree, called *dzáato* (*Virola calophylla*), in order to induce contact with the spirits of the dead in curing rituals. Both the chant owner and shaman are grandfathers whose grandchildren range in age from early childhood to beyond initiation and nearing marriage. They have practiced curing for many years, perhaps as long as three decades, and whatever doubts they might have had about the effectiveness of their healing techniques have vanished by now. Through years of practice, they have come to take on the qualities of the first chant owner and the first shaman in myth, Dzúli and Éeri, and they are well-known as ritual healers in villages along the Guainía-Negro River and throughout the entire region bounded by the upper Orinoco, Atabapo, Casiquiare, and Guainía rivers in Venezuela.

Their fame as ritual healers brings them extra prestige and financial income through the payments received for successful cures. The chant owner and shaman expect to be paid with material goods for providing ritual services designed to reintegrate their patients' two souls. In curing rituals the payment (*dawáinaku*) is conspicuously displayed in order to help the shaman attract the patient's lost soul back to its proper place in the human body. The belief that generosity with material goods influences ritual efficacy is part of a wider sense of openness in which the patient and his kinsmen are expected to confess intimate personal experiences, such as bad dreams, unusual events, or family arguments, to the shaman and chant owner. The specialists listen to these confessions with great attention, for it is through such verbal reconstructions of the unique events leading up to illness that they attempt to diagnose their patients' diseases and begin counteraction. In most cases, the patients' confessions indicate that they have been victims of sorcery, witchcraft, or the violation of a dietary or activity taboo. In cases of serious, life-threatening illness, however, patients and their kinsmen are required to confess every detail of the events preceding illnesses so the ritual healers can unravel the combined effects of witchcraft and sorcery, a phenomenon known as the evil omen (*hínimai*). In such situations, the ritual healers ask everyone in the village to "contribute," or loan, their most valuable possessions in a desperate attempt to attract the patient's lost soul back to this world. The resulting heap of material goods is later redistributed to the original owners, except for the payment made by the patient's kinsmen to the shaman and chant owner. In the event the curing ritual fails to effect a cure, the patient's kinsmen retain the payment, and the ritual healers receive no material goods for their work.

The payments and prestige that accrue to ritual healers do not mean that they are in any way removed from the ongoing cycle of everyday subsistence and social activities. To the contrary, the chant owner and his brother are active manioc gardeners, fishermen, and hunters, and both men take active roles in communal work parties and other social events. They are recognized as charismatic leaders in everyday social contexts precisely because they embody a higher order of sacred and aesthetic values that transcends narrow social ties and economic interests within the local sib and that can cut across phratric and even ethnic boundaries.[6] They acquire a few material valuables that others cannot afford, but they freely lend such items to other members of the village, thereby conferring economic benefits on everyone in the village. In everyday contexts, the ritual healers lead by example and by coordinating group consensus, often carrying over their ritual concern for sacred order through actively participating in collective work activities and imbuing these events with an aesthetic value. Because they are so completely identified with their ritual offices, the chant owner and shaman transform everyday activities such as gardening and eating into categories of symbolic thought that fit into the overall cultural identity of the village. Communal meals, for example, are shared in the chant owner/headman's house once or twice a day and are more than an adaptive mechanism for ensuring that food is shared in the village. They are an expression of cultural etiquette, or "table manners" that contributes to the cultural identities, both individual and collective, or men and women in the village. In short, ritual healers communicate to nonspecialists the transition from a precultural, inchoate past, to a more recent, culturally differentiated past, and they carry this sense of emergent cultural order into their secular lives as model individuals who are at the center of, rather than marginal to, everyday social and economic interests.

In cases of life-threatening illness, the chant owner and shaman may spend up to four or five consecutive days in nearly complete devotion to their curing practices. However, curing rituals are generally brief performances that last only a couple of hours and do not take away much time from everyday social and subsistence activities. Curing rituals are, for the most part, worked into the schedule of everyday activities and do not require any major disruption of that schedule. In most cases, the two specialists separately perform music and other ritual techniques designed to bring the two parts of their patients' souls back together again and to cast out the spiritual and/or physical agents that have caused the separation. Table 8.1 lists eleven curing rituals I observed in 1980, 1981, and 1984. Each ritual is broken down according to the type of illness being treated, the treatment (whether *málikai* or *málirríkairi,* or both), approximate age of patient, sex of patient, and ethnic group(s) of the patient's family. Since diagnosis is based upon the specialists' interpretation of unique patterns of dreams and other intimate experiences, a strict correlation between the type of physiological symptoms and the genre of curing music is impossible to discern from the diagram. However, looking at the cases in which either *málikai* or *málirríkairi* is separately performed, a general tendency is apparent. Performances of *málikai* in isolation appear to be directed at alleviating nightmares, ear infections, and phobias in young children, and disorders of the reproductive system in adult women. Performances of *málirríkairi* in isolation aim mainly at curing diseases of the mouth, respiratory tract, and digestive system.

TABLE 8.1. Wakuénai Curing Rituals Performed during 1980–81 and 1984 Fieldwork.

Problem	Treatment	Age and Sex		Ethnic Group(s)	Results
Severe diarrhea and weight loss	*málikai* and *málirríkairi*	1	F	Baniwa-Guarequena	Death attributed to evil omens
Toothache	*málirríkairi*	14	F	Baniwa nonindigenous	Pains reduced
Cough, fever	*málirríkairi*	1	M	Wakuénai (Dzáwinai)	Symptoms gone within three days
Nightmares and tantrums	*málikai*	4	M	Wakuénai (Ádzenéni)	Child still withdrawn; nightmares and tantrums alleviated
Earache	*málikai*	7	F	Wakuénai (Dzáwinai)	Not effective; pain attributed to toothache
Stomach pains	*málirríkairi*	1	F	Wakuénai (Dzáwanai)	Pains alleviated, no recurrence
Menstrual cramps	*málikai*	45	F	Wakuénai (Waríperídakéna)	Pains relieved; resumed normal diet within two days
Pains when breathing deeply; fever	*málikai* and *málirríkairi*	18	F	Wakuénai	Pains relieved, fever went down
Pains in head and body, fever	*málikai* and *málirríkairi*	57	F	Wakuénai	Pains alleviated, but no total cure possible (evil omens)
Stomach pains, fever	*málirríkairi*	50	F	Guarequena	Recovered within two days
Crying	*málikai*	1	M	Guarequena	Child had been frightened, but recovered well

MUSICAL PERFORMANCE AND RITUAL EFFICACY

From the perspective of Wakuénai ritual healers or their patients, the practical objective of restoring or regaining health is inextricably bound up with the complex series of communications and musical journeys to other regions of the cosmos. Ritual healers thus re-experience the processes of separation that led to their patients' illnesses and link these processes of decay to specific natural and social conditions. Shamanistic curing is not an intellectual mind game of restoring meaningful order to meaningless emotion and bodily pain, but a practical, social process of "musicalizing" speech and action (i.e., chanting, singing, and dancing). The creation of "felt consubstantiality between language music and myth" is grounded in the indigenous concept of "spirit-name" (*liakúna*) (Friedrich 1986, 39). As a verbal, semantic process, shamanistic curing is an activity of reversing the order of creation established in mythic narratives about the primordial human being, Kuwái, whose voice musically named-into-being the species and objects of nature. The naming processes used in shamanistic curing rituals evoke the chthonian space-time of underground and underwater movements, dynamic reversals of creation space-time in which the spirit-names of shamans and their patients are brought into a controlled relationship with the regenerative powers of the mythic ancestors. Shamanistic naming processes are complex, densely metaphorical ways of poeticizing the relations between specialists and their patients, and these naming processes often create ambiguity and higher levels of poetic indeterminacy, as well as images of stability and higher levels of orderliness.

The semantic dimension of shamanistic curing is inextricably linked to two other processes of meaning construction, movements between "places" and musical movements. The indigenous term *liakúna,* or "spirit-name," also means "place." Ritual specialists conceive of these places as simultaneously existing inside the body (i.e., specific organs or body parts), in the social order (i.e., stages in the life cycle, generations, or inherited rankings), and in the surrounding world of forests, rivers, and mythic beings. In other words, shamanic naming processes are not merely representations of a preconceived ordering of experiential realities, but are thought of as a process of movement from one place to another that organically unfolds in the body, the social order, and the surrounding contexts of nature, cosmos, and history. Translation or interpretation of shamanistic naming processes as an exclusively (or primarily) semantic activity of representation would fundamentally distort the indigenous conception of spirit-naming as a set of dynamic movements between places. Shamanistic naming processes are better understood as activities of creating a poeticized space-time of mythic ancestral powers within the bodies of living human beings, the social world, and the cosmos.

Although shamanistic constructions of poeticized space-time make use of elaborate, semantically "thickened" language, the most fundamental dimension of meaning construction is not semantic representation but the projection of semantic meanings into musically organized patterns of verbal, semiverbal and nonverbal sound. In a very direct, sensible way, the movements through musical tones, rhythms, tempos, and timbres are the shamanistic process of movement among distinct places in body, society, and cosmos. The central thesis of this chapter is that Wakuénai shamanistic rituals are, according to the indigeous aesthetics of practicality, generated by musical sound organization. This more naturalized dimension of meaning construction forms a musical aesthetic of ritual curing that has the power to transform bodily, social, and cosmic relations that are grounded in, and to some degree constrained by, the more socialized, lexicalized representation of experience through the semantic functions of language (e.g., naming, metaphor, or other figures and tropes).

The processes of ritually defining illness and recovery through musical performance are highly complex and bring into play a richly elaborated set of symbols, texts, and sounds. The present study of *málikai* and *málirríkairi* songs for curing is not an exhaustive analysis of the many subgenres and specific manifestations that these two genres encompass. The song texts that ritual healers employ can vary almost infinitely in their details according to the different diseases to be treated and differences in the patients' situations. Nevertheless, the analysis below will demonstrate that the contrast between *málikai* and *málirríkairi* is highly significant for understanding the efficacy of Wakuénai curing rituals.

Following T. Turner (1977), Munn (1973), and van Gennep (1960), this analysis of Wakuénai curing rituals will focus on the capacity of ritual symbolism to mediate between inner and outer experience in order to bring about an adjustment of the actor's internal orientation. Turner's reformulation of van Gennep's model of rites of passage is especially helpful for understanding the effectiveness of ritual curing music, since it shows that ritual processes are both models of the social situations in which they unfold, and also dynamic rearrangements of such social situations. The dynamic effects of ritual arise from the hierarchical, asymmetrical structuring of symbols into a number of higher and lower levels in such a way that the "structure of ritual action . . . directly embodies its own principle of effectiveness" (T. Turner 1977, 62). The hierarchical levels of ritual action are defined relative to one another, not in absolute terms.

At the lowest level, a pair of opposing social categories, or roles, defines the structure of ritual action from the "bottom up." Thus, the pair of categories "witchcraft victim/healthy individual" serves to define the chant owner's ritual performances of *málikai,* and the pair "sorcery victim/healthy individual" is the social locus of the shaman's attempts to mediate relations between the living and the dead in his performances of *málirríkairi* songs. At intermediate levels, the musical performances of chant owners and shamans are grouped into symbolic categories, or genres, through classificatory operations, such as binary opposition. Seen from this level, the social situations of witchcraft and sorcery victims are relatively controllable disorderings of the pattern of relations between the individual self and the collective identity of the sib.[7] The structural contrast between *málikai* and *málirríkairi* songs for curing expresses symbolic regulation of the higher level, transcendental power to transform categories that are mutually exclusive at the lowest level. Seen from the bottom up, the two genres of curing music form the common ground within which illness, or "soul loss," becomes intelligible, transformable, and surmountable.

> The upper levels will, in general terms, be seen from the standpoint of the lower levels as standing to them in a relation of becoming to being, generalized potential to specific realization, dynamic to static, and transcendent to immanent (T. Turner 1977, 58).

Finally, at the highest level of structure, the two contrasting genres of curing music are themselves grounded through coordinating operations, such as juxtaposition and interpenetration of categories, which contrast at the intermediate and lowest levels. The "top down" effect of higher level symbolic processes generates the entire structure of ritual action at the same time as the bottom up effects define and locate ritual structure within a specific social context. The dynamic effectiveness of ritual action, its capacity not only to provide a model of social order, but also to shape it arises from the hierarchical, asymmetrical relationship between higher level principles of order and the disorderings of, or transitions between, social categories at lower levels (Geertz 1966, 36; see also Rappaport 1979, 116–26). The hierarchical symbolic structure of Wakuénai curing rituals, and in particular that of curing music, contains within itself the most reliable guide for an analysis of the efficacy of ritual healing.

LEVELS OF STRUCTURING IN WAKUÉNAI CURING MUSIC

The most striking feature of Wakuénai curing rituals is the degree to which the behavior of ritual specialists centers around musical performance. The rituals are essentially musical events around which a variety of other less prominent activities revolve. The strong emphasis on sacred music in Wakuénai curing rituals is grounded in beliefs in the "powerful sound that opened the world" (*kémakáni hliméetaka hekwápi*) emanating from the mythical character of Kuwái. Through ritual enactments of Kuwái's mythical sounds and names in *málikai,* the chant owner taps into indigenous beliefs in the ongoing mythical creation as an eternal coming-to-be of natural species and of human identities. The transcendent powers of Kuwái's musical creation of the cosmos and of the chant owner's reenactments of this process are the highest order principles that regulate and generate the structure of Wakuénai curing rituals from the top down. These musical powers are "postulates in their nature neither verifiable nor falsifiable but nevertheless taken to be unquestionable because mystically known or ritually accepted" (Rappaport 1979, 129). For the Wakuénai, the power of musical sound and language stands above all other classes of communicative events in human society. Contact with the spirits of the dead or with the mythical ancestors is an act of power and beauty when initiated by the owner of *málikai* or his accompanist, the shaman, whereas such contacts result in sickness and death when they happen to individuals who know only the dialects of everyday speech (of which there are five).

Unlike the dialects of everyday speech, the language of sacred music makes use of a system of generic classifiers, or spirit-names, the full meanings of which are known only to specialists. The basic rule of spirit-naming is that each generic category of spirits must be attached to a specific spirit-name. For example, the *palometta* fish (*Mylossoma duriventris*) is called *tsípa* in everyday speech but in *málikai* is named *umáwari máka-ruáduwa* ("anaconda butterfly"). In the sacred, mythical world of Kuwái and his music, human beings and all things in nature have generic, or collective, and specific, or individual, souls. This double aspect of Kuwái's creation gives rise to the two-sided character of Wakuénai sacred music. Depending on the context, ritual specialists can apply the world-opening power of sacred musical sounds in either of two distinct ways, each utilizing different classificatory principles. On the one hand, Kuwái's music can metonymically reenact the creation of the world according to a principle of the Many-in-the-One by emphasizing generic categories that include many distinct individuals, species, and objects into a single, compound entity on the basis of similarity. On the other hand, Kuwái's music can metaphorically "open the world" according to a principle of the One-in-the-Many by highlighting the uniqueness of specific spirit-names that exclude all but a single individual, species, or object on the basis of distinctive qualities.[8] These two opposing, yet complementary, classificatory processes form the conceptual basis for understanding the contrast between *málikai* and *málirríkairi* curing songs, and, at a still higher level, how the two genres form an interrelated pair of symbolic processes for reexperiencing and reversing the breakdown of individual and collective souls in sick individuals. Before going on to discuss the structure of musical sounds in *málikai* and *málirríkairi* songs, a brief consideration of song texts and the physical actions of ritual healers will show how the contrast between the two genres operates in the dimensions of musical language and ritual behavior.

"GOING THROUGH THE CENTER" AND "BRINGING BACK FROM THE DEAD"

The principal means for counteracting harmful effects of witchcraft is the performance of *málikai* songs in which the mythical journey of Iñápirríkuli and his younger brother, Kuwaikánerri, is reexperienced and applied to an actual victim. Kuwaikánerri was the first victim of witchcraft, yet Iñápirríkuli managed to save his life by blowing tobacco smoke over the flowers of many different species of fruit tree and, in doing so, creating the primal curing substances, honey and beeswax. In the song text, Iñápirríkuli makes a canoe out of beeswax for his dying brother and instructs him to lie down inside so that his body can be called and cooled by the beeswax. Iñápirríkuli gathers flowers from various fruit trees as he paddles upstream and turns each species into honey by blowing tobacco smoke over them. The brothers reach Mápawíka, the home of the bee spirits (Kuwáinyai, or "Kuwái People"), and the younger brother eats honey made from all the flowering trees there. As they leave Mápawíka to go up the Isana River, Kuwaikánerri decides that he is well enough to sit up in the canoe and help paddle. Iñápirríkuli makes him a paddle out of beeswax to cool his body, and they set off. They go "through the center of this world" and end up back at Mápawíka. From there, they jump up to Mápakwá Makákwi, the celestial home of the most powerful bee spirits, the "Two Brothers Kuwáinyai" (Dzámadáperri Kuwáinyai). These powerful curers diagnose Kuwaikánerri's illness as the attack of a witch and complete his cure with another dose of honey made from various flowers. Kuwaikánerri walks with his brother to a place on the Vaupés River where he remains hidden from view and protected by a surrogate mother.

As the original victim of witchcraft in mythical times, Kuwaikánerri and his journey to the homes of the Kuwáinyai represent the fate of the collective, animal-shaped soul (*líwarúna*). The two homes of the Kuwáinyai, Mápawíka on the Isana River, and Mápakwá Makákwi, are mythical gateways through which the *líwarúna* soul passes on its one-way journey after death up to the celestial paradise of Iñápirríkuli. The story of Kuwaikánerri parallels the *líwarúna* soul's journey after death, but at the same time brackets the vertical movements up to the Kuwáinyai's celestial village inside of two horizontal journeys in this world. Prior to reaching the bee spirits' home on the Isana, Kuwaikánerri lies down in the canoe made of beeswax, and his illness shows no sign of improvement. After leaving Mápawíka, Kuwaikánerri helps his older brother to paddle upstream, and they cross a threshold at "the center of this world" that sends them back to the place called Dzáwakaná at the mouth of the Isana where they had gathered flowers to make honey immediately before going to the bee spirits' village at Mápawíka. Only after this reversal in time and space do the two brothers travel to Mápakwá Makákwi, the highest point in the *líwarúna* soul's journey after death before reaching the celestial paradise (*likáremi*) of Iñápirríkuli, a place from which there is no return. The mythical return of the two brothers to the point in this world where they went immediately before going to Mápawíka is a highly significant event, since it establishes a direction from the celestial home of the bee spirits back to this world prior to the leap up to Mápakwá Makákwi.

The story of Kuwaikánerri thus replicates the journey of *líwarúna* souls after death to the last point before a return of the soul to this world becomes impossible. The return in time and space prior to leaving for the bee spirits' home applies a concept of reversibility (the capacity to turn around both temporal and spatial movements) to the fate of detached *líwarúna* souls. Placing the unidirectional journey in the context of a reversible mythical space-time effects a partial cure of the witchcraft victim (Kuwaikánerri) and brings the *líwarúna* soul back to the conscious, body-like soul (*likáriwa*). The reunification of the two parts of the soul is apparent in the last part of the story when Kuwaikánerri is able to leave Mápakwá Makákwi walking on his feet.

Shamans' songs (*málirríkairi*) are not based on a single, unified text like the story of Kuwaikánerri's journey in *málikai* songs for curing witchcraft. Instead, shamans have a variety of melodic and textual themes that change according to specific social situations. Early in the ritual, the shaman sits alone on a low bench and faces the eastern horizon to establish contact with the world of recently deceased spirits by snuffing hallucinogens (*Virola calophylla*) and searching the sky for shadows, or spirits. The early period is also used to muster the various supernatural powers, which the shaman later manipulates to effect cures. In his song texts, the shaman "sends" (*hútu*) tobacco (*dzéema*), the power of snuff (*tudáiri*), the attraction of the ritual payment (*dawáinaku*), and the mythical owner of hallucinogenic snuff (Dzulíhwerri).

The other half of this process is the shaman's attempt to "bring back" (*iidiétakawa*) the lost soul of the patient from *íyarudáti,* referred to in songs as the "place where the sun falls" (*liúdza hlíakawa hérri*). In particular, the songs frequently mention the houses of the *lidánam* souls that belong to the two most important sibs in the village. "I bring back from Héemapána" (*nudiétakawa liúdza hémapánadáli káuli*), and "we bring back from where the sun falls" (*wadiétakawa liúdza hlíakawa hérri*) are verses that express the shaman's intent to retrieve the sorcery victim's lost soul. Other verses name the door of *íyarudáti,* called *táuri núma,* which the shaman must open up to let the patient's soul return to the world of the living people.

There remains one last type of spiritual power with which shamans must come to terms in their curing songs: the spirit of sickness itself. The patient and his kinsmen come outside and are seated next to the shaman, who now focuses on restoring their collective bodily strength by blowing tobacco smoke on their heads and by extracting the physical agent of disease from the individual patient's body (fig. 8.1). Having sucked the poisonous substance out, the shaman stands up to scoop in an invisible spirit of sickness (*wáramápwa*) from the air with the feathers of his sacred rattle (*kútirúda*). Then he vomits up the internal and external agents of disease that have mixed together inside his stomach.

The shaman's musical journey does not cross boundaries between vertical regions of the cosmos, but between two areas separated by horizontal space, the world of living human beings and the world of recently deceased persons. In other words, shamans travel away from the center of this world to its edge, to "the place where the sun falls." However, their journeys out to the periphery of this world are controlled by focusing all their energies on "bringing back" (*iidiétakawa*) their patients' lost souls and on opening "the door" (*táuri núma*) of *íyarudáti*. This "bringing back" from the world of the recently deceased expresses the shaman's control over contact with the spirits of the dead (*lidánam*). The proof of his control arrives when he successfully synthesizes the internal physical agent of disease and the external spirit of disease inside his stomach and vomits up the resulting mixture.

BODY POSTURES AND ACTIONS OF RITUAL HEALERS

A consideration of body postures and actions (or lack thereof) that the owner of *málikai* and the shaman display in the course of curing rituals is useful for understanding the musical differences between *málikai* and *málirríkairi* songs. The owner of *málikai* sits in a hammock while performing curing songs and does not stand up until the end of the prayer with which he concludes his performance (fig. 8.2). Since hammocks are places where people usually sleep or rest, the posture of the *málikai* owner is one of sitting up. The shaman, too, performs nearly all his songs in a sitting position, but he sings while sitting down on a low bench after standing up for various reasons. Thus, both genres of curing music are performed in a sitting posture, but the *málikai* owner sits up, whereas the shaman sits down.

Beyond this similarity of posture, the body movements of the two

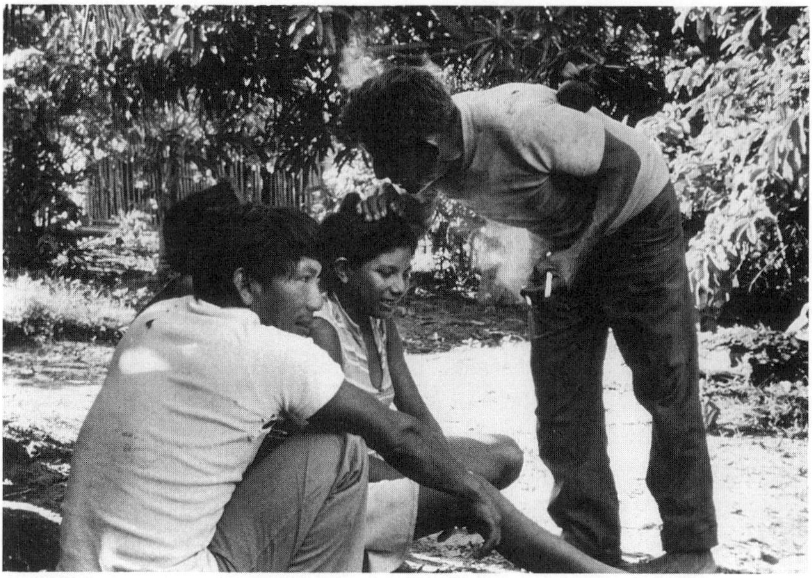

FIGURE 8.1. Shaman blows tobacco smoke onto the head of a patient.

types of ritual healers completely differ from each other. The owner of *málikai* sits rigidly still except for the unconscious, somatic movements of respiration and occasional eye blinking. His mouth and speech organs are the only body parts subject to voluntary movement while singing. In the brief intervals between songs, the chant owner restricts his movements to the minimal hand and body motions necessary for bending over to pick up a pot of manioc drink (*pačáka*), raise the lid, and set it back on the floor. Furthermore, the *málikai* owner sings inside a house. In short, his performances of *málikai* songs in curing rituals are a process of restricting all conscious body movements to a minimum and of temporarily shutting out all sense perceptions except for the sound of *málikai* and the smell of tobacco smoke.

Meanwhile, the shaman working outside is the embodiment of human activity and sensual stimulation. Even in his most inactive movements when he sits down on a low bench to sing, the shaman shakes his rattle in large, slow circles and moves his head and eyes from side to side as

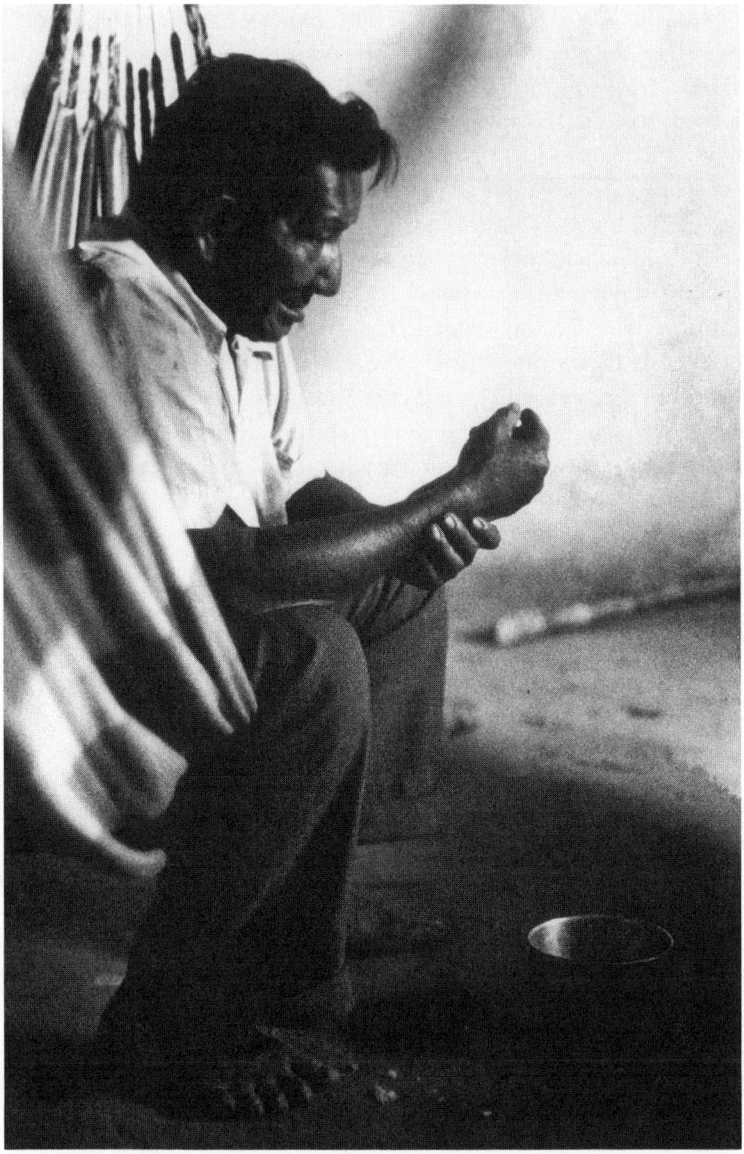

FIGURE 8.2. The owner of the sacred chants (*málikai*) sings the counter-witchcraft myth over a bowl of manioc drink.

he scans the sky for "shadows." The hyperactivity of the shaman is reflected in the great number of spiritual forces that he manipulates, both in *málirríkairi* songs and in physical actions accompanied by a variety of sacred objects: the rattle, cigarettes, stones (both polished red ones and jagged, quartz-like crystals), the *dzáato* snuff, a V-shaped bone tube for snorting, a white tube made of paper, the payment (*dawáinaku*), and the patient's body. Nevertheless, the shaman does not act in a random manner with these objects but uses them in highly structured and redundant sequences of action.[9]

Each activity of the shaman has a clear purpose in terms of the objectives of the curing ritual. Waving a cigarette in the air is done to capture the lost soul of the patient. The shaman tries to bring the lost soul into his arms with the cigarette so he can inhale it into his lungs, carry it over to the patient, and blow it back onto his head. He performs this same action hundreds of times and on occasion blows smoke not only on the patient's head, but also on the heads of every person sitting in the vicinity. The shaman's own view of blowing smoke on people's heads in curing rituals is that he is putting power back into their bodies. The cigarette is a means of capturing the body's power after it has escaped into the sky and putting it back into the head. By blowing smoke over the heads of everyone else present from time to time, the shaman symbolically incorporates the collective body power of all these people into the process of restoring the individual, conscious *likáriwa* soul of the patient.

Capturing and restoring lost souls with tobacco smoke are the only physical activities that bring the shaman into close contact with the entire group of ritual participants and observers. Most of the time, the shaman is either in direct contact with the patient's body or is standing alone in the open space in front of the patient. The shaman searches the sky for the spirit of sickness (*wáramápwa*) while singing, and immediately afterward he sucks the patient's body to remove the physical object that causes sickness. Then he stands up and tries to scoop the external spirit of sickness into his mouth and stomach with the feathers of his rattle. The purpose of his actions is to link together the external and internal, or generic and specific, causes of sickness inside his own body so both disease-causing agents can be vividly expelled into the bushes through vomiting. This moment in the curing ritual marks the shaman's triumph over the evil forces of sorcery and/or witchcraft.

COMPARATIVE ANALYSIS OF MÁLIKAI AND MÁLIRRÍKAIRI SONGS

The contrasts between *málikai* and *málirríkairi* curing songs, in terms of their textual referents and observable behavior during their performances, are summarized in table 8.2. In general, performances of *málikai* curing songs outline a process of internalization, the goal of which is to soothe and calm patients' illnesses in the same way that Iñápirríkuli saved his younger brother, Kuwaikánerri. The symbolism of honey, beeswax, flowers, tobacco, and the bee spirits (Kuwáinyai) are evoked in order to calm fears of illness and death and to cool down fevers. The soothing effects of honey and beeswax are transmitted to patients via tobacco smoke blown into covered pots of manioc drink, the only food allowed to patients undergoing treatment. Later, honey from the forest replaces the pot of manioc drink, beginning a gradual process of return to a normal diet of fish, game, and manioc bread.

Whereas *málikai* performances center around the internalization of the calming effects of honey, performances of *málirríkairi* outline a process of externalization that culminates with the shaman's successful extraction of a harmful substance, his combination of this object with an external, supernatural agent (*wáramápwa*), and his forceful elimination of the resulting mixture into the bush. The shaman's performance is far more active than the chant owner's. Tobacco is not used to quietly transmit the calming effects of honey into patients' food, but to abruptly capture patients' lost souls (*likáriwa*), physically carry them inside the lungs across the arena of curing activity, and blow them back into patients' heads. In addition, all sorts of other substances are physically manipulated in *málirríkairi* performances (fig. 8.3). The sky itself is constantly "pushed" with maraca feathers and sweeping hand and arm motions to give the shaman a clearer view of the shadows, or spirits of the dead (*lidánam*). In short, *málikai* performances minimize physical action and internalize, whereas *málirríkairi* performances emphasize physical action and externalize. The former is a process of "going through the center," whereas the latter is one of "bringing back from the edge."

Málikai songs reconstruct the fate of the patient's collective, animal-shaped soul (*líwarúna*) when it has become detached from the individual, human body-shaped soul (*likáriwa*). The songs place this partial separation into the reversible space-time of the mythical producers of honey, or

TABLE 8.2. Contrast between *Málikai* and *Málirríkairi* Curing Songs in Terms of Their Textual References and Observable Behavior.

MÁLIKAI	MÁLIRRÍKAIRI
"Going through the Center of the World"	"Bringing back from the World of the Dead"
Mythical journey of Kuwaikánerri and fate of *líwarúna* souls after death	Reversal of the transformation of *likáriwa* souls into *lidánam* after death
Controlled contact with the Kuwáinyai, or bee spirits	Controlled contact with the spirits of the dead (*lidánam*)
Relations between vertically separated regions of the cosmos	Relations between horizontally separated regions of the cosmos
No use of hallucinogens	Repeated use of hallucinogens (*Virola calophylla*)
Inside, staring straight ahead	Outside, searching from side to side
Covered pot of manioc drink, no other ritual objects	Sacred stones, payment, rattle, and other ritual objects openly displayed
No direct physical contact with patient or other participants	Direct physical contact with patient and other participants
Minimal movement of body, arms, hands, and legs	Hands, arms, and body used vividly to act out capture of spirits, ejection of illness, and other processes
Sitting up in hammock, no standing	Sitting down on bench, frequent standing

Kuwáinyai. Aside from a few very brief interruptions to blow tobacco smoke into covered pots of manioc drink, the songs are continuous and unchanging. The four tones of the first phrases are repeated over and over without variation of loudness, pitch, rhythm, or tempo. The repetition of this descending phrase over one hundred times has a sort of hypnotic effect on the performer, who at times looks as though he is on the verge of falling asleep. While the song texts are based on imagery of a prolonged journey through space and time, the music conveys a sense of frozen space-time in which the same simple movement unceasingly repeats itself, like a heartbeat or breath of air.

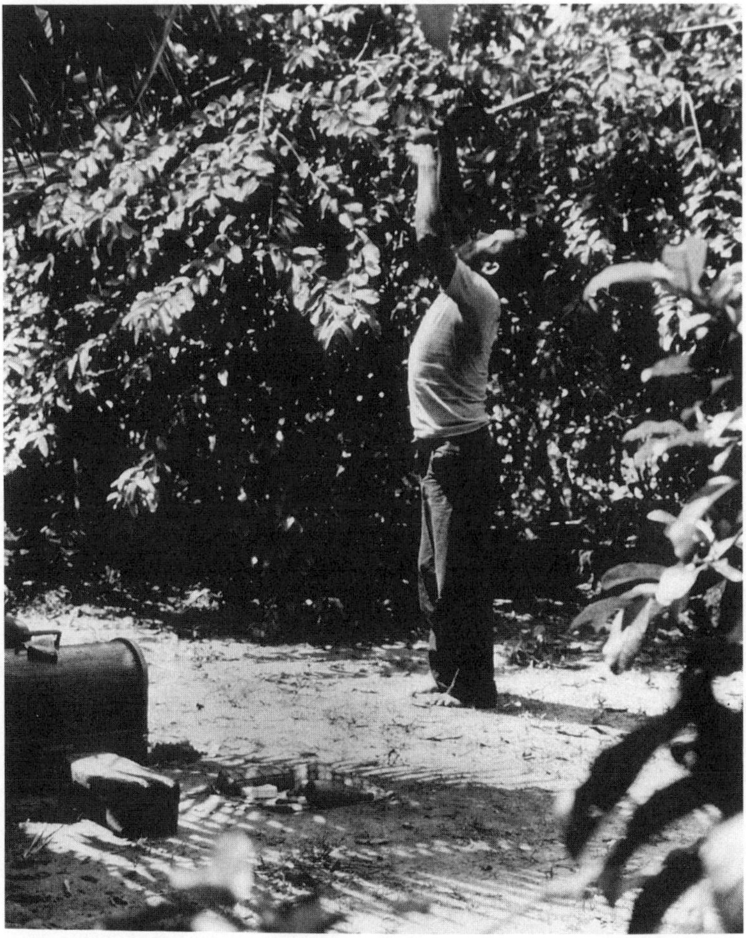

FIGURE 8.3. The shaman (*malírri*) reads the sky for shadow spirits through the feathers of his sacred rattle.

Perhaps the most striking contrast between the shaman's *málirríkairi* songs and the *málikai* songs of the chant owner is the former's discontinuity. Although the shaman's songs sometimes come right after one another, a period of several minutes usually elapses between the ending of one song and the beginning of the next one. These are periods when the shaman is actively using his sacred objects as a way of manipulating supernatural powers, spirits, and souls in the external world, and of bringing these invisible powers to bear on the patient's body and the disease-causing agent inside it. The shaman's songs are, for him, the most relaxing moments of what is otherwise a test of his endurance in the face of increasingly painful overloading of the senses. The songs are the only form of intelligible, verbal communication of the shaman after he has entered into the trance induced by massive doses of *dzáato* snuff.

The tonal and rhythmical organization of the shaman's *málirríkairi* songs are far more varied and complex than the "frozen," unchanging musical structure of the chant owner's *málikai* songs. Whereas *málikai* songs repeat the same four-note melody over and over again to create a hypnotic, dream-like state, *málirríkairi* songs systematically exploit all logical possibilities for musical contrasts out of a small number of principal tones (three or four, depending on the song). A contrast between loud and soft is very noticeable in the shaman's technique of echoing the last words of each phrase in a soft, ventriloquist voice.[10] While the majority of songs are based on descending melodies, a few make very pronounced use of ascending as well as descending melodies, thereby creating a contrast between ascending and descending tonal motion. A contrast between high and low levels of pitch is clearly present in the technique of singing the same melodies on different pitches at different points in the curing ritual, with a general tendency for pitches to rise over time. The first melody is sung on relatively low pitches, the next one on slightly higher pitches, and so forth, until the same melody is sung on pitches that are five chromatic intervals higher than the first song. Within each of the songs, there is a strong tendency toward microtonal rising through a gradual, almost imperceptible ascension of pitch. Finally, the songs display a contrast between a faster and slower tempo. Most of the time, the shaman shakes his sacred rattle at a moderate tempo and in large clockwise circles made with his right hand. At odd moments during his songs, however, he doubles the tempo of his rattling to an extremely fast pace by making smaller circles. This acceleration also increases the sound output of his rattling and further reinforces the vocal contrast between loud and soft dynamics.

The amount of musical variation available to the shaman through exploitation of different musical contrasts is almost limitless, and a complete musical transcription and analysis is beyond the scope of the present study. The importance of musical variation and contrast in *málirríkairi* songs is how it works in opposition to the strictly controlled, unchanging tonal and rhythmical organization in *málikai* songs. The former is a process of awakening the senses and making perception more sensitive to contrasts, whereas the latter is a process of numbing the senses into a frozen, dream-like condition in which the perception of contrasts is either minimized or shut out entirely.

In spite of the opposite effects of *málirríkairi* and *málikai* songs, there is an underlying similarity of tonal organization that allows the two genres of curing music to be understood as two complementary, but opposing, ways of reliving the process of destructuration. Looking beyond the wealth of musical variation and contrast, the shaman's songs are all based on three simple tonal structures that can be grouped into three classes. Using as a sample the nineteen *málirríkairi* songs performed on the second day of a prolonged curing ritual that was held in August 1981, the most frequent tonal structure consists of three tones dividing the interval of a fourth into two unequal, smaller intervals (a whole step and a minor third). This tonal structure, or variant A, is the basis of nine shaman's songs out of the total sample from that day. Variant A is reproduced on four different pitches that are a chromatic half step apart. A second tonal structure, or variant B, consists of three tones in which a minor third is divided into two whole tone intervals. Tonal structure B is the basis for seven songs out of the total sample of nineteen, and it is reproduced at five different pitch levels that are each a chromatic half step apart. Variant B shows the greatest contrast between high and low pitches and is also the tonal structure used for creating ascending as well as descending melodies. The third and least frequent tonal structure, or variant C, consists of four tones that divide the interval of a fourth into three smaller intervals, two whole tone steps and a single chromatic half step. Variant C is the basis of three short songs, all of which are reproduced on exactly the same pitch level. Figure 8.4

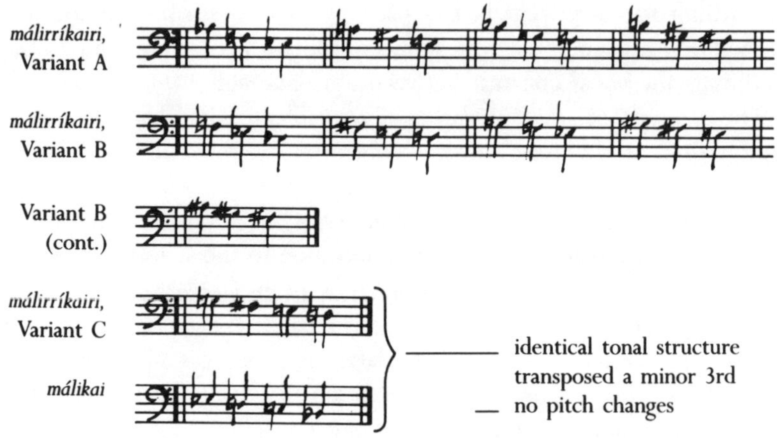

FIGURE 8.4. Transcriptions of tonal structures and pitch changes in *málirríkairi* and *málikai* curing songs; rhythmic and melodic structures not shown. Songs from second day of curing ritual according to tonal structure (indicated by capital letters) and pitch-level (indicated by numerals): B1, B3–B4, A1, B3, B5, A1–A2, C; A1, B4, A2, A2, A1, B5, C; B5, A3–A4, A1, A2, C.

illustrates the three tonal structures, or variants, which form the basis of *málirríkairi* songs and the range of pitch levels spanned by each of the three variants.

Figure 8.4 also shows the four-tone structure of *málikai* songs for curing. An interesting fact that emerges from a comparison of variant C of the *málirríkairi* songs with the tonal organization of *málikai* songs is the identical structure of the tonal organization in the two types of songs. Both consist of four tones in which the interval of a fourth is divided into three smaller intervals, two whole-tone steps and a single chromatic half step at the top. Variant C of *málirríkairi* songs also resembles *málikai* songs insofar as it is always sung at the same level of pitch, whereas variants A and B both rise in pitch in the course of the curing ritual (i.e., they are started on different pitches), and both exhibit microtonal rising (i.e., the entire structure gradually rises during the course of each song). The identity of tonal organization in variant C of shaman's songs and in *málikai* songs is a way of expressing, through musical symbolism, the message that both genres of curing music are interrelated parts of a single myth-ritual nexus that deals with sickness and death as a process of destructuration, or the breakdown of relations between the individual and collective souls.

The four-note melody of *málikai* songs musically anchors the structure of Wakuénai curing rituals, remaining unchanged throughout the duration of each curing ritual and also staying the same from one ritual to the next. A determination of pitches used in *málikai* curing songs performed in two curing rituals that took place in August and October of 1981, respectively, revealed that the chant owner employed exactly the same four pitches on both occasions. After recording the same chant owner singing *málikai* songs in August 1984, a determinatinon of pitches showed that he was still using the same four pitches as in 1981. Thus, the concept of perfect pitch is an important component of Wakuénai curing rituals, despite the apparent lack of technical vocabulary for describing pitch and tone in Wakuénai language.[11] In short, the chant owner (*málikai limínali*) is the keeper not only of sacred names and language but also of the sacred musical tones of Kuwái.

A MUSICAL AESTHETIC OF RITUAL HEALING

The integration of practical-social and aesthetic-cosmological dimensions of shamanistic curing activities is accomplished through the creation of "felt consubstantiality between language music and myth," or a poeticized space-time of mythic ancestral power (Friedrich 1986, 39). The chant owner's singing of the myth of Kuwaikánneri sculpts a complex web of sacred beings, places, and substances into a relatively simple, unchanging melody of four tones. The shaman's musical journeys to the houses of recently deceased persons in *íyarudáti* transpose a relatively simple movement between the living and the dead into a complex, highly dynamic series of movements across the spectrum of vocal timbres, volumes, tempos, rhythms, and microtonal pitches. Practical and aesthetic goals of shamanistic curing are totally interwoven through the interaction of extraordinarily meaningful (i.e., semantically enriched) musical sounds and musically dynamic language.

The contrast between the structure of musical sounds in *málikai* and *málirríkairi* songs directly embodies the differences between the two types of ritual healing. The four-tone melody of *málikai,* sung without any changes in pitch, loudness, or tempo, is a musical expression of the calm, soothing effect that is the goal of the chant owner's performances. The three-tone and four-tone melodies of *málirríkairi,* filled with variations along a number of musical dimensions, express the agitated, active condition of the shaman as he attempts to bring back his patient's soul from the dead. Just as he must visually search all regions of the sky for spirits of sickness and death, so must the shaman acoustically search for his patient's lost soul through actively varying the musical pitches, loudness, tempo, and melodic structure of his songs. The shaman's transformation is based on metaphor: musical and other behavior is employed to go from the known, visible world of living human beings to the unknown, invisible world of the dead. The shaman's songs provide a metaphorical bridge between knowable and unknowable worlds. The chant owner, however, bases his musical curing on metonymy: like Kuwaikánerri, the first victim of witchcraft in myth, the victim of witchcraft in this world will survive due to the calming effects of honey and beeswax. The chant owner places the victim's experience of illness into the symbolic framework of a known mythical reality, a "mystically known postulate," which is ritually accepted when properly cast in the four unchanging tones of *málikai* (Rappaport 1979, 129).

At the highest level of ritual structure, the tones of *málikai* articulate the metonymical and metaphorical healing processes into a single system. In figure 8.5, the identical tonal structure of *málikai* and the third variant of *málirríkairi* is a musical expression of transcendence. At this level, the complementary opposition of the two genres of curing music that form the intermediate level of ritual structure collapses, and the two musical genres are seen as interrelated variants of the same underlying tonal structure. The unchanging four-note melody of the chant owner ritually enacts "the powerful sound that opened the world" (*kémakáni hliméetaka hekwápi*), the aesthetic principle that ultimately generates the structure of musical, ritual action from the top down. The chant owner's unchanging four-tone melody unites the entire structure of the curing from above and, at the intermediate level, divides it through the complementary opposition of metonymy and metaphor. At both highest and intermediate levels, the structure of musical sound acts as a key to understanding the ritual efficacy of the chant owner and the shaman in Wakuénai culture.

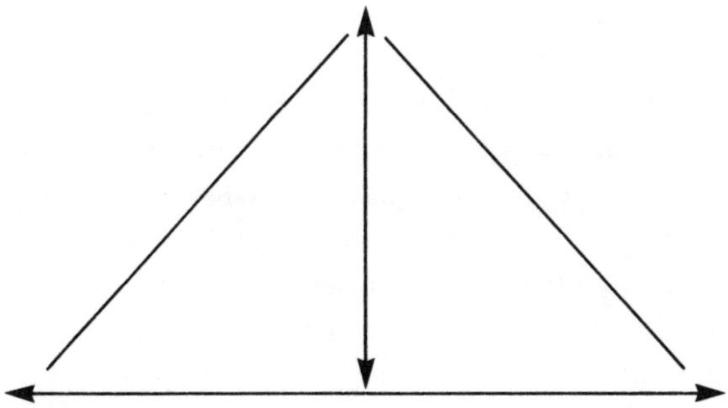

MÁLIKAI

- chant-owner's journey to *Mápakwá Makákwi*
- unchanging tempo
- unchanging pitch
- unchanging loudness
- no instrumental accompaniment
- continuous; small breaks to blow smoke into pot of food but without standing up
- solo voice

MÁLIRRÍKAIRI

- shaman's journey to *íyarudáti*
- acceleration/deceleration of tempo
- different starting pitches and microtonal rising
- loud/soft contrast
- percussive instrumental accompaniment (sacred rattle)
- discontinuous; frequent intermissions for snuffing *dzáato,* reading sky, etc.
- quasi or actual second voice, echoing

FIGURE 8.5. Schematic diagram of the complementary opposition between *málikai* and *málirríkairi* genres of curing music and the higher level, transcendent identity of tonal structures that mediates the two genres.

Given the complexity of hierarchical symbolic processes that make up the musical aesthetic of ritual healing, it is neither possible nor desirable to reduce the Wakuénai system of healing to purely utilitarian, practical functions. Nevertheless, performances of *málikai* and *málirríkairi* songs are always defined from the bottom up in terms of the practical objectives of patients who want to regain physical health. The practical, instrumental function of restoring physiological health is totally integrated with the aesthetic concern for spiritual renewal through musical performance and other ritual action. For the Wakuénai, the spiritual recomposition of the patient must precede any physiological recovery. Without ritual performances of *málikai* and *málirríkairi,* such physiological remedies as honey, wild plant substances, and modern pharmaceuticals would not have any effectiveness in treating disease. Thus, at the same time as ritual performances of music are enactments of aesthetic, higher level principles of order, the same performances are also seen as instrumental means for laying the foundations for physiological recovery.

In conclusion, a radical separation of aesthetic and instrumental thinking inhibits our ability to understand Wakuénai curing rituals as cultural processes that are central to the social identities of individuals and groups who perform them. Wakuénai curing rituals are simultaneously musical, cosmological, social, psychological, medical, and economic events, a multidimensionality that "embarrasses the categories" of Western scientific and artistic culture (Geertz 1984).[12] By focusing on the details of musical performance, closely related ritual behavior, and the larger social and mythical contexts that, as far as the actors are concerned, are the source of ritual efficacy, the study of ritual healing can make a genuine contribution toward a holistic, intercultural understanding of human medical knowledge and practice.

ACKNOWLEDGMENTS

The writing of this study would not have been possible without the fortunate support I have received from a number of people and institutions. I am deeply grateful to the Social Science Research Council and the Fulbright-Hays Program for financially backing my fieldwork with the Wakuénai in 1980–81, and to IVIC, the Venezuelan Scientific Research Institute, and INIDEF, the Interamerican Institute for Ethnomusicology and Folklore, for their logistical support within Venezuela. Special thanks to the Department of Anthropology, Smithsonian Institution for providing me with research facilities and time to rethink my approach to Wakuénai ethnography. I am also very indebted to a number of mentors and colleagues who have provided much-needed and appreciated personal encouragement and intellectual stimulation over the past five years: Anthony Seeger, Nelly Arvelo-Jimenez, Isabel Aretz, Jose Jorge de Carvalho, Robin Wright, Janet Chernela, Norman Whitten, Terence Turner, and Dan

Rose, among many others. I owe special thanks to the Wakuénai men and women who taught me how to listen to, understand, and perform their music. However, responsibility for the opinions, interpretations, and conclusions contained in this study rests solely with the author rather than the individuals and institutions acknowledged herein.

Notes

1. In Brazil, the Wakuénai are known as "Baniwa," whereas in Venezuela and Colombia they are called "Curripaco."

2. The power to bewitch is not accessible to nonspecialists in Wakuénai society, and not even shamans or owners of *málikai* are thought to have such powers. Master shamans, called *dzáwináitairi,* are the only individuals thought to be capable of bewitching. Ironically, the master shamans are also considered to have the strongest curing powers. The master shaman has powers of clairvoyance with which he can instantly tell what people around him are thinking. In curing rituals, the master shaman does not have to spend hours of time searching for the victim's lost soul or dragging confessions out of the victim's relatives, because he can immediately perceive all these things and know within minutes whether or not he can effect a cure.

3. In his analysis of native Amazonian myths on the origins of human mortality, Lévi-Strauss derives two opposite perspectives on death, one prospective and the other retrospective (1969, 162). These two perspectives correspond with remarkable accuracy to the Wakuénai view of the two worlds of the afterlife, the celestial paradise and the netherworld of the dead, respectively.

4. Conversely, honey in great quantities is the most powerful and dangerous evil omen (*hínimái*) for living descendants in this world. A man who cuts down a tree containing a beehive and who finds a great quantity of honey inside is believed to die within one or two years, since he has inadvertently crossed the boundary between this world and the celestial paradise of Iñápirríkuli. Chant owners make extensive use of honey as a curing remedy and of the symbolism of honey, bees, and flowers in their curing songs.

5. The chant owner with whom I studied in Venezuela had learned divination from a Hohódeni father-in-law on the Aiary River in Brazil who had, in turn, learned it from the Desana of the Vaupés River. Tukanoan groups of the northwest Amazon region probably all practice divination, but the Desana are considered the most powerful masters of this art. Since divination is not a traditional Wakuénai ritual practice and has no accompanying musical per-

formances or myths, I will not beleaguer the present study with the chant owner's many stories of successful divinations.

6. Along the Guainía-Negro River in Venezuela, the chant owner and shaman performed curing rituals for Guarequena, Baniwa, Yeral (lingua geral), and criollo (mestizo) families and individuals. Aside from these curing rituals, a Guarequena and Baniwa family came to have the chant owner perform a childbirth ritual for their newborn son.

7. This pattern is established through *málikai* songs and chants performed in rites of passage at childbirth and initiation (Hill 1983). The case of young children who are sick illustrates the interrelations of the two sets of rituals. If a young child is brought to be cured, the ritual healers will first ask whether or not the parents have had the ritual food (*káridzámai*) chanted over. If not, the two sets of chants for newborn infants and their parents are performed before beginning to perform ritual curing music. The same procedure is applied to parents of very young children who have fallen ill.

8. In myth, Kuwái is portrayed as a monstrous creature combining all material elements in one being ("The Many-in-the-One"). After his death in the Great Fire, Kuwái is transformed into a number of distinct flutes and trumpets named after discrete animal species ("The One-in-the-Many").

9. The myth of the origin of *dzáato* snuff emphasizes the importance of the shaman's control while under the influence of the stimulating drug. Four animal-people and a brother of Iñápirríkuli took *dzáato* snuff after the latter sucked it out of the stomach of the daughter of Dzúlihwérri. The four animal-people went crazy from the snuff, but Iñápirríkuli's brother, Éeri, fell asleep and woke up in full control of himself, and he became the first shaman.

10. R. Wright (personal communication) has recorded Hohódeni shamans in Brazil who perform *málirríkairi* songs in groups. The lead singer's voice is constantly being echoed by response singers creating a somewhat disorienting contrapuntal effect, since the echo of the second singer is usually not much softer than the principal melody.

11. The gap between "speech about music" and "music about music" has become an important topic of inquiry in ethnomusicology since the work of Charles Seeger, who called it the musicological juncture.

12. Geertz even suggests that the term "shamanism" is just another anthropological category serving to devitalize the wholeness of religious experience in non-Western cultures.

NINE

NOBODY IS THERE TO HEAR

Desana Therapeutic Incantations

DOMINIQUE BUCHILLET

For the Desana, words are endowed with a physical effect. They are able to affect the intimate experience of an individual in a tangible manner. This power to interfere in the order of things was given to words by the Desana's ancestors. The current ritual specialists, known by the name of *kũbũ,* do nothing but reactivate this power. The potentially creative power of words is particularly evident in the curing rituals that rest fundamentally on the efficacy of the spoken word.[1]

The Desana are one of the several Eastern Tukanoan groups who inhabit the Brazilian-Colombian Vaupés region. This region belongs to the central northwest Amazon culture area whose main features are: extensive cultivation of bitter manioc (*Manihot esculenta* Cranz) combined with hunting, fishing, and gathering; riverine orientation of the settlements; uniformity of social organization and structure; rich mythology whose main lines are common to all Tukanoan groups; and male initiation rites tied to a kind of ancestral cult (Steward and Faron 1959). Within this homogeneous system the Tukanoan are divided into discrete intermarrying groups, mainly differentiated by territorial location, language, and artistic specialization. The Desana occupy the Vaupés River and its affluents, the Tiquié and the Papuri, in a dispersed settlement pattern. Due to the influence of the Salesian missionaries working in the region since 1915, villages composed of individual houses have replaced the ancient communal houses. The abandonment of the communal house, or *maloca* in lingua geral, has profoundly disorganized the ceremonial and ritual life. Serving as more than a living place, the *maloca* was an essential ceremonial center, the true place of the transmission of myths and of their performance during rituals. It was often designated by the expression "house of ceremonies," a denomination that attests to its important ceremonial purpose.

The Desana traditionally recognize several ritual specialists representing different concepts of power who exercise the functions of preventing and curing illnesses:

1. The jaguar shaman *ye:* The term *ye* places emphasis on the shaman's capacity to borrow the form of the jaguar in order to accomplish his goals. The power of *ye* is tied to the use of *paricá* (*Piptadenia peregrina* Benth. or *Virola* sp.), ruled by the Thunder World ancestor, who is also the master of aggressive incantations.[2] The jaguar shamans are described as "able to see the illness in the patient's body," and to "divine the cause of the evil." The role of divination is strictly associated to the intake of hallucinogens in Desana thinking.

2. The *sakaka* shaman: *Sakaka,* a lingua geral term, represents another class of shamans who reside in the subterranean world. By chewing the roots of the *sakaka* plant (probably *Connaracea*), they are able to travel great distances underwater.[3] These shamans, considered the most dangerous by the Desana, are strictly associated with aquatic spirits, "their relatives."

3. The *kũbũ* shaman: The third class of shamans is that of the *kũbũ,* whose power rests on a perfect mastering of incantations, *bayiri,* for protection, curing, and aggression. To recite an incantation is *bayi* in Desana, but this term has also the more generic meaning of "ceremony" or "cure." The Desana generally translate *bayi* "to pray." This term reveals the verbal aspect of the cure, putting the emphasis on the principal activity of the *kũbũ* in every ceremony or cure. In one sense, the term "to pray" is not ill chosen because it illustrates perfectly well the attitudes of meditation and of silence (so appropriate to prayer) during the curing session and illustrates, moreover, the sacred character

of the "texts" and their link with the primordial language of the ancestors. However, the preferred translation of *bayiri* is "incantation," since this term better indicates the pragmatic character of the uttered texts. (See examples later in this chapter.) The therapeutic knowledge that every individual desiring to be a shaman has to acquire is submitted to a strict rule of transmission.[4]

THE METHOD OF TRAINING THE KŨBŨ

"I have learned, seated with my father." This phrase so often reiterated by the Desana *kũbũ,* summarizes perfectly the method of training and the ways of access to the function of *kũbũ* "One learns by listening." Training consists essentially of hearing and memorizing a large number of mythic narratives and incantations. The apprentice *kũbũ, kũbũ pegɨ,* is literally "the one who listens," and his master, *kũbũ bayiri weregɨ,* the *kũbũ* "who recites the incantations." The priority attributed to listening in the process of acquiring shamanistic knowledge is again reflected in the vernacular term that designates intelligence, the faculty to conceive things, *pebãsĩdĩ.* It is formed of *pe,* "to listen," "to hear," "to comprehend," and *bãsĩdĩ,* "to understand," "to know."

One learns by listening. Memorization is facilitated by the intake of emetic potions (unidentified) at dawn in order to purge the body of all the substances that could impede access to knowledge. Beyond this purification for the preparation of the spirit, an "incantation by which one becomes *kũbũ*" (*kũbũ suriye bayiriye*) is recited over a cigar, whose smoke should be exhaled around the apprentice's body.[5] The smoke functions as a stimulant and serves to "fix the individual on his bench," or to "make him sit down in only one place." It helps him to retain his thoughts and prevents distraction. This intimate connection among the Desana of the bench, the thought, and the act of concentration has already been noted by Reichel-Dolmatoff (1971, 110; 1975) who remarks that this association is explicit in certain metaphorical expressions. Thus, of an individual who lacks judgment, in other words, who doesn't think well, one will say "he doesn't know how to sit." The bench is the proper place for concentration and meditation. While seated on his bench, Yebá Bɨro, the ancestor of the world, began to think about creating the world (Panlon and Kenhiri, 1980). It is while seated on their bench that the *kũbũ* effect their cures. This bench has existed since the origin of time, and it is intimately tied to thought and reflection.

Knowledge is never revealed through violent experience. The observations of Reichel-Dolmatoff (1975, 197) on the training of the Tukano shaman apply perfectly here. "A Tukano *payé* does not receive a sudden call to office in an overwhelming traumatic experience, but develops his personality slowly and steadily, the driving force being a true interest in the unknown, and that not so much for the purpose of acquiring power over his fellow men as for the personal satisfaction of knowing things which others are unable to grasp." The notion of physical and mental suffering, so often present in the biographies of South American and Siberian shamans is not, however, absent in that of the *kũbũ*. All insist that those who want to learn must submit themselves to fasting before and during the learning experience. My work sessions with them were frequently studded with reflections that underscore this dimension of power acquisition. "For you, with your tape recorder and your notebooks, it is easy to learn this incantation. For me it was very difficult. I had to fast and remain awake one entire night to learn it."

Knowledge is transmitted patrilineally, and one is *kũbũ* by family tradition.[6] The father generally chooses the one among his sons who by his behavior seems most apt to exercise the role according to his behavior and his interests. The teaching is gradual. The initiation to knowledge, to comprehension of the mythic narratives and the therapeutic and aggressive incantations, is slow. Some are taught first, for example, those incantations destined to take care of problems considered minor (headaches, sores, burns, diarrhea), the knowledge of which is not restricted to specialists. Other incantations are meant to be taught at the end of the learning experience, for example those intended to recapture the soul of the patient. This gradation in the transmission of shamanistic knowledge reflects an increasing difficulty in memorization and in comprehension of sometimes very long passages, a complexity that is generally equivalent to the supposed seriousness of the illness. One of the difficulties encountered in learning these incantations is their length, that is, the number of animals, objects, and substances to be memorized and invoked during a cure. Another difficulty lies in understanding their hidden meanings, the rules of specific word use and their references in the incantations that make them part of a very complex symbolic language.

The apprenticeship is generally composed of two phases. The son first learns all the incantations of protection and curing. When his father judges that he has internalized them, that is to say, when he has perfectly mastered both the literal and the symbolic meanings of the incantations, he begins the second phase of the apprenticeship—when the novice is introduced into the world of aggression. The incantations of aggression are secret, and they can only be taught to a son. Only one who has the hereditary right can benefit from this teaching, a symbol of the spiritual relation that ties a son to his father, and, through the latter, to the ancestors holding this knowledge.

Knowing the incantations of aggression provides, so to speak, the key to the illnesses by disclosing their origin, their essence. To know the origin of an illness gives the holder of this knowledge the power to cure it. Thus, knowledge and apprenticeship of the means of aggression secure the positive efficacy of therapeutic knowledge. The learning experience ends with the cigar ceremony, which consecrates the apprentice in the career of *kũbũ.* Reciting an incantation over a cigar, the father gives the cigar to his son to smoke. This incantation is supposed to put in reserve, or leave dormant in one part of the *kũbũ*'s body, the shamanistic knowledge that will only be revealed in a concrete situation. It is as if the incantation conferred to him a power of oblivion: "He doesn't think anymore about what he knows, he is like a child," the *kũbũ* often says. This ceremony is, in fact, a protection against the untimely use of shamanistic knowledge. It protects the learner from the dangers of experimenting "just to see," which would do nothing but provoke needless illnesses. The danger of experimenting out of context is well-illustrated by a number of myths. For example, one describes how Butari Gõãbɨ, God of Laziness, created numerous diseases just for the sake of checking the worth, either positive or negative, of his knowledge. These myths, in one sense, set up a posteriori, a validation of the real efficacy—negative (cause of illness) or positive (therapeutic)—of the aggression or curing incantations that constitute the shamanistic repertoire current to all *kũbũ.* It is necessary to understand this ceremony as a kind of precaution against a memorized and interiorized knowledge that is conceived as dangerous.

THE CLASSIFICATION OF ILLNESSES

The Desana term that designates illness is *doreri* derived from the verb *dore.* This verb is not limited to the domain of pathology. "To give an order to," "to send to," and "to command" attest to its principal meaning. *Dore* carries, therefore, an idea of order, of commanding, which refers to a scheme of aggression, to an exterior origin of the illnesses. For the Desana, in fact, sicknesses are mainly imputed to animals, spirits, or to humans. In addition to "the illnesses of the whites," attributed to a form of specific sorcery, the Desana distinguish several categories among the "indigenous sicknesses":

1. Catching illnesses, *behari:* these are the common illnesses without a known cause, which cannot be attributed to the work of a spirit nor to that of a sorcerer. These sicknesses are often described by the Indians as "passing from one to another," and "coming by themselves" without one's knowing why. In general they are denoted by the expression *behari* followed by the description of the symptom, *behari etokarikɨri* "passing illness with vomiting," or simply by *behari;* this expression accentuates their benign and transitory character.

2. *Wai bãsã doreri* and *yukɨ bãsã doreri:* respectively, "sicknesses of fish people" (and, by extension, "of the water people") and "sicknesses of the tree people." This category groups all the disorders tied to the life cycle as due principally to the action of animals and spirits. The Desana conceive of the animal world in the image of the human world. The animals are directed by "animal-shaman," *wai bãsã yeri* or *yukɨ bãsã yeri.*[7] The lizard (*Plica plica* L.), the jaguar (*Panthera onça* Podock), the blue morpho butterfly (*Morpho* sp.), the cuckoo bird (*Piaya cayana* L.), and so on, are the principal animal shamans cited by the Indians. These animal shamans are also known as "masters of the illnesses of water people," as well as "masters of the illnesses of the tree people." They are not linked to a specific illness but to all the sicknesses that can happen to a person during certain critical periods (birth, puberty, death), or to any individual after transgression of the dietary taboos that are normal at times of rituals.[8] These illnesses generally appear in an ambiguous fashion through imprecise symptoms such as muscular pains, back pains, fever, swelling of the body, vomiting, and so forth.

Animals by themselves cannot provoke illnesses. The Desana always present them as species inoffensive to man; they have to be manipulated by the animal shamans or by a sorcerer in order to cause sickness, thus becoming the cause of it. The animals then try to strike the individual with their "weapons" (parts of their bodies that become injurious to the individual), thus provoking different troubles. The sicknesses of the "water people" and of the "tree people" are often the result of a personal error (i.e., dietary transgression during a ritual period), or of the errors of others (i.e., *kũbũ*'s forgetting one or several animal or spirit names during the recitation of the incantations of protection).

3. *Goroweori doreri:* sicknesses due to the sorcery of the shamans, the *ye,* the *sakaka,* or the *kũbũ.* These sicknesses are distinguished by their perfectly defined clinical picture. Their effects are restricted to a determined part of the body, and they are, therefore, easily recognized and identified by observation of the dominant symptom (for example, breast tumor, inguinal tumor, menstrual colic, local swelling). These sicknesses can be provoked by the intrusion of a pathogenic object into the victim's body or can be thrown on the body as a garment, a cape.

The connections established here between a symptom, an illness, and a given cause are ideal. In practice, that is in the course of an illness, there can be continuity between different sickness categories. In the beginning, illnesses are always considered benign. After failure of family therapy based principally on plants or incantations the sicknesses are interpreted on a second level of complexity. Indeed, the resistance of the illness to words and plants, the intensity of pain, the patient's social history, his age, the occurrence of other passing disorders, and so forth, can offer complementary information, thus modifying the previous diagnosis and, therefore, the therapy.

THE CURING RITUAL

The cures take place during the day or night in the *kũbũ*'s house if the patient is able to travel, if not, in the patient's house. The ill person comes alone or accompanied by a relative. It is not necessary, however, that he be physically present at his cure. This depends quite evidently on the seriousness of his sickness. At the very most, he should remain within hearing distance of the *kũbũ*'s voice. Seated on his small bench, the *kũbũ* recites an incantation over the opening of a gourd (*Lagenaria siceria* Mol.) containing a liquid, or over a plant.[9] Resting beside him on the ground is a calabash (*Crescentia cujete* L.) containing some green powder of coca, which the *kũbũ* takes frequently.[10] With the aid of a small spoon or stick, he places it for an instant on his tongue so that the coca is impregnated with saliva. After taking a dose of coca to "revive his memory," and "not to sleep," the *kũbũ* begins the cure by drawing out, through his thoughts, all the "defenses" of the individual (defenses placed at the moment of his birth at the time of naming ceremony). Afterward he "opens" the body, the veins, the arteries, the bones, the intestines, and so on, of the patient in order to permit the sickness to run out. Finally, he recites the incantation to himself while exhaling or blowing on the opening of the gourd or on the plant at certain precise moments of the recitation.[11] The incantation is carried by his breath to this object. At the end of the cure, the *kũbũ* hands the gourd to his patient, who is expected to drink the contents. If the object over which the incantation is recited is a plant, the patient should rub it on the sick part of his body. Cures vary in duration proportionally to the seriousness of the sickness. The *kũbũ* generally recites the incantation several times in succession, each time giving to the ill person the liquid to drink or the plant to rub. The cure implies, therefore, a manipulation of an intermediary object or substance. For the Desana, this object, which gives the incantation a material support, functions in the manner of a "medium"; it transfers the incantation to the patient.

SUBSTANCES UTILIZED AS A MEDIUM OF INCANTATION

The intermediary object is, therefore, of two kinds: liquid or plant, chosen in function of the kind of sickness or symptom to be treated. If the sickness is internal, the *kũbũ* will prefer to use a liquid: water; boiled manioc juice (that is to say, detoxified); manioc flour gruel; and so on. Beyond the fact that the liquid carries the words to the patient, once ingested it cleanses him, purges him metaphorically of his sickness. In certain cases, the liquid has a parallel effect to the incantation in that it reinforces the desired effect. Thus, in the case of a difficult labor, the *kũbũ* will recite the "delivery incantation" over a potion prepared from the juice of certain fruits known to be particularly viscous (*Pouteria caimito* L.; *Rollinia mucosa* (Jacq.) Baill.; *Theobroma grandiflorum* [Willd ex Spreng] Schum; *Pourouma cecropiaefolia* Mart.; *Urera uraricera;* etc.).[12] For the Desana the viscous juice of these fruits, once ingested by the woman, lubricates the womb, thus facilitating the delivery. It is clear that this viscous liquid reinforces and reduplicates the incantation's therapeutic efficacy, which aims at the expulsion of the infant or of the placenta (see infra).

On the other hand, in the case of wounds, burns, or local pains, the incantation will be recited over a part of the plant (bark from a tree or vine, leaves, flowers) that will be placed, rubbed, or expressed in liquid form over the affected part of the body. For example, in caring for a wound, the *kũbũ* will recite the incantation over certain particularly bitter barks of a tree or vine, which have been grated or mixed with a little water (*Anacardium ocidentale* L.; *Byrsonima* sp., etc.). This bitterness cleans the wound, removes coagulated blood and impurities, and closes tissue.[13]

The presence of a physical characteristic useful in the cure (as in the two cases cited, viscosity and bitterness) often prevails in the choice of plants used as the medium of incantation. Plants and incantations do not have independent contents. The plants can reinforce the therapeutic efficacy of the language, but they do not replace the action of the latter. Thus, in the case of a difficult delivery, the *kũbũ* will recite the incantation over any available liquid if there is no juice at hand from viscous fruits. This is because "all has been treated by the incantation." In other words, this quality of viscosity necessary to the treatment of the pregnant woman is already transferred to her body through incantation. Words for the Desana are by themselves capable of giving a quality to, or transforming physically, a being or an object. As we have seen, the intermediary object over which the incantation is recited, by its own analogous characteristics, can increase the therapeutic efficacy of the incantation by reduplicating it. Moreover, it seems to confer to the incantation a greater power of penetration by the simple act of ingestion or direct contact with the skin, in other words, of being physically introduced into the body of the individual. Stated another way, "The verbal message is capable of greater precision than the figurative language (one with the help of an object). But the advantage the second has over the first is its permanence and its materiality, which makes it remain always available and that it is possible to receive through other means than those of speech utterances (by absorption, by anointment, by aspersion)" (Lavondes 1963, 110).

Words offer a resistance to time. Once absorbed by the liquid or by the plant, they are always available to the individual without the risk of being changed. Before the arrival of a son who lives in another village, one informant often would recite an incantation of protection over a cigar. According to him the power of the incantation could not weaken even if the son didn't smoke the cigar until some time later.

It is important to keep in mind that the intermediary object over which the therapeutic incantation is recited is not indispensable. The incantations are effective by themselves; that is to say, they have the power, by themselves, to change, to transform a person. The incantations could very well be recited in the direction of the ill person, and it is not the object that gives the words healing power. However, the Desana admit that in this case the actions of the words on the sickness will be slower, the incantation having a lesser power of penetration. When speaking of the liquid carrier of the *kũbũ*'s words, the Indians frequently say "it is like an injection."

THE STRUCTURE OF THE INCANTATIONS

The incantations are not a metaphoric evocation of the state or intimate condition of the patient. (See, for example, the archetypal case of Cuna songs.)[14] They do not implore the help of any spirit and are not addressed to someone in particular from whom knowledge or support is expected. These incantations do not use a language that is injunctive, supplicatory, conjuring, or objurgatory. In their totality, they look like a long enumeration of names of spirits, animals, plants, and substances having direct connection with the source of the sickness, or with the restoring aspect of the cure. In general, they are designated by the name of the sickness (for example, "incantation of the breast tumor"). The incantations always have the same basic structure. They consist of a rather long continuum of sequences with two movements, the interior of each movement having a characteristic overture and end. These two movements can be defined as identification of the protagonists of the shamanic act and restoration of the body or affected part of the individual.

Identification of the Protagonist of the Shamanic Act

By reason of their relation to the source of the evil, of the sickness, the protagonists must be named. This involves identifying, by name, the animals, spirits, plants, and substances; their color (or brilliance, the luminosity of their bodies), and sometimes also their habitats. Then their "weapons" are enumerated, and, finally, the *kũbũ*'s activities to neutralize them are described. The principal "weapons" of the animals or body parts potentially harmful for the individual include: skin, hair, or skin parasites; limbs (paws, wings, fins, tails); teeth; beaks; residual body heat; liquids such as blood, sweat, urine; odor; skin reflection; cries (songs), and so forth. Material objects and plants are considered dangerous by reason of their inherent heat. They are "hot" because they are born from the cindered body of the "master of nourishment." By implication, so are all the objects obtained from these plants, such as bows and arrows, handles of knives or machetes, fishing lines made from the fibers of *tucum* (*Astrocaryum tucuma* Martius), calabashes, and gourds. All the cooking utensils made from different types of earth or clay are equally hot by reason of the cooking processes to which they have been subjected. Likewise, machetes, axe heads, fish hooks, and so on, are hot because they are made of a metal that was smelted and shaped at high temperatures.

The heat inherent in these beings, plants, or objects is supposed to provoke fever, headaches, and also frequent household conflicts. The person is caught in the middle of this hot environment, which excites him and provokes frequent quarrels between him and his neighbors. The danger of these plants resides equally in the parasites that inhabit their different parts (roots, trunks, or bodies, branches, leaves, flowers, or seeds).

The verbs of the incantation offer a detailed account of the *kũbũ*'s activities toward each part of the animal's body, or of the plants that can be dangerous for the person. The *kũbũ* "tears out," "breaks," "pulls to pieces," "chews," "washes," and "cools down."

The incantation presented below, *yarue wẽhẽdã bayiri* (literally, "incantation of the groups of earth worms that kill"), is meant to cure a sickness that affects the newborn when the *kũbũ* forgets one or more names of earthworms in the course of the incantation protecting the bath at the end of the couvade. The latter, not named and therefore not disarmed, are liable to strike the infant with their weapons, provoking fever, rash, inflamation of the body, headaches, or vomiting.

> These earthworms *wãsĩkãbɨ̃,* the black, the greenish, the whitish, I have joined the parasites [literally, "those that inhabit"] of their limbs; I tear their legs; I break their teeth; I break them; I throw them all in the subterranean world ["toward the source"]; I cool them [I "cut" their heat]; I express the fluids of their bodies [I "cut" their liquids]; I catch their smell [I "cut" them]; I wash them from head to foot.

Restoring the Body of the Sick Part of the Individual

The second movement of the incantation consists of invoking certain plants, animals, or powers such as stars, or angels and saints (recently introduced into the incantations), which possess properties particularly relevant to the cure. For example, there could be viscosity for facilitating delivery, bitterness for disinfecting and repairing a wound, black color for making a wound invisible on the surface of the skin, or coolness for refreshing a burn.

The name of the animal or plant chosen is immediately followed by the designation of its required attribute, then by the *kũbũ*'s description, which details the manner in which he instills it or lets it drip into the patient's body, or else how he paints the body with it. In the course of a delivery, the *kũbũ* will shed (through language) a liquid coming from the viscous fruits in the vaginal opening and on the body of the newborn. After having named all the fruits he says, "I pour the viscous liquid of these fruits in the door of the birth canal of this Tukanoan woman who is called X, I pour it [on the body of the infant]. I take it out [the infant]; I take it out. I pull it down."

In the case of burns, the *kũbũ* will invoke the bats, which in their mythology have to do with their origin. "Large or small bats living in the roots, large or small bats living in the trunks, large or small bats living in the holes of trees . . . I collect them, I take from them their coolness, I catch it, I pass it [over the burn], I throw [the bats] over the body of the patient, I cool down [the burn]." The logic of this incantation lies on the observation that, according to the Desana, when bats fly at night over our sleeping bodies, they cool us "by making wind with their wings." The *kũbũ,* through words, throws them and has them fly over the burn to cool it down, thus reducing its heat, its "fire." Then invoking their color he proceeds: "I gather these bats, I catch their color, I pass it [on the burn], I pass it, I paint [the burn], I paint it." This operation is aimed at making the burn invisible on the skin's surface.[15]

The words of the incantation trace sickness to a number of animals, spirits, plants, and substances, and describe the way these animals or these plants—realistically represented down to their finest anatomical details—are collected, put together, destroyed, and expelled from the person. The words then tell how, at the time the person's body is restored, an animal's or plant's attribute necessary to the curing process is transferred to the body through the words of the *kũbũ*. Animals and plants are at all times passive instruments of the shamanistic activity. The efficacy of the incantation depends on the different operations of the *kũbũ* aimed at neutralizing them or at restoring the body of the patient. The verbs of the incantation refer only to the actions of the *kũbũ*. They all are conjugated in the first person singular, in the present indicative of the active form. In so doing, the Desana emphasize the pragmatic value of such statements, which according to them, are uttered to act upon the patient's body. The therapeutic action is set in motion by the words themselves. Thus, when the *kũbũ* wants to pull out the limbs of some parasite, he grants himself the power to do what he says, and this he manages by reciting the appropriate incantation. Animals and plants are named, one by one, and the parts of their bodies or their organs, their "weapons," are carefully enumerated. For the Desana, the incantory formulation of the name of an animal or plant is sufficient in itself to give it both form and existence. The frequent process of denotation by synecdoche (part of the body for the animal, organ for the plant) is meant to reinforce the act of naming, trebling an effect aimed at physically placing animals and plants in the presence of the *kũbũ,* thus giving him a chance to control and manipulate them.[16] This process also confers a supplement of strength to the *kũbũ*'s actions in the phase of the final destruction of the animal or of the pathogenic object.

Desana mythology attests, in the same sense, to the creative powers of naming. For example, in the origin of fish

> The *Diroa* took a large bowl and began to strike the surface of the water to attract the anaconda. Hearing this noise, he soon appeared. They captured him; killed him. Finally they turned the flesh of the anaconda into fish. The first fish that they created in this manner was the carp. Taking up a piece from the anaconda's flesh they gave it the name of *boreka* [*Leporinus* sp.] and decided that it would be "good to eat." To the second fish, they gave the name of *uru,* the *pacu* [*Myloplus* sp.], this time "bad to eat." The third fish, the piranha, was the "fish of envy." When one eats its meat, one feels full of jealousy towards others . . .
>
> Thus they created all the fishes giving them names.

The incantations are infallible in curing illnesses in the sense that their power to cure is never questioned. The nonresponse of an illness to words, the intensification of symptoms, or the appearance of additional ailments are never attributed to any failure or defect inherent in the incantation. The lack of reaction of the illness to the *kũbũ*'s words is, in fact, understood as nothing less than a forgetting of one or several animal or spirit names during the recitation of the incantation, or of an inaccurate diagnosis. The effect of the cure is immediate. The repeated absorption of the same words should immediately produce a decrease of the symptoms.[17] An indicator of this belief in the rapid efficacy of the words is provided by the use of an expression that generally ends all curing incantations, *siyɨ̃, siyɨ̃bea, siyɨ̃doa;* respectively, "I calm it down," "I have him sit quiet," and "I leave him quiet and peaceful." In the last words of the incantation, the sick person must be calmed, reassured. These expressions are the signal that the words of the *kũbũ,* once they are absorbed by the patient, have already left an effect on the illness, in other words, that the *kũbũ,* by these words, dominates the sickness. So we can say that, for the Desana, the words reel off in the body of the patient like the beads of a necklace.

CONTEXT

As we have seen, the incantations are recited secretly over an intermediary object (a liquid, a plant). One should now examine the symbolic function of this speaking under the breath, of this silence. One hypothesis is that this inaudible aspect, which is the mode appropriate to the cure, confers to the *kũbũ*'s language a particular power. One myth insists that incantations ought not to be heard.

> The *Diroa* were dead. Then the old woman began to stop up their mouths, the noses and all their body openings with leaves. Then she recited the incantation but the *Diroa* were very smart. They had pretended to be dead so they could see what the old woman would do, to learn all her words. Simulating death, they went out of their own bodies and settled on each side of the old woman to watch all her gestures, to listen to all her words. This is how they learned the incantations.

A little later, the myth tells how, in order to bring the old woman back to life, the *Diroa* reproduced the gestures they had just learned; they closed her ears to prevent her from hearing their incantation. Thus, this myth insists on the fact that therapeutic language is not meant to be heard, or better, *to be listened to.* Therefore, the cure doesn't present any didactic aspect either for the patient or for anybody who might attend. "Nobody is there to hear," the *kũbũ* often say, which means that, on one hand, the curing session is not thought of as a means of acquiring knowledge. An individual cannot, therefore, hope to receive training by attending curing sessions, as is often the case in many indigenous societies. On the other hand, the session is in no way expected to fashion the shape of the mind (see in particular the analysis of Lévi-Strauss [1958] of the Kuna chant Mu-Igala). In fact, the silent aspect of the cure doesn't as much explain the secret character of the incantations as it insists on the necessity and importance of their social circumscription. The acquisition of shamanistic knowledge is thus dependent on a spiritual genealogy. This knowledge can only be transmitted and applied by certain people who "are distinguished . . . not by their 'natural' characteristics and capacities but by their social relation to others: namely by standing in a continuous line of legitimate succession to an original founder" (Skorupsky 1976, 149). The private character of the cure responds to a practical necessity: this is a protective measure against a knowledge that is perceived as dangerous when it is used out of its specific context or when it is applied by laymen.

A rapid survey of the recent ethnological literature on the efficacy of speech in magico-religious rituals shows two major orientations: some explain the efficacy of speech by the particular construction of magical discourse (rhetorical mechanisms and the performative aspect of magical language), others by the evocative power of the sound of words.

Two articles by Tambiah (1968, 1973) perfectly illustrate the first orientation. According to Malinowski (1974), the incantations are recited over an intermediary object, which transfers the incantation to the specific person by the magical act. In spite of the insistence of the Trobrianders that "the strength of magic lies in the incantation," Tambiah shows that the intermediary object and incantation cannot be considered separately. Austin (1962) states that certain utterances are enunciated not to inform or account for a state of things, but in order to realize an action, what he terms the performative aspect or the "illocutionary force" of language. Tambiah, adapting this theory to the analysis of ritual, shows how object and incantation operate jointly.

> . . . in terms of predication and reference the words exploit analogical associations, comparisons and transfers (through simile, metaphor, metonym, etc.). The illocutionary force and power by which the deed is directed and enacted is achieved through use of words of commanding, ordering, persuading, and the like. . . The action can be similarly analysed. The objects manipulated are chosen analogically on the basis of similarity and difference to convey meaning. From the performative perspective, the action consists of an operation done on an object-symbol to make an imperative transfer of its properties to the recipient. Or to put it differently, two objects are seen as having resemblances and differences, and an attempt is made to transfer the desirable quality of one to the other which is in a defective state (1973, 222).

The second orientation is illustrated by Stoller, who shows that, for the Songhay, the sound of the words carries the magical efficacy: "Sounds of magical praise-names, magical words, and magical sacred instruments create an auditory presence that can transform a person morally, politically and magically" (1984, 559). In order to be efficacious, the words must therefore be pronounced, listened to, and heard: "Sound penetrates the individual and creates a sense of communication and participation" (ibid., 563).

The conclusions of Tambiah apply perfectly to the Desana example: one has seen the function of the synecdoche as a rhetorical means that confers more strength to the manipulation of the pathogenic object by the *kũbũ,* the importance of the substances, chosen for their analogous characteristics, which were introduced into the patient's body through the *kũbũ*'s words, and the effect of reduplication of the meaning of the incantation by the substances used as a medium. Nevertheless, it seems difficult to account for the power of the incantation (according to the indigenous theory) on the sole basis of the construction of the incantation. The positive efficacy, that is to say the therapeutic efficacy of an incantation, also depends on the respect of certain conditions in formulation of therapeutic knowledge that narrowly define its accessibility (importance of the spiritual genealogy) and its use: the therapeutic knowledge cannot be used except in two contexts, each being characterized by an appropriate mode of recitation (inner recitation in the curing situation, or audible utterance in the situation of apprenticeship).

The therapeutic speech of the Desana is a silent speech and without an addressee. Its mode of operation violates the principal functions of language perceived as a means of communication and translation of thought. Under this private and silent aspect, the therapeutic ritual of the *kũbũ* differs from the shamanistic cures usually described as a sort of dramatization, by gesture and/or voice, of the combat that the shaman wages with the spirits. Lévi-Strauss (1958) has shown that the efficacy of the cure depends on a triple experience—that of the shaman, that of the patient, and that of the attendants (participating or not)—and also on the key role of the audience, which, by its participation, stimulates and reinforces the curing powers of the shaman. On the contrary, the cure carried out by the *kũbũ* is a solitary ritual: the *kũbũ* doesn't give anything to see, nor does he give anything to hear. "Nobody is there to hear," the Desana insist. The shamanism of *kũbũ* is a shamanism of silence, and in this lies its originality.

NOTE ON TRANSCRIPTION (DESANA)

consonants	voiceless	p, t, k, s, h, '
	sounds	b, d/r*, g, y
		w

*Kaye (1965) interprets /d/ and /r/ as allophones in complementary distribution with the phone /n/: the first two appear only in oral context, the last one in nasal context.

vowels	i	ɨ	u
	e	a	o

At the phonemic level we find nasal consonants and nasal vowels. Kaye (1970) showed that nasality is a feature of the entire morpheme and not only of one of its components. The nasality affects consonants and vowels in a nasal morpheme. It is a feature of morphology. The voiceless consonants p, t, k, s, h are not sensitively affected by the nasalization process. According to Kaye, the phones m, n, ñ, ng are nasal realizations, respectively, of the phones b, d, y, g, and not particular phones. b is pronounced (m) before or after a nasal vowel, d is pronounced (n), y is pronounced (ñ) as in the Spanish "mañana" and g is pronounced (ng) as in the English "tongue." In this article the nasalization is represented with a (~) disposed over the vowels of the nasal morpheme.

ACKNOWLEDGMENTS

Translated by E. Jean Matteson Langdon and Alroino B. Eble. A shorter version of this article was presented in the symposium "Lenguajes y palabras chamánicas" at the Forty-fifth International Congress of Americanists (Bogota, July 1–7, 1985) under the title "The conditions of performance of the therapeutic language among the Desana."

I wish to express my thanks above all to Batista and Raimundo V. for the depth of their teaching. I would also like to thank P. and F. Grenand, P. Menget, B. Albert, and S. Hugh-Jones for their critiques and valuable suggestions, M. Menget and M. J. Robert for their revisions of the translation. The plant and animal identification was made with the collaboration of A. Gely and P. Grenand, whom I thank. The data on which this article is based were collected during several trips made in 1984 and 1985 in the region of the Brazilian Vaupés and realized within the agreement on scientific cooperation between Brazil and France (Agreement CNPq/ORSTOM). Finally, I thank the Fundação Nacional ao Indio (FUNAI) for having given me research authorization in the upper Rio Negro region.

Notes

1. Two works present similar material: one by Reichel-Dolmatoff (1976) who studied metaphors of the spells and their relationship with Desana society and culture; the other one of T. Langdon (1975) who examined food prohibitions in the context of Barasana and Taiwano ritual and the preventive and curative spells of illnesses provoked by food transgression.

2. The identification of this plant is not certain (see Wassen and Holmstedt [1963] on this subject).

3. According to P. Grenand (personal communication), the hallucinogenic effect of this plant is not yet proven, but its toxic effect on the organism is certain.

4. The research was realized until now with *kũbũ*. There are practically no *ye* or *sakaka* shamans still existing on the Tiquié where I am doing research, both because they have fled the intolerance of the Salesian missionaries, who upon settling the Tiquié in 1945 hastened to condemn all shamanistic practices, and because they have not found anyone to whom to pass on their knowledge. The quiet character of the *kũbũs'* therapeutic ritual, however, undoubtedly contributed to maintain their practice and permitted them to resist better the missionary intolerance. Their activity, which depends on the interior recitation of an incantation, is solitary. It doesn't require any of the aspects of the collective ritual in the traditional shamanistic sessions. The existence, at the heart of Desana society, of three ritual specialists responsible for the functions of prevention and cure of illnesses poses some interesting problems. It would be

necessary, in particular, to analyze the relations between these different specialists and their actual social function. Have the *kũbũ* always taken care of the illnesses, or is this function recent, following the disappearance of the *ye* and of the *sakaka?*

5. "Without this incantation, I would have never been able to learn," the *kũbũ* often say. There exists another incantation, stronger because it invokes the hallucinogenic *paricá,* which permits them to learn through dreams. Finally, one can learn from a hallucinogenic vine "that makes *kũbũ*" (*Banisteriopsis* sp.). It is, for the Desana, the rope or vine of understanding, of knowledge. The individuals subject to the power of this vine or of the incantation must respect certain food restrictions (avoid fat food, roasted or smoked meat). Disrespect for this rule results in madness.

6. It is necessary to distinguish the true shamans from those who know only some incantations. In one sense, every adult man is a little *kũbũ.* Many of those who are married and are fathers seek to learn from their fathers or from their fathers-in-law (or even from an unrelated *kũbũ*) a few incantations that might help them face certain problems of daily family life (delivery or minor ailments). The embarrassment of having to ask a nonrelated *kũbũ* to attend to their family problems, more than a true interest in learning, motivates them in this case. Their protection and curing activities are limited, in any case, to the family sphere. There are very few who use their knowledge and their competence to help others. The social character of the function is a fundamental element.

7. The exact nature of these animal shamans is still unclear. Are all the animal species of the dolphin, of the jaguar, etc., the animal shamans? Are there individuals not marked spiritually? And are these animals animal-shamans or spirit-shamans? Finally, it is necessary to ask about the exact nature of the manipulation of the animals by these animal-shamans.

8. The Desana, like many other indigenous groups, mark the different phases or states of human development (birth, puberty, death) with particular ceremonies. These rites, which express the corporeal and spiritual transformation of the individual, comprise a certain number of dietary and activity restrictions. The nonobservance of the alimentary restrictions (consumption of "dangerous" food during a "bad" period, or food insufficiently purified by the shaman) is supposed to provoke (in the consumer, as well as in certain persons who are directly affiliated to him such as parents or sons) different troubles that vary with the nature of the food item ingested: digestive problems, sores, consumptive illness, etc. For the Desana, see Buchillet (1983); for the Barasana, Taiwano, and other Tukanoan groups, see T. Langdon (1975) and S. Hugh-Jones (1979).

9. Protective incantations that aim to guard the biological family during

periods of crisis or to protect the local group during rituals are recited over tree resin or cigars. In the food decontamination rite that marks the end of dietary and activity restrictions characteristic of these periods, incantations are recited over a sample of food (fish, meat).

10. Coca is the only stimulant with tobacco used by the Desana *kũbũ* in order to effect a cure. Coca has several functions: consumed in a regular manner, it reinforces physical endurance and it diminishes hunger; it increases concentration for the *kũbũ* and reinforces the acuity of his thought and memory. When not taking the hallucinogenic *paricá,* the *kũbũ* often have difficulties in establishing the diagnosis of a sickness. They declare themselves "incapable of seeing the illness in the body of the ill person," a capacity strictly associated in the Desana conception with the intake of hallucinogens.

11. The *kũbũ* breathes the incantation over the opening of the gourd or over the plant either at the end of each sequence or at the end of the entire text of the incantation.

12. A difficult labor includes: wrong position of the infant, "impossibility to be delivered" (the woman feeling the pains without succeeding in expelling the infant), or difficulty in rejecting the placenta. These are attributed to the act of a sorcerer or to an individual fault of the mother or her husband.

13. The barks that contain tannins are hence chosen for their astringent and healing properties.

14. See the analysis of the chant in Lévi-Strauss (1958).

15. In order to hide a sore the *kũbũ* invokes the plants with a "black body." Because of the dark color of the Indian's skin, the *kũbũ* will always opt for animals and plants with black bodies. If the person to be treated is a white he will invoke the whitish plants.

16. See "synecdoque de la partie" in Fontanier (1968).

17. The repetition can operate on two levels, joining the particular words—names of animals, of spirits, of plants, and of action verbs—or the entire text of the incantation. The repetition confers more force to words, it makes them act more rapidly on the sickness. The frequent usage in the incantation of the synecdoche by referring to the pathogenic object in its whole adds to the redundant character of the incantation.

TEN

ICAROS

Magic Melodies among the Mestizo Shamans of the Peruvian Amazon

LUIS EDUARDO LUNA

The Amazonian provinces of Peru, like those of all other countries sharing the Amazonian basin, have experienced great socioeconomic changes during the last decades due to the intense and chaotic exploitation of jungle products, heavy migration from the Andean and coastal regions, and indiscriminate deforestation. Many native groups have disappeared—physically or culturally—while others are being subjected to a rapid process of acculturation. However, there are many elements of native cultures still present in the mestizo population. Among them is the persistence of a rich shamanic tradition, which probably originated through the contact, often extremely violent, between white or mestizo rubber collectors and Indian groups during the last decades of the nineteenth century and the beginning of this century (San Román 1975, 142–49; Taussig 1984; Whitten 1981, 140–41).[1]

Distinctive elements of Amazonian native shamanism still persist among people who do not identify themselves with any particular tribal group. Practitioners locally known as *vegetalistas,* or simply *maestros,* still cure and perform other shamanic tasks through the use of tobacco and psychotropic plants, through magic chants or melodies called *icaros,* with which they communicate with the spiritual world, and with the help of a magic substance variously known as *flema* (phlegm), *mariri, yausa,* or *yachay.*[2] As is the case in native Amazonian shamanism, shamans acquire their powers from spirits of nature—plants and animals—or from deceased native or mestizo shamans, and by means of periods of isolation, food restrictions, and the ingestion of psychotropic plants. Native ideas of the supernatural cause of illness are still ubiquitous in the mestizo population, coexisting with modern Western concepts (see Andritzky 1989; Dobkin de Rios 1972, 83–88; Mabit 1988; Regan 1983, 2:31–34).

Among the psychotropic plants used along with tobacco, most important are those employed in the preparation of *ayahuasca,* a psychotropic brew known under such names as *yagé, natem, caapi, Santo Daime,* and so on, which is ritually used by large sections of the populations of the Amazon and Orinoco basins (Friedberg 1965; Schultes 1982; Uscategui 1959). (The area where I have carried out most of my fieldwork is the departments of Loreto and Ucayali.) In the Peruvian provinces of Loreto and Ucayali this brew is prepared by cooking the stem of *Banisteriopsis caapi,* (Spruce ex Griseb.), Morton (Malpighiaceae), a jungle vine, and the leaves of *Psychotria viridis* Ruiz and Pavon, or *Psychotria carthaginensis* (Rubiaceae). Only one informant used *Diplopterys cabrerana* (Cuatrecasas) Gates (Malphighiaceae) instead of *P. viridis.* This plant was brought to Iquitos by his wife, who purchased it from Huambiza Indians in Rio Santiago, near the Ecuadorian border. Other species of *Banisteriopsis* have also been reported, and also a large number of additives (Luna 1984b; McKenna, Luna and Towers 1986; Pinkley and Lindgren 1972; Schultes 1957, 1982). These plants belong to a series of species called *doctores* by local practitioners, because if ingested under certain conditions they are believed to be able to "teach" the shamans (Luna 1984a, 1984b). During the initiation period, which may last from some months up to several years, these plants are ingested periodically and successively, while a very strict diet and sexual continence are observed. The informants affirm that the spirits, or *mothers,* of the plants present themselves to the initiated, either during the visions they elicit, or during dreams, and teach the shamans how to diagnose and cure certain illnesses, how to dominate evil spirits of the earth, water, or air domains, how to travel through time and space, and how to perform other shamanic tasks (Chaumeil 1982, 1983, 74–89; Chevalier 1982, 346; Kuczinzki

1947, 28; etc.). These powers are acquired mainly through the memorization of magic melodies or songs, called *icaros,* which the future *vegetalistas* learn from the spirits of plants, animals, stones, lakes, and so forth, either during the visions produced by *ayahuasca,* or in dreams. The number and quality of his *icaros* is the best gauge of the knowledge and power of a shaman. All the informants claim to know dozens of them. I taped almost all the *icaros* (totaling about seventy) of Don Emilio Andrade Gómez, a practitioner who lives 12 kilometers from the city of Iquitos, and also a number of the *icaros* of other *vegetalistas.*

Herein is a preliminary attempt to make a survey of the most important functions of the informants' *icaros,* and a presentation of some of the ideas that are intimately linked to the learning and use of these magic melodies. More fieldwork should be carried out in order to clarify this interesting and little-studied aspect of mestizo shamanism.[3]

ICAROS AND PLANT TEACHERS

The word *icaro* seems to be a castilianism derived from the Quichua verb *ikaray,* which means "to blow smoke" in order to heal (Park et al. 1976, 45). This term seems to be used in various parts of the Peruvian Amazon, both among the mestizo and among Indians of the Ucayali (cf. Kamppinen 1989, 103; Karsten 1964, 204–5; Regan 1983, 2:27–29).[4] *Vegetalistas* of Iquitos and other areas of the Peruvian Amazon also use the verb *icarar,* which means to sing or whistle an *icaro* on a person, object, or preparation to give them power.[5] *Icaros* are used ritually, but not only in *ayahuasca* sessions, as has been stated (Dobkin de Rios 1972, 131; Katz and Dobkin de Rios 1971, 325). They are used also during the preparation of certain remedies, during healing sessions that take place independently of *ayahuasca* ceremonies, and even during activities such as fishing for certain species.

All the informants claim they learned their *icaros* by ingesting plant teachers, and by keeping a diet consisting mainly of smoked fish and plantains without any salt, sugar, or any other spices (Chevalier 1982, 346; Dobkin de Rios 1972, 70; Karsten 1964, 202; Luna 1984b, 145; Tessman 1930, 116, 229; etc.). Sexual abstinence, isolation—in the case of men, total separation from women in their fertile age—and certain requirements of ritualistic character are also necessary.

Each plant has its *icaros,* so the repertoire of the shaman apprentice

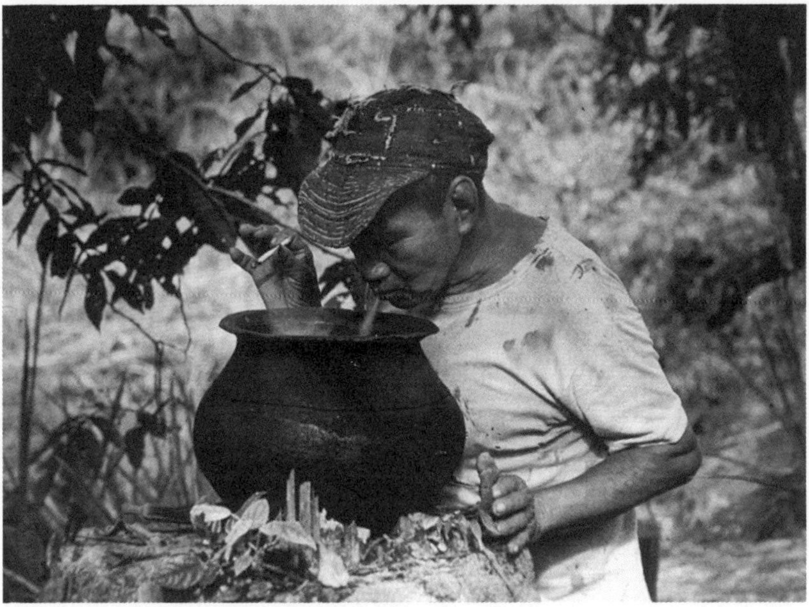

FIGURE 10.1. A Peruvian mestizo shaman blowing tobacco smoke over the *ayahuasca*.

expands as he adds other plants to the basic *ayahuasca* preparation (*Banisteriopsis caapi* plus *Psychotria viridis*), or as he ingests other plant teachers that are taken by themselves. The acquisition of magic chants or melodies and the memorization of myths during shamanic initiation seems to be a widely reported phenomenon (cf. Halifax 1979, 29–33). The association of the learning of magic chants or melodies with the absorption of psychotropic plants is quite common (see Dobkin de Rios 1976, 69–70). It is found among the Huichol who ingest *peyotl* (*Lophophora williamsii*) and other psychotropic plants (Juan Negrín, personal communication; La Barre 1969, 49–52; Myerhoff 1974, 97; Myerhoff 1975, 425). This relationship is also found among the Mazatec who take mushrooms of the genus *Psilocybe* (Estrada 1977, 82; Wasson, Cowan, and Rhodes 1974). It is also found as well among mestizo practitioners using *San Pedro* (*Trichocereus pachanoi*), among the Yanomama of southern Venezuela and northern Brazil who use *epena* (*Virola theiodora* or *Virola calophylloidea*), and among Mataco Indians who use *hataj* snuff (*Anadenanthera colubrina*) (Altschul 1972, 64; Donner 1984, 171–74, 187; Gonzáles Viaña 1979; Palavecino 1979, 72; Schultes and Hofmann 1980, 122–23; Seitz 1979; Sharon 1978). The association of the learning of chants with psychotropic plants is also found among numerous tribes using tobacco and *Banisteriopsis* (see Baer 1984, 210–13; Bellier 1986; Chaumeil 1983, 131–32; Elick 1969, 206–7 cited by Wilbert 1979, 21; Gebhart-Sayer 1985, 1986, 1987; Goldman 1963, 210–11; Illius 1987, 173–78; Kensinger 1973, 11; Langdon 1979b; Ramírez de Jara and Pinzón 1986, 180; Reichel-Dolmatoff 1972, 104; Siskind 1973a, 24; etc.).

A connection is also found among the mestizo population. Dobkin de Rios (1972, 120), for instance, reports that patients under the effect of *ayahuasca* see a very large snake entering the circle where they are sitting. If they are not frightened, the snake begins to teach the person his song. The idea that certain plants teach magic melodies seems intimately linked with the use of *ayahuasca* among Indian and mestizo populations of Caquetá, in Colombia, and in the provinces of Loreto, Ucayali, and Madre de Dios in Peru. In the state of Acre, in Brazil, there are communities who ingest the brew under the name *Santo Daime.* All these communities possess *himnarios,* collections of songs inspired by *Santo Daime.* Some community members have memorized up to three thousand *himnos* (cf. Monteiro da Silva 1983, 1985).[6]

Don Emilio Andrade Gómez, the main informant, related that, during his initiation to *ayahuasca,* an old man appeared both in the visions produced by the beverage and in his dreams, in order to teach him *icaros.* When he took other plants he learned more *icaros.* On occasions, while sleeping, he dreamt of being taught *icaros,* which he brought back and memorized perfectly during *ayahuasca* visions. There are similar descriptions from other informants. It should be observed, however, that learning *icaros* is not synonymous with being a shaman. Several persons have learned a few *icaros* from *ayahuasca,* but do not consider themselves qualified for curing or performing other shamanic tasks. On the other hand, knowing a number of *icaros* is a prerequisite to becoming a *vegetalista.*

When a *vegetalista* is keeping the diet, he may learn not only how to perform acts that may be considered positive or morally neutral, but he may also learn *hechicería* (witchcraft), how to cause harm. The informants claim that the spirits or "mothers" of the plants offer, first, the ability to cause harm through gifts in the form of thorns, bones, insects, or razors. If the shaman apprentice accepts them, he will then become a brujo or evil shaman. Later the spirits will teach him how to cure and other shamanistic activities. Don Emilio said he never learned witchcraft. In fact, only one of the informants acknowledged knowing how to cause harm. However, all of them affirm that their powers are embodied in their *icaros.* Don Alejandro, another informant, put it in these words: "A man is like a tree. Under the appropriate conditions he grows branches. These branches are the *icaros.*"

By singing *icaros* obtained from plants, animals, stone, metals, and so on, *vegetalistas* are capable of using some of the qualities or properties of these objects in their shamanic practices. In fact, it seems that one of the central ideas is that certain qualities or properties of plants, animals, minerals, or metals can be incorporated either by the ingestion of some part of this object, or by other means unknown. The *icaro,* which is the result of this absorption, is like the quintessence of the corresponding object, and can be used by the shaman for healing or causing harm, to protect himself against evil shamans or spirits, to make journeys into various cosmic realms, and so on. Here are some examples from Don Emilio's repertoire.

Icaro de la Bobinzana

Bobinzana is a beautiful tree (*Swartzia arborecens* (Aubl.) Pittier) (Leguminosae) considered a plant teacher by the *vegetalistas* of Loreto (Soukup 1970, 332). According to Don Emilio, the smell of the flowers of this tree has healing properties. Birds, monkeys, and insects use it as "their medicine," and it has the virtue to "clarify" the mind of human beings. The spirit of this tree is a prince, who presents himself dressed in beautiful garments and with a sword. The tree is in his palace, and this is why it always has flowers. Emilio says the *icaro* of this tree is used both for healing and as a melody to win the love of a woman.

Icaro de la Catahua

Catahua (*Hura crepitans* L.) (Euphorbiaceae) is considered to be a very strong and even dangerous plant teacher. It is possible to "learn" from this tree if a few milliliters of its latex are consumed, after a good *vegetalista* has cooked it carefully, and has sung a powerful *icaro* during the preparation. A strict diet of several months is required, otherwise the tree "can kill the person." Don Emilio explained that a mixture of the latex of this tree, together with *patiquina* (*Dieffenbachia* sp.) (a genus containing very toxic constituents) and *pucunucho* (unidentified) is used to destroy lakes where there are *yacuruna,* or evil inhabitants of the water often identified with huge boas, *bufeos* (freshwater dolphins), and mermaids (Arditti and Rodriguez 1982; Dobkin de Rios 1972, 80; Karsten 1964, 197; Luna 1986, 80–86; Regan 1983, 2:176–85; Valdizán and Maldonado 1922, 11).

As a matter of fact, this plant contains strong piscicidal and other biodynamic compounds (Evans and Soper 1978; Pere, Pere, and Rouge 1981; Sakata and Kawasu 1971). According to Don Emilio, the *icaro de la catahua* is whistled before one enters dangerous lakes. If this is not done, diabolic spirits can produce heavy winds and rain, and the person runs the risk of being devoured by a boa.

Icaro del Doctor Ojé

Ojé (*Ficus anthelmintica* Mart.; *F. insipida* Willd.; *F. glabrata* HBK) (Moraceae) is a large tree, whose latex is widely used in the Peruvian Amazon as an anthelmintic (Hansson 1986). Species of this genus are rich in biodynamic compounds (Eidler, Genkina, and Shakirov 1975; Elgamal; El-Taiwal and Fayez 1975; Venkatachalam and Mulchandani 1982). Don Emilio considers *Ojé* a powerful plant teacher. The spirit of this tree is supposed to be a big, fat, elegant white man (wearing a hat, and carrying a walking stick), who instructs the shaman in the cure of certain illnesses. The *icaro* of this tree is a powerful defense against evil shamans. By whistling this melody, a dense fog will be created around the witch, rendering him incapable of seeing where he is and causing any harm.

Don Emilio's repertoire includes the *icaros* of several other plant teachers such as the *icaro del Clavohuasca* (*Tynnanthus panurensis* [Bur.] Sandwith) (Bignoniaceae), *icaro de la rayabalsa* (*Montrichardia arborecens* Schott) (Araceae), *icaro del ayahúman* (*Couroupita guianensis* Aubl.) (Lecythidaceae), and others. He explained that it is also possible *dietar* (a term that means to ingest, keep the diet, and learn from) perfumes, certain minerals like *pedernal* (flintstone), and even metals, such as steel, so that one will be able to learn their *icaros*. By adding some drops of a perfume to the *ayahuasca* beverage during its preparation it is possible to learn *huarmi icaros* to attract women. By putting a piece of flintstone or steel in a glass of water for several days, drinking the water, and keeping the diet, it is possible to assimilate certain qualities of these objects. The *icaro del pedernal* is used by witches to cause destruction by fire. The *icaro del acero* (*icaro* of the steel) makes the body strong enough to resist rains and heavy winds. In Yarinacocha, near Pucallpa on the Ucayali River, the son of a well-known Shipibo shaman, Don Guillermo Arévalo, who was also a practitioner and seriously engaged in the study of the medicinal flora of his ethnic group, said it is also possible to learn from gasoline and certain acids, not by ingestion, but by inhaling them and keeping the prescribed diet.

The spirits of the plant teachers, in their turn, teach the shaman apprentice other *icaros* during his initiation by which some qualities of certain animals can be incorporated. Here are some examples.

Icaro del Pelejo

The *pelejo* (sloth) (*Bradypus tridactylus*), according to Don Emilio, is a very clean and strong animal. It is not disturbed by rain or heavy winds. It never eats meat or fruit, but only the shoots of certain trees. The *icaro* of this animal is used for curing children with digestive disturbances, or those affected by illnesses "produced by the water." (See appendix.)

Icaro de la Pinshe

The *pinshe* (toucan), according to Don Emilio, is a bird that sings in the evening to attract females. Its song is sad and beautiful. By singing the *icaro* of this bird, one can make a woman cry and win her love.

Icaro del Flautero-Pinshe

The *flautero-pinshe* is another bird (unidentified) whose *icaro* is used as a defense against the *Yashingo, Chullachaqui,* or *Shapshico,* a mythological being who has some of the characteristics of a "master of game animals," and who is generally considered evil because an encounter with it may cause madness (Kuczinski 1947:22; Luna 1986, 75–76; Valdizán and Maldonado 1922, 11–12).

Icaro del Ninacuru

According to Don Emilio, the *ninacuru* (from Quechua *nina* = fire, and *curu* = worm) is an insect whose eyes look like the headlights of a car. By singing this *icaro,* one is able to look for a person that has been stolen by the *yacuruna* (people from the water). The shaman, projecting light out of his eyes, will become like one of these insects and will more easily find the person in the underwater world.

Invocations to other animals are frequent, as established through conversations with other practitioners. Animals such as the eagle, the condor, the boa, the eel, and the jaguar, are called upon for healing, for protection, or, in the case of evil shamans, for causing harm. All the informants claim to be good hunters and are extremely good at imitating animals. Don Emilio says he "understands" the language of certain animals. While the novice is keeping the diet, one of his tasks is to carefully watch the animals and plants of the jungle to learn from them. According to Calvo (1981, 232) and Lamb (1985, 21–24), when taking *ayahuasca* Don Manuel Córdoba Ríos is able, through imitation, to bring the visions of birds and animals to people so that they are able to study their behavior. Through the *icaros* the shaman is able to "become one" with the animal and see the world accordingly. This idea is admirably expressed in Lamb's (1985, 24) narration based on interviews with Córdoba Ríos, who is a *vegetalista* from Iquitos.

Apparently, in certain cases an animal can become the teacher of a novice during the novice's initiation. On one occasion, a young man who had been keeping the diet was asked who his teacher was. "A hawk," he said. Another one, a well-educated man of about thirty-six, told how, years ago, he kept the diet for several months. During this time his mentor told him to observe the animals and plants very carefully. When talking about taking *ayahuasca,* the older *vegetalista* asked the younger man which, of all the animals he had been observing, had impressed him most. "The *isula* [a large ant]," he said. During his visions he felt himself becoming very small. An ant appeared in his visions, communicated with him in a tridimensional language, and invited him to visit the place where it lived. He did so, and remained with this ant several days, and was able to learn all about its habits (see Luna 1986, 47–50).

In many cases, the healing process comprises an awareness of, and integration with, the ecological setting through imagery. In the summer of 1990, while in Tachshitea, a small town by the Ucayali River, a beautiful example of this idea was found. There Don Williams Vásquez, a *vegetalista,* allowed the taping of some of his *icaros* in Quichua language. Don Williams used to sing one of them when a women in labor had difficulty giving birth. Several animals and plants are invoked—and visualized—in the song: First, a ray is invoked. The ray is ovoviviparous (the egg hatches within the mother) and, according to Don Williams, gives birth to living young in any position, be it sideways, or with the head or the tail first. Then Don Williams invokes a *shuyo* (*Hoplerythrinus unitaeniatus*), another fish, which has the property of being able to jump out of the water and transport itself with the help of a phlegm it regurgitates (cf. Tovar 1966, 186). He then invokes a boa that is so slippery that it can get into any hole or cavity, and a *paiche* (*Arapaima gigans*), a huge fish with a slippery skin. He finally invokes three trees, *cacao* (*Theobroma cacao*), *cetico* (*Cecropia* sp.), and *topa* (*Ochroma* sp.). Don Williams characterizes them as *flemosos,* containing phlegm. The *icaro* is sung on a glass of water that the mother has to drink. By invoking and visualizing the slippery qualities of these animals and plants, the mother is supposed to be able to give birth with ease.

FUNCTION OF THE ICAROS

The material collected so far does not allow great generalizations nor closed classifications. However, there are certain *icaros* (described below) that seem to have specific functions.

Icaros for Calling the Spirit of a Person, Plant, or Animal

Implicit in the cosmovision of the informants, as is also the case among most if not all South American Indian tribes, is the belief that plants, animals, human beings, rivers, lakes, mountains, and perhaps other inanimate objects, have a spirit (cf. Karsten 1964, 26–49). It seems the preeminent mode of communication between the shaman and the spirits is through magic chants or melodies. The spirits often present themselves to the shaman while singing or whistling a particular *icaro.* When the shaman learns these *icaros,* he can use them to call on the spirits when he needs them. By singing or whistling the *icaro* of the plant teachers, the shaman invites the spirits to present themselves. Also the guardian spirits, which may be anthropomorphic or theriomorphic, that all informants claim to possess are called through *icaros*.

By calling the spirit of a man and a woman through an *icaro,* they can be attached emotionally. Men in love with women who do not return their love frequently ask Don Emilio for his help. In an *ayahuasca* session Don Emilio whistles the *icaro de la piedra,* by which he can call the spirits of the man and woman. A black stone rotating very rapidly on an axis also made of stone then appears. He attaches the spirits of both the man and the woman to the stone so that the woman will feel dizzy and afraid, and will embrace the man who stands at her side. The *icaro* will unite them forever.

Through the *icaro de la arañita,* Don Emilio says, a similar effect can be accomplished. By whistling this *icaro,* a little spider appears that will spin its web around the spirit of the man and the woman, uniting them for eternity. These sessions always take place during the night. The woman, who at this time is supposed to be sleeping in her home, dreams of the man. When she wakes up she feels sad and thinks of the man and tries to get in touch with him.

Don Alejandro, a *vegetalista* who lives in the city of Iquitos, explained that there are witches who are able to cause harm with the help of the spirit of the *bufeo colorado* (pink freshwater dolphin). The dolphin, in the mythology of the area, is an intelligent and evil being, able to transform itself into a person in order to steal a partner to its underwater world (cf. Camara Cascudo 1983, 139; Reátegui 1983, 40–43; etc.). By removing the penis of a dolphin it is possible to call its spirit during a special session, and attach it to the spirit of a woman with the purpose of causing her harm. She will then have an insatiable sexual appetite and will have sexual intercourse with any man. Only through an appropriate *icaro* is it possible to neutralize the effect of the *icaro* used by the witch to call the spirit of the dolphin (cf. Karsten 1964:197–98; see also Dobkin de Rios 1972, 81 for a similar report).

Icaros to Modify the Effect of Ayahuasca and Other Plant Teachers

By using *icaros* the informants claim to be able to modify the hallucinations produced by *ayahuasca* and other psychotropic plants. There are *icaros* for increasing or diminishing the intensity of the visions produced by the plants, for changing the colors perceived, for directing the emotional content of the hallucinations, or for bringing specific visions. During the ceremony, the first *icaros* sung or whistled are usually for *subir mareación* (for calling the hallucinations). If any of the participants becomes frightened by the visions, there are specific *icaros* that will diminish the effects—*icaros para sacar mareación,* literally, *icaros* to take out the hallucinations. In fact, their visions are sometimes described as some sort of electromagnetic phenomena that comes in waves and can be attracted, modified, or sent away.

When several *maestros* or persons that know *icaros* are present at a ceremony, they all often sing their *icaros* at the same time. The effect is highly suggestive, and indeed it contributes to the enhancement of the emotional state of the participants, and may even alter or intensify the content of their visions. There are, however, cases in which a master *vegetalista* and one or several disciples sing the same *icaro,* which increases the effect of the song.[7]

Icaros Arkana

Once the *vegetalista* has entered into that other reality, he needs defenses. Through the *icaros arkana* the *vegetalista* protects himself against attacks by witches or evil spirits of the air, water, or earth. When a *vegetalista* is healing, or when he enters the other dimensions through the ingestion of psychotropic plants, he is particularly vulnerable and exposed to the attack of the agents who caused the illness.[8] If the *vegetalista* does not possess stronger *icaros* than those of the witch who caused the illness, he runs the risk of being killed by him. One way a witch attacks a rival shaman is by darkening his visions through an *icaro.* But there are also *icaros* to counteract this effect and to recover the clarity of the visions produced by *ayahuasca* or other plant teachers.

Arkana is, apparently, an abstract concept meaning protection. It includes guardian spirits (some of whom are ingested symbolically during *ayahuasca* ceremonies), magic melodies, and also an invisible "shirt," which covers the body of the shaman to protect him from magic darts (Luna 1984b, 143–44). The idea of a magic garment is also found in certain tribes, for example among Jivaro and Yagua shamans, where it is made out of the magic darts the shamans keep in their bodies (Chaumeil 1983, 125–230; Harner 1973, 24). As Métraux clearly pointed out in his discussion on Amazonian shamanism (1967, 91), the magic substance that shamans keep in their bodies, the pathogenic darts that they use to cause harm, and the guardian spirits, are three different aspects of the same magic power. Perhaps the magic melodies are also another manifestation of the same power.

Here is an example of an *icaro arkana* from the repertoire of Don Pablo Amaringo, a painter and former *vegetalista* whose religious iconography the author is currently studying (cf. Luna 1989a, 1991; Luna and Amaringo 1991).

Maimandara shamurimun
yana puma chicunaca
Urcu puntamantashia
Shamuirimun paicayari
Allpatashi chuchuchimun
Shamuipana paicayari.

Huashantashi shamuicuna
Otorongo pumacaya
Atunsacha ucupishi
Caparisha shamuricon.

Huashantami shamuricon
Mesticita pumacaya
chaimiyari tingunanchi
Huashantami shamuricon.

Huashantami shamuricon
Chai lluicho pumanchica
Caparishpa shamuricon
sinchi sinchi tingunanchi.

(Where are you coming from/ offspring of the black jaguar./ You nourish the earth with the milk of your breasts/ In this way you come forth.

Behind it comes,/ the otorongo [jaguar] is calling him/ in the midst of the great forest/ it comes screaming.

Behind him it comes/ the jaguar already tamed/ my tinguna[9] *is likewise/ it comes behind him.*

Behind him it comes/ the red jaguar,/ it comes screaming/ my tinguna *comes likewise.*

Icaros for Healing

Some examples have already been described above. According to Don Alejandro, *icaros* are especially effective for curing illnesses caused by witchcraft or by the actions of evil spirits. There are also *icaros* to cure other illnesses, for example snake bites. The following point should be stressed: it is believed that it is the melody itself that has curative powers. One example may illustrate this idea. During fieldwork in August 1984, this author met Don Manuel Ahuanari, an eighty-year-old man who lived with his second wife near the city of Iquitos. He was a *vegetalista* but did not practice anymore, since he had become seriously ill. In an *ayahuasca* session at the home of Don José Coral, one of the informants, Don Manuel said that when he was twelve years old he was bitten by a *jergón* (*Bothrops atrox*), a dangerous snake. When he was near death, a young man happened to visit the plantation on which he lived with his family. The young man heard about his case, and said he was going to try an *icaro* he had learned against snake bites. By singing and blowing smoke over Don Manuel he managed to cure him. Don Manuel learned this *icaro* during the healing process, and said he had cured many cases of snake bites during his long life with the help of this magic melody.

Don Emilio once said something very significant: "If you have learned from *ayahúman* [one of the plant teachers, also used in the extraction of the *virote* or magic dart thrown by evil shamans], you do not need to go out to the forest to bring its bark, because you already know its *icaro*." This shows that, at least in certain cases, the very essence of the tree is thought of as being in the magic melody, and therefore it can be used instead of the tree itself. In other cases, the *icaros* are used to reinforce the effects of medicinal plants. All the shamans interviewed always sing or whistle an *icaro* during the preparation or application of medicinal plants.[10]

Huarmi Icaros

Huarmi means "woman" in Quechua. There are *icaros* for winning the love of a woman. One of the most important tasks of the shaman is the solving of emotional conflicts in his community. The people of Iquitos and its vicinity, as with those of many other Amazonian settlements, have characteristically a very unstable emotional life. Couples break apart

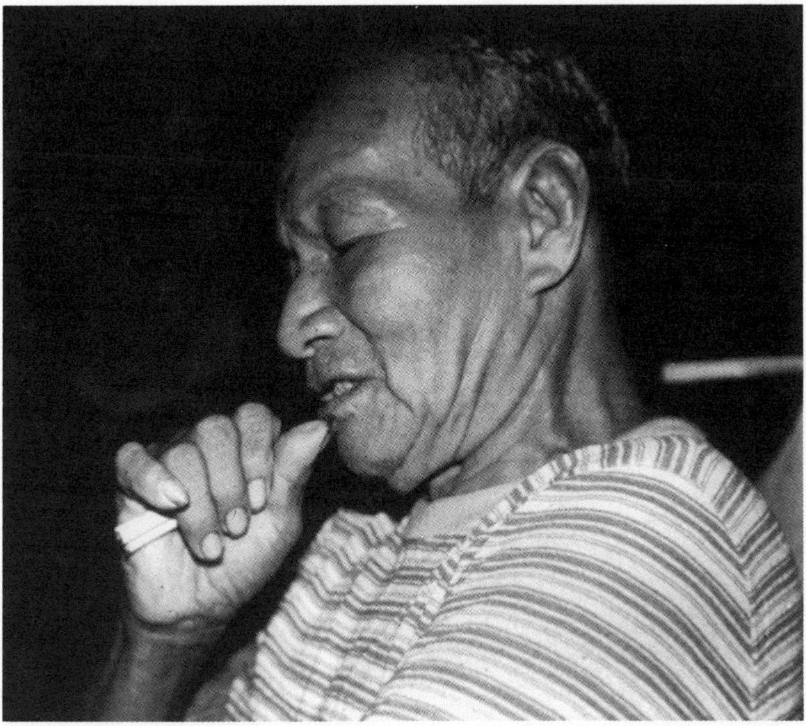

FIGURE 10.2. A shaman singing an *icaro* over some cigarettes before curing a patient.

easily. Many women with large families are abandoned by their husbands, or, conversely, men coming back from work in the jungle find that their wives have left their homes. Many of the clients of Don Emilio and other *vegetalistas* are men and women looking for advice or help to recover or retain their partners. Love *icaros* are extremely important in this context. Some of these *icaros* are sung or whistled in association with ritual baths with the plant *sacha ajos* (*Mansoa alliacea* (Lam) A. Gentry). These baths, very popular in Iquitos, are believed to bring good luck in work and love.

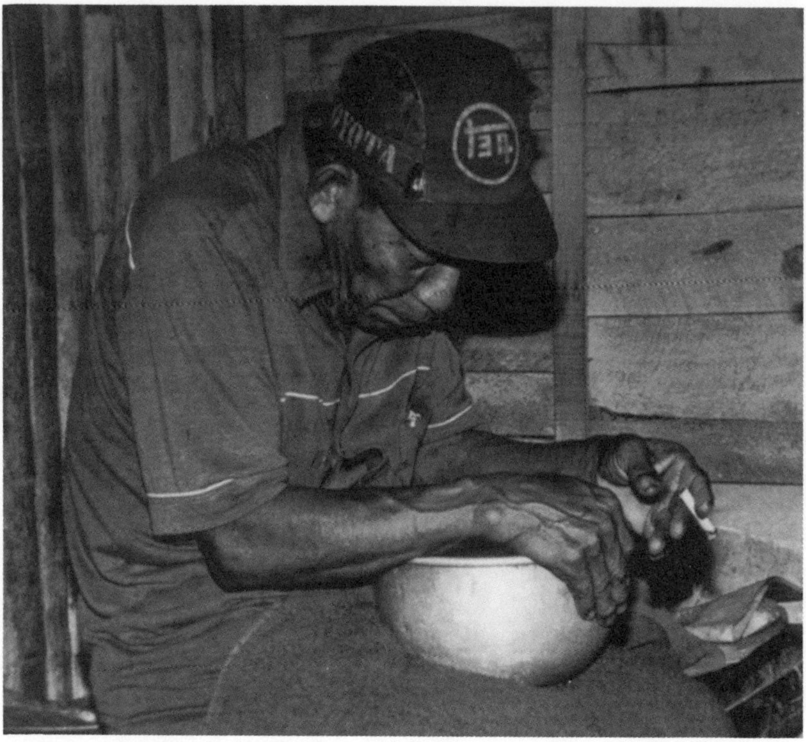

FIGURE 10.3. A shaman whistling an *icaro* over a preparation of *sacha ajos,* a remedy used in baths for good luck in love and work.

Other Icaros

In the repertoire of the informants there are other *icaros,* which are not easily classified. Don Emilio, for instance, has a beautiful *icaro* to wish farewell to a "good person" (*icaro para despedir a un personaje bueno*). There is one *icaro* by which he is able to attract a *paiche* (*Arapaima gigas*), a huge fish much appreciated for its delicious taste. Through the *icaro del alcanfor* (*icaro* of camphor) Don Emilio is able to make a witch fall asleep, so he can try to convince the witch in his dreams to stop doing harm to people. Camphor, an organic compound extracted from *Cinnamomum camphora* is widely used in the Peruvian Amazonas by shamans and curanderos. It is normally present in healing sessions and in *ayahuasca* ceremonies. Like tobacco, it is used for helping the shaman to regurgitate the magic phlegm, which is used as an aid for subtracting magic darts or *virotes* from the body of a victim. The psychotropic properties of camphor have been pointed out by Lewin (1980, 303–5). This is probably one of the reasons for its use among the *vegetalistas* of the Peruvian Amazonas.

Don Emilio also knows an *icaro* (*icaro para llamar a un indio Yagua*) by which he calls a Yagua Indian, who presents himself playing a *llupana,* a pan flute. Through the *icaro del Jívaro* Don Emilio is able to cure illnesses caused *en idioma,* that is, caused by chants or recitations in native languages. It is interesting to observe that anthropomorphic spirits may adopt the form of Indians, foreign entrepreneurs (the spirit of *Doctor Ojé* above), black men (one of Don Emilio's guardian spirits is a huge black Brazilian with wings), in other words, modern inhabitants of the jungle. Or they may also adopt the form of angels or princesses. Chevalier (1982, 352), describing the cosmology of a highly acculturated Campa shaman, reports how the spirits communicate with each other via radio frequencies (!). All this bears witness to the incorporation of new elements in Amazonian shamanism, and is probably of interest to the religions historian.

There is a certain hierarchy among the *icaros* of a shaman. Each shaman possesses a main *icaro,* which represents the essence of his power. Don Alejandro says that if a *vegetalista* manages to learn the main *icaro* of another practitioner, he will inherit his knowledge on his death. There is also a hierarchy among the shamans, depending on the *icaros* they know. Both Don Alejandro and Don José Coral value the fact that their *icaros* are difficult to memorize. *Icaros* in Indian languages, in contrast with *icaros* in Spanish, are considered especially powerful. The language most frequently used is jungle Quichua, a Quechua dialect, which is the mother tongue of several tribes of the Ecuadorian, Peruvian, and Colombian Amazonas (see Whitten 1981, 125). Don José also sings in Cocama and Omagua, and sometimes in a mixture of all three languages, with the purpose of impressing and confusing rival shamans. Don Manuel Ahuanari, on the other hand, states that the *icaros* should be clearly intelligible, so that everybody is aware of the animal spirits being invoked.

What I have presented here is only a brief and incomplete survey on the subject of the *icaros* of the *vegetalistas* in the Peruvian Amazonas. The learning of *icaros* is a condition for becoming a *vegetalista.* They are materializations of the shamanic powers received from the spirits, and are constantly used by *vegetalistas* in their practice. Communication with the spirit world is always done by means of the *icaros.* It is important to document this tradition as soon as possible. Only in the area where this author's fieldwork was conducted, there are dozens of *vegetalistas,* each with his particular repertoire. There are literally hundreds of chants and melodies that should be recorded and studied before the bearers of this tradition disappear. The work to be done is enormous and fascinating, and should be carried out with urgency, before our old wise men are carried away by time.

ACKNOWLEDGMENTS

This work was supported in part by the Finnish Academy of Finland and by Donnerska Institutet för Religionshistorisk och Kulturhistorick forskning, Turku, Finland. I wish to thank Dr. Timothy Plowman (Field Museum of Natural History, Chicago), Dr. Gerrit Davidse (Missouri Botanical Garden), Dr. Bronwen Gates (University of Michigan Herbarium) and colleagues for identification of plant material; Dr. Ilkka Kukkonen (Botanical Museum of Helsinki University), for supporting the transportation and preservation of vouchers and living specimens; Prof. Åke Hultkrantz (Institute of Comparative Religion, Stockholm), Prof. Bo Holmstedt (Karolinski Institut, Stockholm), and Prof. Richard Evans Schultes (Botanical Museum of Harvard University), for their inspiration and guidance; Mr. Alfonso Padilla (Department of Ethnomusicology, Helsinki University) for the transcription into musical notation of Don Emilio's *icaros.*

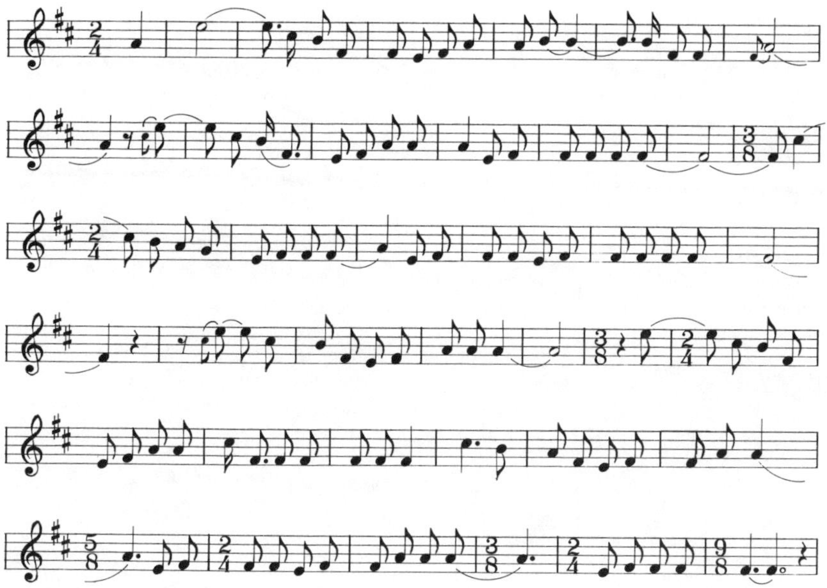

FIGURE 10.4. An *icaro* to call a spirit.

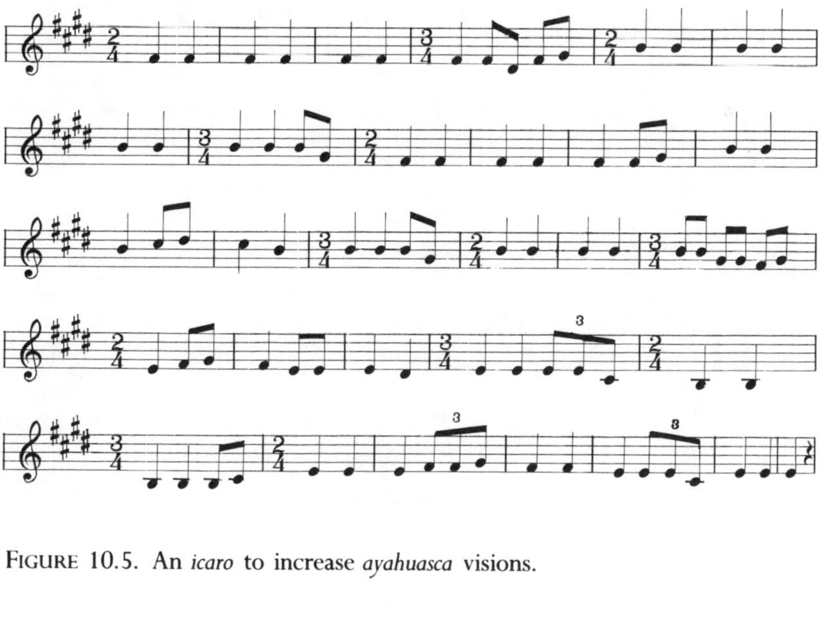

FIGURE 10.5. An *icaro* to increase *ayahuasca* visions.

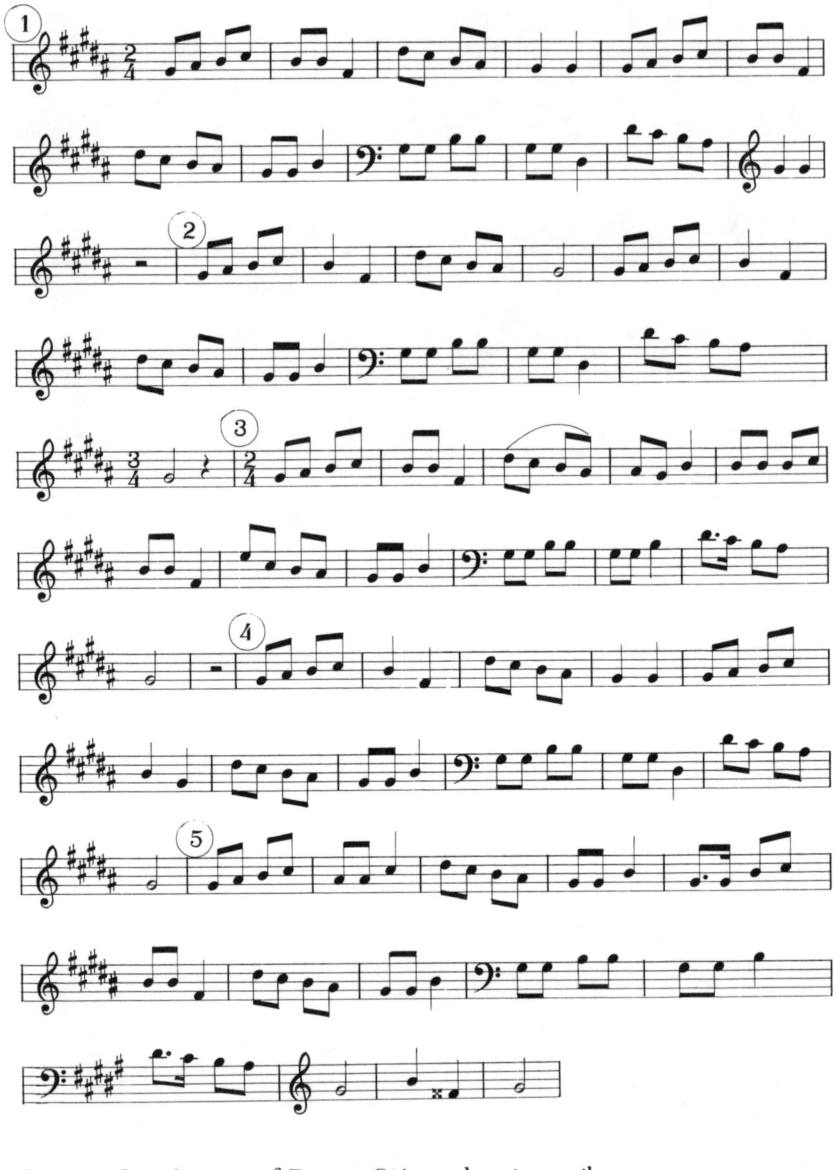

FIGURE 10.6. An *icaro* of Doctor Ojé, used against evil sorcerers.

Notes

1. An earlier version of this paper was presented at a conference on shamanism at the Santa Sabina Center, San Rafael, California, on 11–13 May 1984 and later published as a chapter of my book *Vegetalismo: Shamanism among the mestizo population of the Peruvian Amazon.* Stockholm: Almquist and Wiksell International. 1986. Out of print.

2. *Yachay,* a Quechua term, is also found among Lamista shamans, who used it both to refer to the magic substance and to a "ritual knowledge giving rise to spiritual power" (Scazzocchio 1979, 178–83). This magic substance, reported among several Amazonian tribes (Karsten 1964, 178; Nimuendajú 1919–1920, 1002–39; 1921–22, 367–406; Tessman 1930, 229, 406, 472, 520) is known among the Siona as *dau* (Langdon 1979b), among the Shipibo-Conibo as *quenyon* (Arévalo 1986, 158; Gebhart-Sayer 1986, 195), among the Jivaro *tsentsak,* "a brilliant substance in which the spirit helpers are contained" (Harner 1973, 17–20), etc.

3. In 1965 Rosa Alarco published a brief article, "Análisis musical de las canciones del *ayahuasca* usadas por los brujos de la tribu de los orejones del río Napo y por los curanderos de Iquitos. Informe.," which is to be found in Chiappe et al. (1985, 135–36). Two papers have been written on the magic melodies of the *vegetalistas* of the Amazonian provinces of Peru. They both analyze only the *icaros* taped during one *ayahuasca* session (Katz and Dobkin de Rios 1971; Stocks 1979). A. Padilla (1984) wrote a paper on the melody, harmony, rhythm, and expressive features of seven of Don Emilio's *icaros,* based on the material I gathered during my first period of fieldwork. Until now no attempt has been made to undertake a systematic survey of the whole repertoire of a mestizo shaman. It is to be hoped that ethnomusicologists will carry out new studies in this interesting area.

4. When I questioned a Shipibo shaman living in Yarinacocha about the origin of this term, he confirmed the Quechua origin of the word: the Shipibo terms for the magic melodies are *taquina, mashá,* and *cusho* (to work through blowing). Angelika Gebhart-Sayer distinguishes six classes of songs used in therapy among the Shipibo-Conibo. *Icaro* songs serve for diagnosis; *huehua* songs feature the content of the visions and the actual treatment; *mashá* songs enhance the patient's *shina* (mind, awareness); *shiro-huehua* (fun songs) animate the patient, induce joy and hope; *manchari* (sometimes thought identical with *mashá*) is sung to lead an abducted soul back to its owner; *muchay* songs used to be sung during eclipses of the moon (Gebhart-Sayer 1986).

5. In Cesar Calvo's novel on Manuel Córdoba Ríos and other shamans of the Peruvian Amazon, the following definition of *icarar* is given: "Icarar es

devolverle a las cosas los poderes que no les vinieron de natural en esta su vida. Icarar es magnetizarlas con fuerzas que las cosas no aprendieron, no saben. . ." (Calvo 1981, 104).

Rafael Karsten, referring to the Shipibo of the Ucayali, writes: "*Icaro* is also the name of a special formula of incantation which the demon teaches those who have taken the narcotic *nishí*. There is a special *icaro* for every animal or, more correctly speaking, every animal demon conjured" (Karsten 1964, 205).

6. The Centro de Iluminação Cristã Luz Universal "Alto Santo" published *Livro dos Hinários,* with the text of the songs of Raimundo Irineu Serra and some of his disciples. See also Polari de Alverga (1984, 334–42).

7. I would like to point out that a trance state can be achieved alone without the consumption of psychotropic plants by singing or whistling certain *icaros*. During the summer of 1982 I spent one month in the home of Don José Coral, who at that time was treating two very sick women. He took *ayahuasca* approximately once a week, but conducted healing sessions three or four times a week. On those occasions he entered into a trance state merely by singing and smoking one or two cigarettes of *mapacho* (a local variety of tobacco normally employed by shamans). The trance state cannot be attributed to tobacco, because he did not inhale large quantities. I would rather say that it was auto-induced through concentration and the whistling of magic melodies. He engaged thereafter in long conversations with the spirits in a language he told me was Cocama. These observations are in accord with those of Olsen (1975) among Warao Indians, and certainly reinforce his hypothesis that altered states of consciousness may be also reached through music alone.

8. In Cesar Calvo's novel on Manuel Córdoba Ríos and other "brujos" of the Amazonas, there is the following paragraph: "'When one takes *ayawashka,* one becomes like a crystal,' said Ino Moxo. One becomes like a crystal exposed to all spirits that live in the air, evil and good ones. It is for this reason we have icaros, icaros to protect oneself, icaros to heal, songs that call a certain spirit to counteract others. . ." (Calvo, 1981, 208) (My translation).

9. The term *tinguna* is a word probably related to the Quechua verbs *tincuni, tincunacuny,* "to quarrel," "to compete" (González Holguín 1989, 342). *Tingunas* are described by Amaringo as some sort of electromagnetic emanations, which shamans control with their songs, and which may adopt any form according to the shaman's wishes. *Tingunas* are particularly used as a means of defense.

10. In the healing sessions in which I participated, in the area of Iquitos and Pucallpa, the *vegetalistas* usually combined several elements: *icaros,* tobacco blowing, sucking the afflicted parts, and the use of plants, both for healing and for returning the illness to the person who caused it. This is not always

the case among some of the native groups of the area. For example, in Yarinacocha I participated in an *ayahuasca* session conducted by Don Benito Arévalo, a Shipibo shaman, and his son Guillermo. They were treating a young man suffering from *paludismo* (malaria). During the whole session they never physically approached their patient, who was lying under his mosquito net. At a distance of two meters they sang their *icaros* in his direction. They told me that he had been near death a few days earlier, but was now recovering. I witnessed the same procedures while spending a month with Don Basilio Gordon, another Shipibo shaman living in Santa Rosa de Pirococha, a small settlement by the Ucayali River.

For an in-depth study of the role of Shipibo chants in therapy, and their connection to the design art found in textiles, ceramics, and body painting, see Gebhart-Sayer (1985, 1986, 1987). On the use of magic chants for curing among the Sharanahua, see Siskind (1973a, 31).

PART FOUR

SHAMANS AND RESPONSES TO CHANGE

ELEVEN

VENANCIO KAMIKO
Wakuénai Shaman and Messiah

ROBIN M. WRIGHT
JONATHAN D. HILL

On the Acque River, a tributary of the upper Rio Negro (Guainía) in the northwest Amazon, there is an abandoned village site where Venancio Kamiko, the famous Wakuénai shaman and messiah of the mid-nineteenth century, made his home. Today, Venancio's tomb, preserved in concrete and marked with a cross, is regularly visited by the Indians who continue to worship him, placing candles before his grave and asking him through prayer for luck in hunting or for special favors. For the Wakuénai, the memory of Venancio Kamiko, immortalized in this shrine and in several legends, serves as a powerful reminder of a historical struggle, and of the Wakuénai's millenarian beliefs in saviors who guide and protect them.

Over one hundred years after Venancio, many of the approximately three to four thousand Wakuénai living in the border region of Brazil, Venezuela, and Colombia are Protestant evangelists. This is the result of New Tribes Mission proselytism among them, beginning in the early 1950s. At that time, the missionaries unwittingly sparked a resurgence of millenarian activities (Hill 1983; R. Wright 1981; R. Wright and

Swenson 1982). For the Wakuénai who chose not to follow the ways of Protestant evangelism because it meant the destruction of some of their central beliefs, there were, and are still, powerful shamans around who, like Venancio, are considered to be saints and messiahs.

Wakuénai millenarianism and beliefs in messiahs have frequently been mentioned in the ethnographic literature (e.g., Galvão 1959; Koch-Grünberg 1967). But until recently, there have been no systematic efforts to analyze their historical contexts or their basis in indigenous ritual and shamanism (Hill 1983; R. Wright 1981).

Herein is a documentation and interpretation of the life of Venancio Kamiko and the politico-religious movement organized by him in the late 1850s. This interpretation is based on historical documents from the eighteenth and nineteenth centuries, published works by explorers, scientists, missionaries, and government officials whose work took them to the upper Rio Negro region in the colonial period, as well as ethnographic fieldwork with northern Arawak-speaking peoples of the Isana-Guainía (Içana-Guainía) drainage area of Brazil and Venezuela in the 1970s and 1980s (Hill 1983; R. Wright 1981). Venancio Kamiko's millenarianism is intelligible only through simultaneously grasping the impact of critical events in the colonial history of the northwest Amazon region and the structural frameworks of significance within which Venancio and his followers formulated a strategy of resistance to colonial domination.

Contextualizing Venancio's millenarianism in both colonial history and Arawakan culture demonstrates that Venancio's movement was a historical rite of passage in which native peoples were struggling to reorient their social and economic activities in accordance with indigenous beliefs and practices. This reorientation was a historical rite of passage in a double sense. For individuals, Venancio's movement was a call to take stock of the history of relations with white men and to seek ritual purification through ceasing to participate in the white men's plans for economic development and political control. At the same time, the movement was a call for collectively deciding to stay together and act in opposition to the external forces of colonial domination that threatened indigenous societies of the region with total annihilation.

In a perceptive article on messianic movements during the early post-Conquest period in the northern Andes, J. Rappaport criticized functionalist and psychological typologizing of messianic movements for failing to acknowledge that "it is the structure, or the relations between the total configuration of symbols forming the movement itself, that defines the movement as a manifestation of messianism" (1980, 368, authors' translation). Messianic leaders are cultural innovators whose powers derive as much from their creative ability to extend indigenous symbolism into new, contradictory sets of relations, as they do from political and economic conditions or psychological stress and anxiety (Wagner 1972). Several recent studies have begun laying the foundations for a deeper theoretical understanding of messianic movements in South America as historically situated, cultural processes of innovation (Carneiro da Cunha 1973; W. Crocker 1967; Melatti 1972; Ossio 1973; Wachtel 1977). Our interpretation of Venancio Kamiko's millenarianism is based on a similar assumption that the dynamic, messianic quality of his movement, its expressive force, was a process of improvisation upon central symbols of indigenous Arawakan cultures of the northwest Amazon region.

Although many of the symbolic elements and activities making up the messianic movement were taken directly from Catholicism, the underlying structure of the movement was organized around indigenous mythical concepts and shamanic practices. Instead of viewing Venancio's millenarianism as an illustration of religious syncretism, the argument put forth here is that Venancio and his followers radically selected from Christian symbolism only those key symbols, activities, and contexts that made sense in terms of the regional Arawakan cultures and the historical experience of indigenous peoples during the eighteenth and nineteenth centuries. In this view, Venancio's selection of Christian symbols and activities was not so much a rediscovery of autochthonous messianic ideology triggered by the introduction of Christian symbolism as a discovery that the Christian symbolism of the colonizers could be strategically used to ritually protest the profoundly alienating effects of colonial domination (Ossio 1973, xxi).

THE WAKUÉNAI OF BRAZIL AND VENEZUELA

The Wakuénai, or "People of Our Language," are a northern Arawakan society of three to four thousand people inhabiting the Isana-Guainía drainage area of Brazil, Venezuela, and Colombia. Like the Eastern Tukanoan societies of the neighboring Vaupés river basin, the Wakuénai organize themselves into several exogamous, patrilineal phratries, each consisting of five or so named patrisibs ranked in a serial order. The phratries are named exogamous units associated with specific territories (Hill 1984a). There are five dialects of Waku, which are mutually understandable. The Wakuénai attribute less significance to dialect differences than to the basic contrast between the sacred, musical language (*málikai*) of ritual and the language of everyday social life. This contrast is, in turn, part of a much wider social and cultural distinction between, on the one hand, a hierarchical system of ritual specialists and ranking of sibs according to mythical order of emergence and, on the other hand, the strongly egalitarian character of everyday social and economic activities (Hill 1984b).

Missionization by the New Tribes (a fundamentalist Protestant group) and by Salesian Catholics, the division of Wakuénai lands among three nation-states, and a variety of other factors have set in motion a complex array of change processes. Wakuénai adaptations to these extralocal factors range from the formation of phratry-like, pan-Arawakan ethnic identity along the lower Guainía in Venezuela, to total conversion to evangelical Christianity along the upper Guainía in Colombia and in parts of Brazil, and finally, to emigrations to urban and semiurban locations such as São Gabriel, Manaus, San Fernando de Atabapo, and Puerto Ayacucho (Hill 1983; Journet n.d.; Wright and Swenson 1982). These transformations are too complex for an interpretation of any length here (see Galvão 1959; Hill 1984c; Journet 1981; Oliveira and Galvão 1973; R. Wright 1981, 1983). They are mentioned only to give a somewhat clearer understanding of Wakuénai culture in the late twentieth century and the rapidly changing sociohistorical contexts as evidenced by our fieldwork with the Wakuénai in the 1970s and 1980s.

THE MILLENARIANISM OF VENANCIO CHRISTU

Venancio Aniseto Kamiko was a Baniwa man born in Tsipinapi, a village on the lower Guainía between Maroa and San Carlos.[1] Although little is known of his early life, there are two points worth mentioning about his religious upbringing. Documents state that he was raised by a Don Arnao, a famed preacher of San Carlos, whom Spruce in 1853 described as "an old man, a Zambo, resident in Balthazar, whose tlent for singing masses and litanies, and strict attention to religious observances, have given him great influence, and gained for him the name of Padre Arnaoud" (Spruce 1970, 451).[2] Wakuénai legends of Venancio describe him as a powerful shaman, capable of transforming in order to escape his enemies, and with a remarkable gift of clairvoyance. Venancio's religious upbringing thus combined a deep knowledge of Christian and indigenous religions.

As most Indian men did in the 1850s, Venancio hired himself out as a woodcutter in the boat-building industry around San Carlos. It was common practice in this trade for men to be hired by their employers with an advance payment in cash or trade goods for the amount of work they were supposed to do. They were thus in debt before the work actually started, and on occasion, employers were also expected to pay back debts of their employees (Spruce 1970, 377). Venancio was unable to pay his work debt to several employers, including officials at San Carlos and Maroa in Venezuela and to a Brazilian trader, Manuel Gonçalves Pinto who lived at São Jose do Arara on the Isana River. Undoubtedly, the weight of all his debts contributed to an acute sense of oppression, which many Indians of the Rio Negro felt at this time.

After being sent to trade for manioc cereal and sarsaparilla on the Isana, Venancio lived at Santa Ana de Cuiary, a large village of Muriueni (a Wakuénai sib name meaning, "Children of the Anaconda") near the mouth of the Cuiary River. While there, he began to explain some of the Christian teachings he had learned from Arnao—often, as the documents say, in the presence of a cross. At some point, Venancio was struck with a serious illness, known as catalepsy. Early documents from the upper Rio Negro describe catalepsy as "a type of paralysis in which the body becomes rigid and immobile, the jaw bone and teeth clench together, convulsions are universal, and those afflicted with it die if not treated by the appropriate remedy" (Rodrigues Ferreira 1885, 144). This sickness was reported among the Indians of San Carlos in 1853 and was apparently aggravated by excessive consumption of alcohol (Spruce 1970, 378–89).

Venancio miraculously survived his sickness, however, and attributed his salvation to a divine calling. According to the trader, Pinto:

> One day he began to say that he had gone to heaven, had spoken with God, and other similar nonsense, and the Indians believed him, above all when he had attacks of *gota* from which he suffered, for he said after that he had died and God had called him and ordered that he give orders so that no one should cut wood and that they should give him

> chickens, this or that pig, etc., and that he had orders to pardon the debts of those who gave him what he asked for. (Joaquim Firmino Xavier, Director dos Indios, 1/1/58, in *Arquivo do Amazonas* 1(4): 116). (Hereafter cited as *AA*. All archive translations are the authors'.)

Pinto's report was later confirmed by a priest, Father Romualdo Gonçalves de Azevedo, who was sent to find out about Venancio (Azevedo-Furtado, 2/10/58, in *AA* 2(5): 14).

The powers of a Wakuénai shaman are substantially enhanced by surviving a critical illness, which is frequently interpreted as a divine calling. Venancio's experience went beyond the expected, however, for not only had he overcome death, he was also divinely ordained with the responsibility of eliminating people's debts, absolving their sins, and protecting them from harm. This power is more like that of a saint whom one asks for assistance in a crisis. In fact, shortly after his first experience of the divine, Venancio began to call himself a saint (Romualdo-Furtado, 10/2/58, in *AA* 2(5): 14). The orders given him by God to transmit to the people were derived, in large part, from the practices of saint cults on the upper Rio Negro at this time. Presents of animals, such as chickens and pigs, were promised or given to particular saints in order to obtain their protection and redemption from sin (Wallace 1890, 186). In Amazonian saint cults today, people are expected to follow the orders of the saints, for these are as good as the word of God, and in fact, people are punished if the orders are not obeyed or respect not given to the saint (Galvão 1955; Wagley 1968, 220).

At some point, Venancio began to call himself Christu. Like Yaperikuli, the mythical creator of the Wakuénai, Baniwa, Guarequena, and other northern Arawakan societies of the region, Christu is considered to be a savior who rids the world of dangerous and threatening forces, or overcomes them by his incredible knowledge and miraculous powers.[3] Powerful shamans (*dzáwináitairi,* "jaguar owners") similarly are believed to have miraculous powers for eliminating trouble, and hence are equated with Yaperikuli and Christu.

Throughout 1857 and the early part of 1858, Venancio preached in Isana villages; word of his miraculous powers spread to the Rio Negro and Guainía. Indians of the Vaupés soon heard about him, but Venancio's following mainly consisted of several hundred Indians and *caboclos* (Indian-white mestizos) from about ten villages of the middle to lower Isana and upper Rio Negro basin.

With time, his closest followers assumed titles within his movement. Three old people—Nazaria Josefa, Narciso José, and Venancio José Furtado—for example, became known as Santa Maria, São Lourenço, and Padre Santo (Pinheiro, 24/11/57, *AA* 1(2): 62). While he preached and received those who came to visit him, Venancio sent his followers to other villages to encourage them to visit him and bring him presents.[4] He organized mass meetings during which he preached and his "priest," Padre Santo, heard public confessions and assisted at marriages and divorces. Following these rituals, there would be festivals in which people would dance, sing, drink, and eat—in much the same spirit as saint festivals and indigenous exchange ceremonies (*dabakuris,* lingua geral; *pudali* or *kwepani,* Waku), which all Indians of the upper Rio Negro celebrated.

As the momentum behind his following increased, Venancio then announced that the end of the world was at hand. He prophesied that on St. John's Day (24 June 1858), the world would end in a great fire and that God would descend to earth to realize the final judgment.

> From the general burning, the Rio Isana would be excluded and in it, those who followed his dicta which consisted in dancing in rounds to the lugubrious and monotonous sounds of the words—"Heron! Heron!" without any significance. . . With all veneration and frequency they repeated it night and day . . . some arriving at sacrificing life in consequence of the continuous motion and absence of food (*Arquivo Histórico Nacional* (*AHN*): "Objetos Diversos" 3: 62–65).

People probably danced with crosses, a practice common in other millenarian movements around this time.

In the ritual calendar of Catholic Amazonas at that time, St. John's Day was one of the principal saint days. People celebrated elaborate festivals, and, in the evenings, made large bonfires. The celebrants walked or danced around the fires and occasionally jumped through in order to purify themselves from sickness and social ills. On the upper Rio Negro, St. John's Day had particularly strong—potentially explosive—political connotations, for it was believed that at that time the dominant political and economic relations would be annihilated. In June of 1853, the English biologist Richard Spruce, living in San Carlos, noted that the Indians were planning a revolt against the dominant white population to commence on St. John's Day, when "old scores would be paid off" and white governance would end (1970, 348–49). Four years later, Venancio prophesied that the time had arrived when popular hopes for radical change were to be realized.

In order to guarantee an uncompromising group of followers, Venancio required a "tribute payment" from the dancers.

> Another condition for escaping the burning and the purified ones ascending to heaven consisted in paying a tribute for marriages, baptisms, and confessions, the rule being that the more generous would more quickly enjoy the fiery exemption and the celestial ascension, . . . for Venancio advised them that in Heaven, they would not need gardens, nor what they possessed in the world. For it is notable the hunger and the misery which today the Isana and Vaupés are feeling again (*AHN* "Objetos Diversos" 3: 62–65).

In exchange for material goods, Venancio offered a way of breaking the political and economic stranglehold in which the Wakuénai and other indigenous people were ensnared. Instead of being caught in an endless spiral of debt bondage and dependence on material goods, Venancio asked that people give the fruits of their labor as "tribute" to him, in return for which he promised eternal salvation and happiness. The hunger that people experienced—in large part due to the exploitation of the traders—would be overcome by ritual fasting and rejecting their gardens altogether, for their needs would be taken care of in Heaven. By casting his orders in the form of Christian symbolism, Venancio created a new sense of religious authority and power among indigenous peoples of the region. They were able to conduct their own marriages and baptisms, and, hence, they no longer had any use for Christian missionaries.

Probably the first Brazilian official to learn about Venancio's movement was Frei Manuel de Santa Ana Salgado, the vicar of São Gabriel and Marabitanas. In September 1857, Salgado went to São José do Arara and summoned the messiah who was then preaching at Jandu Falls. He ordered Venancio to quit teaching and to leave immediately for Venezuela, threatening him with police reprisal should he fail to do so. Word of the millenarian movement had reached the Director of the Isana

Indians, Captain Mathias Vieira de Aguiar, who quickly dispatched a large military force to the Isana. Some twenty canoes of soldiers went to the lower Isana, and when they arrived, they broke up a dance festival in progress, "sacked" the longhouse, killed chickens and pigs, robbed the best handmade goods they found, and took the three leaders, Padre Santo, São Lourenço, and Santa Maria, as prisoners. On their way back, they terrorized several other Isana villages, warning people that a second military force was on its way to kill everyone (*AA* 1(3): 62–67; 1(4): 111–25; 2(5): 11–15).

As a direct result of the military depredations, the Indians of the Isana, lower Vaupés, and upper Rio Negro fled in fear to shelters in the woods, to the headwaters of the Isana and its tributaries, and to Venezuela. In early November, upwards of four hundred Indians had been seen going in forty-five canoes via the Cuiary River to Venezuela (*AA* 1(4): 111, 115, 125). Four large Wakuénai settlements were totally abandoned, and one, Tunui, had been burned to the ground.

Some of these incidents are remembered by members of the Hohodene phratry, for it was a time when many Hohodene left the Isana River and relocated to the Aiary River. According to the oral history, the Hohodene were living at São José do Arara, when a mestizo trader came to live with them and make canoes. One day he began to tell the Hohodene that it was very "poor" on the Isana and they should all move to the Rio Negro. The Hohodene held a large council meeting near the mouth of the Aiary River—many canoes arrived full of people and bushels of manioc cereal. One of the Hohodene chiefs then questioned the others: "What is this pain?" he said, "So it was with our ancestors. They killed our ancestors, we lost nearly everyone, there is no more Hohodene chief. Now they want to finish us off. . . How are your hearts? Shall we follow the white man?"

One man replied that he did not want to go, for he was building a new house and had much work to do on his gardens. Other men replied in a similar fashion. It was then decided that they would part ways. Most of the Hohodene, led by three elders, went to the Aiary River to settle, while only a few followed the trader to the Rio Negro.

The Hohodene village of São José do Arara was one of the four Isana River villages that was completely abandoned after the military raid on the lower Isana. The merchant Manuel Gonçalves Pinto had been living in this village for several years and cooperated with the military in sending Indian laborers to "public service" on the Rio Negro. According to two reports, after the military raid the Hohodene abandoned São José do Arara and went to the Aiary River; despite later efforts by the military to persuade them to resettle in São José, the Hohodene refused to do so (Xavier-Furtado, 1/4/58, in *AA* 2(5): 17; "Relatório" in Avé-Lallemant 1860, 130). As the Hohodene state, they refused to follow the white man because the white man had nearly finished them off once before, and because their own work had greater meaning for them than an illusion of prosperity on the Rio Negro. It was the Hohodene's collective decision to stay together—in opposition to the outsiders, the white men—that enabled them to survive and retain their political and economic autonomy.

Despite efforts by the missionaries and Director of the Indians to reunite the Indians of the Isana, they were unable to persuade more than a handful of people to engage in "public service," or to send manioc cereal, or even to leave their refuge settlements in the forest. By early 1858, the millenarian activities and rebellions had spread to the Vaupés and Xie rivers. Large-scale millenarian dance festivals were reported in a half-dozen locations, led by Tukano and other Indians of the upper Rio Negro. These movements became much more militant and determined in their resistance of the intrusion of outsiders. Until late 1858, when a military force was sent from Manaus to "quell the rebellions," the Indians of the upper Rio Negro managed to pursue their millenarian activities and keep outside officials away.

After the military raid on the Isana, Venancio fled to San Carlos, where, apparently, one of his creditors took him and several other leaders prisoner and sent them to San Fernando de Atabapo. Venancio escaped and sought refuge on the Acque River, where he continued his millenarian activities among the people of the Tiriquem, a tributary of the Guainía (*AHN*: 62–65; Xavier-Amaral, 20/11/57, in *AA* 1(2): 62). For many years after, Indians of Venezuela and Brazil visited the messiah, bringing him presents and seeking his guidance and protection.

BRIEF HISTORY OF THE WAKUÉNAI PEOPLE: PRECONTACT TO THE 1850S

In precontact times, traditional Wakuénai territory encompassed a large part of the upper Rio Negro valley, the greater part of it being in the

Isana and upper Rio Negro or Guainía river basins. This territory was in the center of a much larger area occupied by northern Arawak peoples that extended from the middle Orinoco, homeland of the Maipure people, to the Manao and the Arawak on the middle and lower Rio Negro. The Wakuénai principal subsistence activities were bitter manioc cultivation, fishing, gathering, and hunting. In areas where food resources were scarce, neighboring phratries frequently made reciprocal arrangements to utilize resource areas.

Neighboring phratries also frequently formed social and political alliances for the purposes of trade, marital alliances, and warfare. Oral histories of the Wanana, a neighboring Tukanoan people of the Vaupés, indicated that the Wakuénai sometimes sent war parties to the Vaupés and that, at least in some areas, supralocal organizations formed under paramounts, or "war chiefs" (Chernela 1983, 50–51). Wakuénai oral histories also recount wars against "cannibal" tribes, and, as in their mythology, these stories recall a primordial conflict between kinsmen and outsider groups.

European penetration of the upper Rio Negro valley began in the first half of the eighteenth century with the slave trade (see especially, Hemming 1978; Sweet 1974; R. Wright 1981). As many as twenty thousand Indians of the upper Rio Negro were taken in slavery during the height of Portuguese activities between 1740 and 1755.[6] By the 1760s, several very large nations of the Rio Negro had been exterminated and vast sections of the river depopulated. The Wakuénai, however, appear to have remained numerous throughout this time and probably absorbed refugees from other tribes into their number (R. Wright 1981, 134–35).

Throughout the latter half of the eighteenth century, the Spaniards and Portuguese began colonizing and laying claims to territory in the upper Rio Negro and Orinoco valleys. Spanish efforts were, for the most part, limited and unstable because the missionaries and military were scarcely able to establish a permanent colonial structure. One important industry, boat building, was introduced to the Spanish Rio Negro in the late eighteenth century, but outside of that, the region remained economically marginal and its commerce limited (Primov n.d., 13–38; R. Wright 1981, 163).

Similarly, forced relocation of Indians to mission settlements *(reducciones)* met with little success. Very few missionaries were available to work in the region until the late eighteenth century, and their efforts to convert the Indians often met with resistance (R. Wright 1981, 160–67).

Portuguese colonialism was more systematic and its impact more widely felt. Throughout the latter half of the eighteenth century, hundreds of upper Rio Negro Indians were relocated to colonial settlements where they worked in plantations and in the extraction of forest spices. In the 1780s, major epidemics devastated vast sections of the Rio Negro and Japura, putting a heavy strain on the *descimento* (descent, relocation) system to replenish the settlements. Frequently, soldiers used armed force to relocate the Indians (R. Wright 1981, 149–53). At the end of the eighteenth century, the Rio Negro government at Barra (Manaus) underwent a virtual political and economic collapse, leaving the Indians to return to their homelands and recoup their losses.

During much of the early nineteenth century, the Brazilian upper Rio Negro remained a source of labor, forest spices, and certain staples for the sustenance of colonial settlements. The provincial government attempted, with little success, to institute a labor system and taxes on manioc cereal, which were to be enforced by government-recognized Indian chiefs. In the 1830s, Brazilian traders (*regatões*) began operating around São Gabriel and Marabitanas, and by the 1850s, when the merchant system had become firmly established, they were conducting a prosperous business with their Venezuelan counterparts (Primov n.d., 40; R. Wright 1981, 210–11).

The territorial government at San Fernando de Atabapo in Venezuela essentially left the administration of the Rio Negro basin area in the hands of local officials, or commissaries, who were usually the local criollo merchant class. As in Brazil, Indians were exploited in trade and often forced to provide free labor (Primov n.d., 42; R. Wright 1981). The abuses of this system became so flagrant that, by the early 1840s, the Venezuelan government attempted unsuccessfully to introduce reforms. Indians again sought refuge from the harassment and exploitation in the forest.

By the 1850s, the Rio Negro basin of Venezuela had become the most active economic center of the territory, primarily due to the flourishing boat-building industry at San Carlos and Maroa, the rope-making industry, and trade with Brazil. Riverine settlements had an air of prosperity and were attracting many non-Indian settlers, both Venezuelan criollos and Brazilians. Yet, despite their apparent prosperity, the permanent settlements were barely able to sustain themselves, suffering chronic shortages of food and a lack of currency. Indian laborers were often in severe debt to the criollo boat makers and were apparently kept at work only by liberal supplies of alcohol (Spruce 1970, 377–78, 475). Ethnic relations between Indians and non-Indians were based on class differences in which the non-Indian merchants and local officials oppressed and exploited the Indian population and those of Indian descent.

In the early 1850s, the newly formed state government in Manaus launched a major program for the "civilization and catechization" of the Indians of the upper Rio Negro valley. The government revived the system of Directorships of the Indians, increased its number of missionaries, and instituted a program of "public service" labor, in which government-recognized chiefs were expected to send laborers and children, who could be raised into "civilization," to Manaus (R. Wright 1981, 228–32). Official government policy classified native peoples into forest Indians (*gentios*), settled Indians (*indios aldeiados*), and "civilized Indians." The Directors and missionaries were charged with the responsibility of attracting forest Indians to the main rivers, where they were more accessible, while settled Indians supplied the labor for "public service" programs (R. Wright 1981). To accomplish these objectives, the Directors relied on the support and alliances of the traders and several powerful chiefs of the Vaupés River, who acted as middlemen in negotiating resettlement, providing children and adult laborers, and organizing punitive raids against tribes who resisted.

This system proved to be extremely abusive: "Macus" of the forest were hunted and sold to the military; children were kidnapped and sold to the military; periodic raids on villages were conducted to obtain laborers and manufactured goods; and in 1852–53, a massacre was perpetrated against the Carapana Indians of the upper Vaupés in retaliation for a Carapana attack on the military to avenge the kidnapping of their children. The Directors of the Indians frequently used armed force to persuade the chiefs of forest tribes to settle on the main rivers and to accept "the order of the government" (R. Wright 1981, 239–75).

Compounding these abuses, the traders and the Directors exploited Indians in boat building, extraction of forest products, and public service works. Consequently, the Indians of the Vaupés and Isana were unable to provide for their own subsistence needs. In 1853, Richard Spruce reported a situation of near-famine on the Vaupés, while in 1857, the Wakuénai of the Isana complained to the authorities of their extremely miserable conditions, exploitation by merchants, military abuses, and hunger. The time was clearly ripe for rebellion.

CULTURAL CONTEXT OF WAKUÉNAI MILLENARIANISM

Venancio Kamiko's millenarianism emerged at a critical transition in the colonial history of the northwest Amazon region. The growth of non-native political and economic institutions had been temporarily halted in the early nineteenth century, allowing indigenous Arawakan societies time to recover from severe population losses and to regain a sense of sociopolitical order and autonomy. However, mid-nineteenth-century development of the region in the newly independent states of Brazil and Venezuela became much more sustained and systematic. Venancio Kamiko's life coincided with the implementation of increasingly abusive programs in Brazil and with the expansion of an oppressive Indian labor system in Venezuela in the 1840s and 1850s. As the Hohodene oral histories clearly indicate, the mid-ninteenth century was a time when Wakuénai of the Isana were evaluating their previous historical experience and deciding what to do about it.

Although Venancio Kamiko's millenarianism outwardly embodied Christian symbols of Amazonian folk Catholicism, the symbolic structure of Venancio's movement was organized around mythical concepts and shamanic activities, which were deeply rooted in the indigenous Arawakan cultures of the Isana-Guainía basin. The following discussion relies on fieldwork with Wakuénai ritual specialists of the Hohodene phratry along the Aiary River in Brazil and of the Dzawinai phratry along the lower Guainía River in Venezuela (Hill 1983; R. Wright 1981). Among the cultural beliefs and practices that are central to an understanding of Venancio Kamiko's millenarianism are: (1) the mythical space-time of the trickster-creator in the distant past and its transformations during the mythical life cycle of the monstrous, world-opening, primordial human being, (2) Wakuénai concepts of immortality, (3) the cultural significance of ritual fasting and inactivity as expressions of control over basic psychological needs, (4) the belief that sickness and death are processes in which individual and collective souls split apart, and (5) the belief that payments of material valuables must be offered to ritual specialists in exchange for spiritual cures and other services.

Wakuénai mythology outlines a complex cosmic history, organized into several cycles of myths that describe different stages of creation. The first of these cycles is about a distant and remote past in which the world began as a small area around Hipana, a place on the Aiary River. This miniature world was chaotic, for cannibalistic animals walked about killing and eating all people. Then, Yaperikuli, the Wakuénai culture hero and trickster, came into the world and proceeded to rid it of the dangerous animals by taking vengeance against them. Despite the animals' unceasing attempts to kill Yaperikuli, he repeatedly subdues them, and, through his extraordinary divinatory powers, creates order in the world. Underlying Yaperikuli's struggles is a fundamental social conflict between kinsmen (Yaperikuli and his brothers) and affines, or "others" (the animals; Yaperikuli is married to a woman of the animal tribe), the resolution of which is the basis of human society (Hill 1983, 39).

The second major cycle of myths goes beyond the first to explain how human society is reproduced over time. The central characters of this cycle are Yaperikuli, Amáru, the first woman, and Kuwái, the son of Amáru and Yaperikuli. Kuwái is an extraordinary being whose body consists of all wordly elements and whose humming and singing brings into being all animal species. His birth sets in motion a rapid process of growth in which the miniature world of Yaperikuli opens up into the life-sized world of forests and rivers inhabited by human beings and the various species of forest animals, birds, and fish. Kuwái teaches humanity the first sacred rituals of initiation; yet, at the end of these rituals, Yaperikuli "kills" Kuwái by pushing him into a bonfire, and the world then contracts back to its miniature size. Out of Kuwái's ashes grow the plant materials for making the sacred flutes and trumpets played in initiation rituals and sacred ceremonies today. Amáru and the women steal these instruments from Yaperikuli, setting off a long chase in which the world opens up for a second time as the women play Kuwái's instruments throughout the world. Eventually, the men regain the flutes, and Kuwái, Amáru, and Yaperikuli leave this world to go live in the various celestial regions from whence they are invoked in ritual.

The Kuwái myth contains a wealth of religious symbolism that is open to a wide range of interpretation. The Wakuénai are aware of the diversity of this symbolism and often use it as a conceptual vehicle for intellectual speculation. The myth is frequently told, for example, to explain the beginning of initiation rituals and the cult of the sacred flutes; the beginning of sickness and misfortune that Kuwái left in the Great Fire; the relationships among people, animals, and spirits; and the transmission of culture from ancestors to descendants. In effect, this myth cycle bridges the gap between the distant, miniature, and eternal past of the Beginning at Hípana and a more recent, life-sized, and dynamic past beginning with Kuwái and Amáru. In short, Wakuénai mythology outlines a very dynamic version of an expanding and contracting universe in which the notion of time depth is centrally important. The myths about Kuwái and Amáru essentially carve out a more recent, human past that is both differentiated from the precultural, chaotic past and brought into the experience of living people in rituals.

The narrative of Venancio Christu's movement in 1858 provides unambiguous evidence that Venancio and his followers were evoking the mythical being of Kuwái and the transformation of the world after the fiery death of Kuwái at the first initiation ritual. Venancio's order that his followers dance "in rounds to the lugubrious and monotonous sounds of the words 'Heron! Heron!'" (see above) was certainly a significant symbolic act. The words "Heron! Heron!" are a translation of *"Maariye, maariye,"* a pan-Arawakan musical verse that refers, among other things, to the white heron feathers used to decorate the sacred flutes and trumpets of Kuwái and worn as a sign of prestige by ceremony owners. *Maariye* is a refrain word sung at the beginning and end of each verse in a genre of sacred dance music called *kapetiapani* (whip dance). The mythical origins of *kapetiapani* are found in the Kuwái myth cycle that describes and explains the first initiation ritual. Kuwái explains to Yaperikuli that his body is virtually indestructible and that it consists of all things that can be used to kill people—shotguns, machetes, poison arrows, vines, and so on. The only element that can destroy Kuwái is fire. Yaperikuli then prepares a bonfire and leads Kuwái—old, drunk from a night of dancing and chanting, and nearly blind—in a dance (*kapetiapani*) around the great fire. At the end of the ritual, Yaperikuli kills Kuwái by pushing him into the fire, creating an "inferno" that scorches the earth, causing it to contract to miniature size. Thus, when Venancio's followers danced to the words "heron, heron," they were evoking that very moment in Wakuénai mythology when the great, fiery transformation of the world was about to take place. At the same time, Venancio and his followers evoked Christian beliefs in immortality by performing *kapetiapani* in the context of a patron saint festival, St. John's Day, and by adopting Christian symbols in place of dance whips (*kapeti*).

Venancio promised spiritual salvation and eternal happiness to his followers, provided they obeyed his orders to abandon all subsistence and commercial activities. These orders, in effect, translated into the idiom of the millenarian movement, indigenous beliefs in the importance of ritual fasting and abstention as necessary preconditions for participating in the creative and transformative powers of Kuwái and his music. Ritual fasting and abstention is a form of voluntary suffering to which individuals must submit if they are to demonstrate that they are fully cultural beings capable of controlling their own destinies, rather than social animals caught up in a perpetual cycle of violence and revenge. Abstention from everyday activities of production, sharing, and consumption of food forms an essential part of the relationship between shamans and their clients on sacred occasions. A client's failure to observe proper restrictions on diet and daily activities is believed to undermine attempts by shamans and chant owners to effect orderly transformations or restorations of the client's identity. Venancio's orders that his followers abandon all economic activities in 1858 were thus deeply embedded in indigenous myth and ritual as they were historically situated in the political and economic stranglehold of debt bondage and "public service" labor in the mid-nineteenth century.

Ritual fasting is also important as a means for restoring health whenever the vital processes of growth and development have broken down. In cases of serious, life-threatening illness, both the patient and the patient's kinsmen must fast on manioc drinks over which the chant owner has blown smoke and sung *málikai*. Regardless of its cause, serious illness among the Wakuénai is seen as a process of disintegration in which the individual, human body–shaped soul (*likaale,* or *likáriwa*) becomes alienated from the collective, animal-shaped soul (*lidzarúna,* or *líwarúna*). Similarly, when groups of people have been displaced from their ancestral lands, they experience a painful separation equivalent to sickness and death.

Chant owners and shamans seek to restore the connection between the two parts of their patients' souls by using their ritual powers to travel to the two worlds of the afterlife: the chant owner journeys in his *málikai* songs to the celestial home of the Kuwáinyai (Kuwái People, or bee spirits), whereas the shaman travels in *málirríkairi* songs to the dark netherworld (*íyarudáti*) of recently deceased persons (*lidánam*). The musical journeying of ritual curers acts as a means for symbolically controlling relations between living human beings in this world (*hekwápiríko*), mythical ancestors in paradise (*likáremi*), and recently deceased persons in *íyarudáti*. Through fasting and ritual music, the two souls of sick individuals, or the souls of collective groups of individuals, are reintegrated, and proper relations between the living, the dead, and the ancestors are renewed.

Spiritual transformation and renewal in the world of living people has its counterpart in the belief that the souls of recently deceased persons (*lidánam*) transmigrate to rejoin their respective sib ancestral souls in celestial paradise after a period of painful separation in *íyarudáti*. The Wakuénai concept of immortality arises from a juxtaposition of two opposing views of human mortality: the continuous, vertical journey of collective *lidzarúna (líwarúna)* souls to paradise and the discontinuous, horizontal transformation of individual *likáriwa* souls in this world into *lidánam* souls in the shadowy world of *íyarudáti*. The period of time during which individuals must remain in a limbo status as recently deceased souls depends on the manner of death rather than behavior during life in this world (Hill 1983, 209; Matos Arvelo 1912, 95).

Once the *lidánam* souls have been purified in fire and have transmigrated to the celestial paradise of Yaperikuli, they enter into a state of eternal bliss where all souls are brilliantly white, live in beautiful houses, eat only the purest food (honey in great quantities), and bask in eternal sunlight (Hill 1983; R. Wright 1981). Like the Kuwái myth cycle and the rites of passage through which it is enacted in the human life cycle, the soul's journey after death is a twofold process of cumulative, irreversible transformation from which there is no turning back. Once the *lidánam* souls have transmigrated into paradise, they never return to the world of living people (Hill 1983, 201). Thus, Wakuénai eschatology explores the dichotomy between individual death and collective continuity in order to construct a belief in individual immortality and salvation in a celestial paradise, rather than attempt to short-circuit this essential paradox through beliefs in the reincarnation of individuals as living members of this world.

Wakuénai ritual specialists are living representations of the idea of immortality and salvation. They are recognized as charismatic leaders in everyday social contexts, precisely because they represent a higher order of sacred and aesthetic values that transcends the narrow social ties within the local sib, and that can cut across phratric and even ethnic boundaries. Ritual leaders communicate to nonspecialists the transition from a precultural, inchoate past to a more recent, culturally differentiated past, and they carry this sense of cultural order into their secular lives as model individuals who are in no way exempt from the practical concerns of everyday social life and subsistence activities. They are men living in this world who assume the heroic powers of mythical beings in their struggles to relieve human suffering.

Shamans are usually graded by their peers in terms of their knowledge and abilities to cure. The highest grade are known as *dzáwináitairi* ("jaguar peoples' owner") and are able to attain the highest level of the cosmos (where Yaperikuli resides) continuously in their dreams and cures. These few shamans have extraordinary abilities to foretell and affect events, send their souls great distances, and cure any sickness. They are considered to be "saviors" whose powers, like those of Yaperikuli, are able to overcome or eliminate dangerous and threatening forces in the world (R. Wright 1981, 62–64). Among Christian Wakuénai, Yaperikuli is equated with Jesu Christu, and the *dzáwináitairi* are equated with both saviors.

The narrative of Venancio's movement indicates that the messiah's recurrent attacks of catalepsy enhanced his power among the Indians of the Isana basin. To the Wakuénai, an individual who survives repeated attacks of serious illness, in effect, demonstrates an extraordinary ability to carry out the ritual journeys of shamans and chant owners to the two worlds of the afterlife, as well as the renewal of life in this world—through safely returning from the other realms of the cosmos. Life-threatening or fatal illnesses, such as the seizures suffered by Venancio Kamiko, are sometimes linked with powerful forces of the cosmos, especially evil omens (*hínimai*). Venancio's miraculous survival from recurrent seizures no doubt elevated his ritual status beyond that of shamans and chant owners to the level of *dzáwináitairi* (jaguar peoples' owners).

Venancio's calls for displays of generosity from his followers arose from the indigenous system of exchange between ritual specialists and their clients, who include not only sick persons but also newborn children and their parents, young men and women at puberty, and other individuals undergoing transitions in the life cycle (i.e., the ritual equivalents in Wakuénai culture of the Christian rites of baptism and marriage). Ritual specialists, called chant owners (*málikai limínali*) and shamans (*malírri*), expect to be paid with material goods for providing ritual services. In curing rituals the payment (*dawáinaku*) is displayed in order to help the shaman attract the patient's lost soul back to its proper place in the human body. This belief that generosity with material goods influences ritual efficacy is part of a more general openness in which the patient and his kinsmen are expected to confess intimate personal experiences, such as bad dreams or family arguments, to the shaman. In situations of life-threatening illness, shamans ask everyone in the village to "contribute," or loan, their most valuable possessions in an attempt to attract the patient's lost soul back to this world. Venancio's request that his followers give generously in order to escape the cataclysmic fire, elevated the indigenous system of exchange between ritual specialists and patients to a new level: the messianic leader sought to renew the spiritual integrity of the Wakuénai by ridding them of the social disorder brought by the white outsiders.

LEGENDS OF VENANCIO CHRISTU

Several legends of Venancio Christu recorded among the Wakuénai of the Guainía and the Aiary provide crucial evidence for understanding Wakuénai messianism (Hill, field notes; Wright, field notes). As might be expected from the analysis of Venancio's movement in the previous section, Wakuénai legends about Venancio embody indigenous concepts, which are firmly rooted in the mythology of Yaperikuli and Kuwái and in the ritual activities of shamans, chant owners, and master shamans. Two legends of Venancio will be summarized and interpreted in this section.[7] Both legends were told to Hill in response to his questions about Venancio; the first legend was also told to Wright in the context of a discussion about powerful shamans who are "like Yaperikuli."

Legend One: Venancio Christu and Tomas Funes

A man who knew that Venancio Christu was a saint told Funes about him. Funes sent a commission of soldiers to fetch Venancio from his home on the Acque River. They took Venancio up to Funes's house in San Fernando to interrogate him. Venancio denied that he was a saint, since a saint is a person who does not eat bread and meat. Then Funes asked him if it were true that he had many followers who brought gifts to him in payment for cures. Again Venancio denied what the others had told Funes. Funes ordered Venancio to be put inside a coffin, which was nailed shut, tied with a cord, and weighted with a rock. The soldiers threw the coffin into the Rio Orinoco and left it there for one hour. Then they raised up the coffin and took it back to Funes. When they opened the coffin, it was totally empty inside. The soldiers explained that Venancio must have escaped because the cord was not strong enough and the nails had not been placed close together.

Again the soldiers fetched Venancio from his home on the Acque River and brought him to Funes in San Fernando de Atabapo. This time they tied the coffin shut with a rope instead of a mere cord and spaced the nails only three fingers' width apart. They threw it into the same deep part of the river, but again Venancio escaped and the coffin came up empty.

The third time, they put nails very closely together, only one finger's width apart, and tied the coffin shut with a very thick rope made of rawhide. After waiting an hour, they raised up the coffin and untied the stone. This time, they felt that the coffin was very heavy and were certain that they had finished off Venancio. When they opened the coffin, there was a huge anaconda inside. Venancio was seen on the other side of the river, dancing and chanting. At that moment, Funes decided that Venancio was really a saint and that he could never kill him no matter how hard he tried.

After several months, Funes sent his soldiers to fetch Venancio from his home on the Acque River so that he could apologize to him. However, Venancio pronounced a punishment on Funes, saying that he would be killed one day in a revolt by his own soldiers. Funes felt guilty about what he had done and lived in great fear until his death.

This legend explicitly focuses on the political struggles between Venancio and the territorial government. More generally, the legend can be interpreted in terms of the political and economic struggle between the Wakuénai, whose source of power is represented in Venancio, and the white man, whose power is represented by the military and an oppressive government. Tomas Funes, in fact, was a governor of the Venezuelan Amazon territory in the early twentieth century and not the mid-nineteenth century; hence the legend conflates two very similar time periods, for the Wakuénai were faced with a tyrannical government under Funes just as they had been in the mid-nineteenth century. According to Hill, "During the 1920s, Wakuénai groups living along the lower Guainía fled from the terrorism of the Funes regime up the Guainía and its tributaries, such as the Tomo and the Acque. . . The rise and fall of the rubber baron turned dictator, Tomas Funes, was the culmination of rubber boom politics that decimated whole indigenous societies almost overnight" (1983, 336). Venancio's prophesy that Funes's government would come to an end in a revolt is similarly accurate not only for Funes's regime but also for the late 1850s, when there were four attempted revolutions in the territorial government (Tavera Acosta 1927, 183–84).

Funes's efforts to kill Venancio can be also interpreted in light of the Wakuénai myths of Yaperikuli's struggles against the animal tribes who try to kill him. One key symbol found in both this legend and the myth of the beginning of Yaperikuli is the *container* (R. Wright 1981, 536). In the myth, Yaperikuli's father-in-law tries to kill him by sending him into the middle of a new garden and setting fire to the garden periphery. Yaperikuli transforms and enters a small *ambauba* (*Cecropia* sp.) tree trunk. When the fire reaches him, the tree trunk/container bursts apart and Yaperikuli flies out, unharmed, declaring that he is immortal and cannot be killed.

As the object of legendary narratives, Venancio is a multivocal symbol who simultaneously calls to mind both the creator, Yaperikuli, and the primordial, monstrous, and world-opening human being, Kuwái. Venancio's ability to escape the combined forces of wood (coffin), metal (nails), vines (rope), water (river), and stone similarly evokes the mythical figure of Kuwái, whose body consists of all wordly elements with the exception of fire. Like Kuwái, Venancio cannot be killed by any of these elements. Finally, the container as a symbol of the primordial womb is a major theme throughout the Kuwái myth cycle. In the beginning of the cycle, Kuwái is stuck inside his mother's (*Amáru*'s) womb and has to be forcefully let out by Yaperikuli. Later, Kuwái himself transforms into a container when he eats the three boys who prematurely break their ritual fast. In both cases, whether it is the womb of Amáru or the belly of Kuwái, the myth cycle focuses attention on the narrow escape from the container.

In the legend, the container as a mythical symbol of womb, death, and rebirth is extended to a new object, the coffin. Three times the coffin is closed, each time with a stronger rope (cord, rope, rawhide rope) and more nails (spaced widely apart, three fingers' width apart, one finger's width apart). As a representation of historical reality, the rope and the nails can be interpreted as a metaphor of the white man's economy—specifically, the rope-making industry and carpenters' nails, both important in the mid-nineteenth century—while the tightening of the coffin evokes the increasing economic oppression and stifling of the Indians at the time of the movements. Venancio escapes each time through his shamanistic abilities to transform: like Yaperikuli, he is immortal, and like Kuwái, he is all wordly elements combined into one being.

On the final try, the coffin is pulled out of the water and is found to contain an enormous anaconda (*umáwari*). The anaconda continues to evoke the imagery of increasing constriction, since the anaconda kills its prey by squeezing it to death with its coiled body (see Drummond 1981). In addition, the anaconda is a mythical figure of great importance throughout the northwest Amazon. Among the Wakuénai, the anaconda is connected in numerous myths with the concept of adulterous, dangerous sexual relations and a reversal of the container/womb symbolism found in the Kuwái myth cycle. Instead of expressing the theme of narrow escape from the womb through fasting and other ritually controlled processes, the anaconda represents the child who refuses to come out of its mother's womb for fear of permanent separation, or death. The appearance of an enormous anaconda inside Venancio's coffin expresses a similar theme: the anaconda is stuck inside the container, whereas Venancio, like Kuwái and Yaperikuli, has escaped unharmed.

Legend Two: Venancio's Annual Death and Resurrection

In Holy Week, on Friday afternoon, Venancio Christu told his followers that he was leaving this world for his house in the sky but that he would return soon. Privately, he told his wife to take care of his body and to pray for him while his spirit went to the sky. "We have to wait for Venancio two days, until late Sunday afternoon," his wife told the people after Venancio had "died." She told the people that they would all pray for Venancio and take care of his body during his spirit's two day absence.

Some soldiers and other white people arrived and asked what the people were doing, for many indigenous people had gathered to follow their leader's instructions. Venancio's wife explained to the outsiders that everyone was praying for Venancio and that they would continue to do so until Venancio came back in two days. There would be no dancing or drinking *aguardiente* until Venancio had safely returned.

But the woman broke her promise to Venancio and started a dance on Saturday while she was supposed to be leading the people in prayer. She told everyone that they could pray on Sunday and that would be enough. When Venancio came back, he would see that everyone was praying as they were supposed to be doing. She danced with the soldiers and other white men until she had danced in all the households of the village and with each of the men.

On Sunday, she led the people in prayer until Venancio returned in the late afternoon. Venancio's body rose and he asked his wife what she had done while he was away. "We prayed the whole time," she claimed. But Venancio had seen that she danced with men while his spirit had been away. He punished his wife by waiting until she fell ill and, instead of curing her disease, handing her a piece of paper with instructions on it. The paper told her that she was permanently refused access to God through prayer. Then a devil with no legs or lower body came and made love to the woman. When they finished, the woman was also minus her legs and lower body. She went on dancing with the devil forever, using her forearms as feet.

Each year, Venancio died for two days during Holy Week. He told his followers never to cut any wood during his spiritual journey since to break even a little twig would break their souls in half. Three brothers were sitting around talking the day after Venancio had left for the sky, and one decided to test Venancio's claim by going outside to break a piece of wood. He went to sleep thinking that Venancio had lied, since he had broken wood and found it to be harmless. But the next day Venancio returned and called his followers up to be examined, family by family. When he got to the three brothers who had broken wood, he told them exactly what they had said and done the day before. The three were silent and afraid to answer Venancio. Venancio told them that a group of men would come to kill them as punishment for their deeds, and later that same day they were killed.

The second legend may again be read for its specific historical references: the documents do state that Venancio claimed to have "died" and gone to heaven while his followers prayed for his return, and Venancio did order his followers not to cut any lumber. We also see more evidence of Venancio's articulation of Wakuénai shamanism and Christian millenarianism: his death and return, which are characteristic of shamanistic journeys, are brought into line with Christ's death and resurrection during Holy Week. Venancio is at once a curer and a saint to whom promises are made, prayers offered, and respect given, who can punish disobedience and failure to carry out vows and ritual proscriptions.

As with the first legend, the second can be seen to focus on a larger historical issue: how Venancio exercised spiritual authority over his followers and managed to keep his movement together despite the persistent weakness of his following. The success of Venancio's spiritual journey to obtain orders from God or the protection of his following depended on their respecting his ritual rules and proscriptions to remain spiritually pure through prayer, free from the debilitating influences of drinking *aguardiente,* dancing with whites, and physical labor for the white people. In other words, the principal threats to Venancio's spiritually based movement were to be found in social and economic relations with outsiders.

In the first episode, Venancio's wife succumbs to moral weakness. She did not only break her promise to the saint to guard his body, she also lies to him and dances with the soldiers and other white outsiders, and all of the men of the village—suggesting that sexual relations were another source of weakness. In the legend, Venancio's wife is eternally banished from paradise for dancing and, implicitly, mating with the soldiers and other white outsiders. She is "refused access to God through prayer" and condemned to dance eternally with the devil with whom she has sexual relations. In the second episode, one man is a disbeliever, who "tests Venancio's claims" by breaking an injunction against physical labor. For this he and his brothers were punished with violent death.

In both episodes, body and spirit, or soul, form a central dichotomy, which is symbolically manipulated to underscore key themes in Venancio's millenarianism. As discussed above, the Wakuénai believe that in illness, the individual human body–shaped soul becomes alienated from the collective, animal-shaped soul. Shamans seek to restore the connection of the two souls through their cures. Without this restoration, souls of recently deceased persons are unable to transmigrate to paradise. They must wander about eternally in the world as shades. Ritual prohibitions, such as fasting, are essential, not only for demonstrating individual control over destiny, but also are a way to reintegrate body and soul. Breaking the prohibitions brings about ritual and physical degeneration and, ultimately, death. Thus, when Venancio's wife succumbed to bodily pleasures during a time when she was supposed to be leading the community in prayer, her transgression set off a process of complete separation of her soul from her body. She was denied a cure (i.e., the two parts of her soul remain permanently alienated) and was ultimately denied salvation in paradise (i.e., she was forever alienated from her collective sib ancestral soul). She was forced to dance with the devil in a transfigured and inverted body (she danced with her forearms).

In the second episode, Venancio's ritual proscription was against cutting lumber, for even a little twig would break men's souls in half. Again, the message is that Venancio's followers were expected to remain spiritually whole during their savior's journey to the heavens. Venancio sought, perhaps, in this way to revitalize the souls of those men who constantly labored for the white traders. While the first episode emphasizes the importance of respecting promises in marital relationships, the second focuses on consanguineal ties. All three brothers were equally punished for the transgression and disbelief of one. Failure to observe Venancio's interdiction against labor was, in a sense, equivalent to a failure of the men to control their own destinies. It would bring about a situation where men killed each other, which ultimately degenerates into a perpetual cycle of violence and revenge.

Underlying this second legend is a fundamental connection to the Wakuénai myth of Kuwái and Amáru. Like Venancio Kuwái establishes the laws of ritual observances, such as fasting during sacred ceremonies, and punishes with death those who fail to observe his proscriptions. In the myth of Kuwái, three brothers undergoing initiation break an injunction against eating roasted food. As a result, Kuwái devours them, but spares one who goes on to complete the initiation. In the legend, three brothers are prohibited from cutting lumber; when one of them tests Venancio's claims to sanctity, and cuts wood, all three brothers are killed.

As the Kuwái myth explains how social groups are reproduced over time and cultural norms passed from ancestors to descendants, so this legend explains how Venancio suceeded in keeping his movement together. As the Kuwái myth and related beliefs about death and immortality focus on the proper relationships of body and spirit, which are kept in balance through ritual observances, and which ultimately ensure the soul's safe passage to paradise, so Venancio's teachings emphasized that his followers had to remain spiritually pure, free from the corrupting social and economic influences of white outsiders, and had to respect his laws in order to gain salvation.

The millenarianism of Venancio Kamiko was a historical rite of passage in which Venancio and his followers analogically linked select Christian symbols to the underlying metaphors of shamanism and religious ideology: the cross and the whip as symbols of ritual suffering, St. John's Day, and the sacred dance of Kuwái as symbols of purification through fire, and Christ the Savior and Yaperikuli/Kuwái/powerful shaman/Venancio as symbols of salvation and immortality. The mythology of Yaperikuli and Kuwái and the ritual activities of shamans, chant owners, and master shamans render intelligible the selection of symbols in Venancio Christu's movement and in current narratives about Venancio.

In arguing for the importance of symbolic analysis in understanding revitalization movements, the implication is not that the symbolic processes in Venancio's movement or its interpretation in legends are in any way autonomous things, or reifications which serve to mask underlying social relations. Although Venancio's movement had its roots in indigenous religion, it was not merely a passive reenactment of cosmogonic mythical realities, but a historically situated praxis in which key symbols were strategically employed to resist the external imposition of alien political and economic systems (Taussig 1980b; Whitten 1978). The analogic linking of Christian symbols with the paradigmatic imagery of Yaperikuli/Kuwái/powerful shaman/millenarian leader illustrates a creative process of mediating the social and historical transitions of the nineteenth and twentieth centuries through directly embodying these same transitions in symbolic forms. Thus, in the legend, Venancio escapes the tomb made for him by the whites, while in history, the Wakuénai escaped near annihilation at the hands of Funes in the early twentieth century and the oppressive debt bondage of the mid-nineteenth century.

What was at stake in Venancio's movement was the kind of transformation that Arawakan societies of the upper Rio Negro region were to follow: whether to become totally dominated tools of the external ruling classes, or to seize hold of the historical moment and carve out a ritual space-time in which a degree of spiritual and political freedom was possible. Wakuénai oral histories and legends portray the mid-nineteenth century as a time of choice between two starkly opposed alternatives: either stay together in opposition to the outsiders' plans for development or "become the white population" of the emerging towns and cities of Amazonas. The specific cultural forms in which the Wakuénai cast this historical dilemma are drawn from the mythology of Kuwái, sacred ritual, and shamanism: control over hunger through ritual fasting leads to orderly growth and development, whereas failure to control hunger (i.e., premature breaking of the fast) leads to death and destruction. The mythology of Kuwái and sacred shamanistic rituals are centrally concerned with the mediation of internal and external experience within Wakuénai society, and in Venancio's movement these same cultural processes became the principal means for mediating between an external order of domination and the disruptive effects of that order on the internal social order.

What Venancio Christu's movement accomplished was a reorientation of social and economic relations in which the refusal to cooperate with the external, dominating order of the white men became elevated to the status of a sacred cosmological postulate. Writing some fifty years after the climax of Venancio's movement, Martin Matos Arvelo recorded the following statements made by Wakuénai ritual specialists in their advice to male initiants: "The white men are thieves who buy our wares cheap and sell them to us at high prices. That is why they are rich and we are poor. Hide your hatred of the white men, for it is strong, and know that they are traitors" (Matos Arvelo 1912, 86, authors' translation). Thus the transformation that Venancio Christu and other millenarian leaders of the nineteenth century effected was a redefining of the indigenous ancestor cult into a cult of historical opposition to external domination. Today, the Wakuénai continue to evoke Venancio Christu as a symbol of their own historical rite of passage and cultural survival.

ACKNOWLEDGMENTS

Hill's fieldwork among the Wakuénai of Venezuela was made possible by doctoral dissertation grants from the Social Science Research Council (*SSRC/ACLS*) and Fulbright-Hays in 1980–81, and by a faculty research grant from

Fulbright-Hays in 1984. Wright's fieldwork with the Wakuénai of Brazil was made possible by a doctoral dissertation grant from the National Science Foundation. The authors would like to thank Jean Jackson, Lawrence Sullivan, and Renato Rosaldo for their comments on an earlier draft of this paper. We also wish to thank the Wakuénai of Brazil and Venezuela for their hospitality and cooperation.

Notes

1. The Baniwa are an Arawak-speaking people whose ancestral lands centered around the lower Guainía River and tributaries (Acque, Pimichin, and Tirikin). Although the Baniwa language is mutually unintelligible with Waku, Baniwa mythology and ritual are quite similar to that of the Wakuénai. In Brazil, the Wakuénai are known as "Baniwa," whereas in Venezuela and Colombia they are called "Curripaco." The term Wakuénai can be glossed as "People of Our Language."

2. "Zambo" is a Black, probably a Black/Indian mestizo.

3. In 1900, the German ethnographer Koch-Grünberg was told by an Oalipere shaman that Christu and Yaperikuli were one and the same (1967, 200). Probably this identification had been thought of by Wakuénai shamans well before Venancio.

4. Little information emerges from the documents about opposition to Venancio's movement by other Indians, except that the chief of Santa Ana de Cuiary is reported to have expressed resentment at the messiah's activities and "wished to kill him because he ordered people to steal chickens and pigs to eat" (Xavier-Wilkens de Mattos, 1/1/58, *AA* 1(4): 115).

5. Padre Santo, Santa Maria, and São Lourenço were all suffering from sicknesses but were sent to Marabitanas and later to Manaus. They had in their possession the following items: one nailed box; two bundles, one wrapped in old rags and the other in a bag of bark cloth; three old shotguns; and two old violas (Pinheiro-Furtado, 24/11/57, *AA* 1(2): 62). The significance of these items remains obscure, although we may suppose that all were used in the dance festivals and cult activity. The three old people were taken to the new president of the state of Amazonas, Francisco José Furtado, who was very concerned that all of the commotion on the upper Rio Negro might be the work of a political agent disguised as a missionary, who was encouraging the Indians to rebel and to emigrate to Venezuela in order to undermine Brazil's control of the region (Furtado-Xavier, 11/13/57, in *AA* 2(5): 8–12). Furtado's questioning, however, failed to reveal any such motives of the messiah, whom

the old people called "the patriot." Furtado put them to work in "public service" and sent a missionary, Father Romualdo Gonçalves de Azevedo, to try to persuade the Indians of the Isana to return to their villages.

6. From the rapids of Corocubi (modern-day São Gabriel) to the confluence of the Orinoco and Guaviare rivers, the limits of Portuguese exploration. No estimates are currently available for the Spanish slave trade.

7. Unlike the myths of Yaperikuli and Kuwái, the legends about Venancio Kamiko were narrated in the local Spanish and Portuguese dialects of the upper Rio Negro. The summaries provided here are highly abbreviated translations of narrations that lasted over ten minutes.

TWELVE

SIBUNDOY SHAMANISM AND POPULAR CULTURE IN COLOMBIA

MARÍA CLEMENCIA RAMÍREZ DE JARA
CARLOS ERNESTO PINZÓN CASTAÑO

This is a study of how shamans among the Indians of the Sibundoy Valley have resolved the question of external influence.[1] Sibundoy strategy for cultural survival consists of integrating foreign elements without denying their own beliefs by establishing mediations that match native thought structure, which is based on a movement of complementary opposites. This integration yields a great cultural plasticity, whose fundamental principle achieves a dynamic equilibrium in those institutions, such as shamanism, on which their cosmic vision is based. It is the shaman who mediates the diverse contradictions experienced by the Indians.

As traders since precolumbian times, Sibundoy shamans have incorporated different cultural codes and elements from other groups into their own shamanic structure, thus widening their magical power over these other groups. This dynamic allows them to resist potentially disruptive influences. Even though new forms may be introduced, the traditional content prevails and continues to respond to their cultural specificity. This strategy was used first in order to achieve a synthesis of highland and lowland cultures, later to resolve the contradiction between Indian and Spanish cultures, and currently to confront the national society with its diverse manifestations of popular culture.

The importance of the lowland shamanic systems for highland cultures of Colombia has been documented by various scholars. Reichel-Dolmatoff (1975) investigates manifestations of the lowland shaman jaguar complex among the precolumbian Muisca (Chibcha) of the highlands, as well as its presence in extant highland groups (Paez and Kogi) and those of the Pacific lowlands. In particular, southwestern Colombia is indicated as an important area for such migrations, although extensive archaeological research is lacking for the Putumayo and Caqueta river basins. In his study on coca, Henman (1981) discusses the probability of the upper Magdalena river basin of Cauca as an entrance for lowland cultures. He calls attention to the fact that the first formative groups of the Cauca region must have entered from the western and eastern lowlands around 700 to 200 B.C. During this period, a group known for its large painted tombs established itself on the eastern slope of the central chain of the Andes. The vivid geometric designs in these tombs have close parallels with those made by Amazonian Indians using hallucinogens. He speculates that, as in the case of Peru, the introduction of coca among the early agricultural groups of the upper Magdalena came from the Amazonian lowlands (Henman 1981, 48).

The Sibundoy Valley is quite likely another important migratory pathway. It is located in the northwestern end of the Putumayo Intendencia, known as the Upper Putumayo, a mountainous zone in the Andean chain. A semitropical, humid valley, its altitude ranges between 2,000 and 2,500 meters above sea level, with surrounding peaks of 3,000 to 3,500 meters. The valley forms a passage between the highlands and lowlands, giving it importance as a strategic intermediate location in migrations. In addition, the intermediate position of the valley has important implications for the role of Sibundoy shamans in the southwestern cultural region of Colombia, particularly in popular medicine.

Two Indian groups occupy the Sibundoy Valley: the Kamsá, whose linguistic affiliation is not satisfactorily established, and the Inga, speaking a Quechua dialect. According to the 1980 calculations of the División de Asuntos Indígenas (Indian Affairs Division) 4,000 Inga, and 4,419 Kamsá occupy the valley, along with approximately 12,000 whites (Zambrano 1985). The Indians inhabit primarily the rural areas, while ninety percent of the white population lives in the four townships along the road linking the valley to Mocoa in the lowlands and to Pasto in the highlands. Most of the Inga live near the townships of Santiago, Colón, and San Andrés, while the Kamsá are nearest Sibundoy. Even though these two groups recognize each other as different, they in fact become one by sharing various cultural traits without losing their individual ethnic identities. Because of this common ground, particularly in the shamanic system, we shall refer to both groups as the Sibundoy, considering them together. When necessary their individual designations will be used.

SHAMANISM AND YAGÉ

The Sibundoy shamanic system has been investigated by both anthropologists and ethnobotanists (Bristol 1964, 1966a, 1966b, 1968, 1969; Langdon 1991; Langdon and MacLennan 1979; Seijas 1969a, 1969b; Taussig 1980a). The primary role of the shaman is to cure illnesses and other misfortunes believed to be mystically caused. Although there are other health practitioners in the valley representing both scientific and popular medicine, the Sibundoy shaman is the only one believed capable of curing diseases originating from mystical causes. As a consequence, the shaman has been important in maintaining the Sibundoy worldview as well as ethnic identity.

Sibundoy shamanic practices are inseparable from *yagé* (*Banisteriopsis* sp.), a jungle hallucinogenic plant.[2] When a Sibundoy shaman discusses his conceptions of the world, he will affirm that they are learned only under the effects of *yagé*.[3] *Yagé* leads to a transcendental experience of comprehension of the world's essence. This is not gained through simple ingestion. A long training process must accompany it, enabling the contents of the experience to be handled and deciphered. As one of our shaman informants states:

> *Yagé* is a force that has power, will, and knowledge; with it we can reach the stars, enter the spirit of other people, know their desire to do good or bad; we can foresee the future of ours and others' lives, see illnesses and cure them, and with it we can travel to heaven or hell.

The process of becoming a shaman entails exhaustive training that demands courage, decisiveness, and above all, mental stability: repetitive intakes of *yagé* may lead one to lose mental equilibrium due to the multiple realities that must be managed simultaneously. The hallucinogenic journey requires the handling of emotional conflicts, repressed emotions, past affections, and all kinds of fantasies and visions as one acquires a greater understanding of the world.

The initiation and learning process generally lasts from four to six years. The first step consists of knowing the *Yagé* Spirit and its predisposition toward the novice. If the *Yagé* Spirit accepts the novice, a master shaman begins his training.[4] The first ceremonial contact with *yagé* requires a special preparation called *andaki*. It differs from others in the use of *Borrachero* flowers as an additive (identified as *Datura Andrés* by Bristol [1969]).

After four to six years have passed and the novice has ingested many varieties of *yagé*, experiencing the basic repertoire of sacred visions, the master shaman awards him with instruments and signs corresponding to the hierarchy of acquired knowledge. The first awarded is the *pichanga*, a whisk of dry leaves; then follows a small feather crown, which signifies that the novice can now fly with his thoughts, as birds do, and that he has traveled to heaven. Subsequently, he continues adding more bead strings to his necklace. The greater number of beaded strings and the greater variety of colors signify his status as shaman, since they represent the number of trips taken in each color of *yagé* visions. Later he receives a quartz crystal, implying that he has become a "Thunder Shaman." As of this moment, knowledge becomes a matter of perfection and the most visible symbols of prestige are strings of jaguar, bear, and tapir teeth, as well as the number of feathers added to the crown (fig. 12.1).

The decisive test in the passage to master shaman occurs when the apprentice confronts and endures the same number of uninterrupted *yagé* ingestions as his master. This ceremony is held during the full moon, after four days of fasting and sexual abstinence. The ritual is generally performed after the master shaman has tested the apprentice's healing powers on his patients, covering the entire range of diseases from the most benign to the most serious.

The Sibundoy shamans have various ways of preparing *yagé* in order to alter the nature of the visions. Three species of *Banisteriopsis* used by the Sibundoy have been identified as *B. caapi*, *B. inebrians*, and *B. rusbiana* (Bristol 1966b). Gates (1982) has reclassified *B. rusbiana* as *Diplopterys* Malpighiacae. Ethnobotanical and ethnochemical research has demonstrated that all the known species of *Banisteriopsis* require an additive to

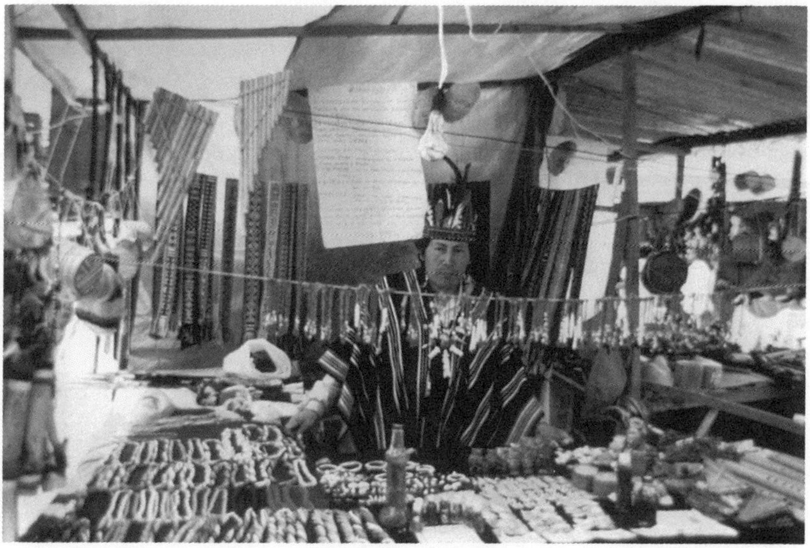

FIGURE 12.1. An Inga shaman in his stand of botanical remedies at a Bogotá trade show. Similar stands are found in various localities of Colombia.

activate the chemical compounds. Although the jungle groups, such as the Siona, tend to rely most heavily of *Diplopterys* Malpighiaceae and other additives to vary the visions, the Sibundoy appear to rely more on *Datura*. According to one shaman, it is the addition of *Datura* that introduces variations in the visions, and also "there's a type of *Borrachero* to mix with the *yagé* and cause the *pinta* (hallucinogenic episode) that is desired, *yagé* by itself does not produce fine *pintas*." The Sibundoy employ *Datura candida, D. sanguinea,* and *D. Andrés* (Bristol 1969).

ETHNOHISTORY AND SHAMANISM

The Kamsá and the Inga have a common origin. Both come from the south, possibly from Peru and the lowland jungles. The most accepted theory is that the valley was first conquered by the Kamsá. Shortly before the Spanish conquest, the Quillacinga followed a route on the eastern side of the Andean slopes and crossed the Sibundoy Valley before settling in northeastern Nariño (Groot et al. 1976, 162). Ethnohistorians and archaeologists suggest that the Kamsá are related to the Quillacinga and probably were part of the migration.

The Inga had not arrived in the Sibundoy Valley before the sixteenth century (Romoli 1978, 16). It is suggested that they might have migrated from the Peruvian tropical rain forest across the eastern flank of the Andes, reaching Colombia through the San Miguel River (Friedemann and Arocha 1982, 108).

Seijas (1969a) and Taussig (1980a) assert that the Sibundoy established their role as intermediaries between the highlands and lowlands before the conquest and that they maintained this role throughout the colonial period. According to archaeologists and ethnobotanists, medicinal plants were an important commercial item. Frank Solomon cites studies that make it possible to date commercial links as early as 400 B.C. (in Taussig 1980a, 291). Seijas (1969a, 71–72) states that active commerce was carried out during the eighteenth century between Pasto and the valley. Among other things, the Indians traded the jungle resin to make the famous Pasto *verniz.* Medicinal plants continue to be an important commercial item, and their trade is maintained by the Inga of the valley, particularly those from Santiago.

Of course this trade has always included more than medicinal plants. Shamanic healing rituals passed along the trade routes (Langdon 1981), as lowland shamans journeyed to the highlands to demonstrate their powers. Taussig (1980a, 231) affirms that tropical forest master shamans continue to receive great respect from highland Andean healers. The Sibundoy shamans form part of this important network of healing. In the past, they journeyed to the lowlands to contact the Siona and Kofan, two groups famous for their curing powers. There they were taught the use and preparation of the jungle *yagé,* as well as the use and preparation of other medicinal herbs. They were trained and initiated as shamans, and they returned to the valley with *yagé* to continue their shamanic practices.

Today the Sibundoy obtain *yagé* from the Inga in Yunguillo in the lowlands. They also treat whites from many parts of Colombia who journey to the valley seeking cures. Many Inga and some Kamsá travel farther into the highlands and to the lowlands of the Choco, as well as to some of the major Colombian cities to sell herbs and perform cures with *yagé.*

Given that trade in general, and in particular that of medicinal plants, has been important since ancient times, and taking into account that it is the Inga who continue to maintain the trading tradition, we posit the Inga as a hypothetical link between the lowland and highland. It should also be noted that the Quechua language was the lingua geral at the time of the conquest, allowing them to dominate the region and relate to the various indigenous groups.

The Spanish arrived in Sibundoy in 1542 and began a deculturation process that still continues. This "Christianization" was initially undertaken by the Franciscans. The Dominicans arrived in 1577, to be followed by mercenaries, Augustinians, and Jesuits. In 1893 the Capuchins began their ecclesiastic hegemony, which lasted until 1969 and their replacement by the Redemptorists (Bonilla 1972).

The four-century ideological domination is noticeable in Sibundoy oral tradition, which records discontinuously the relevant events and people from within and without native culture. Such histories demonstrate a mediation strategy that clings to historic events by coupling and solving the contradictions and influences that have threatened their ethnic identity. For instance, the elderly recall Carlos Tamoabioy, an eighteenth-century governor, as a mythological hero whose dying wish allowed the Indians to recover ownership of their land. He is referred to as Saint Carlos Tamoabioy. From the opposing culture, Fray Bartolomé de Igualada, a missionary working in the area during the early part of the twentieth century, has become a legendary character, highly respected and remembered for his participation in *yagé* ceremonies with the Indians. He accumulated enough shamanic knowledge to reach the sacred Patascoy summit, although the spirit dwelling in the mine there prohibited him from entering.

Thus, a member of their own culture, such as Carlos Tamoabioy, is magnified by a Catholic title, though in fact he was central in the struggle against the Church for recovery of native land. The contradiction between Christian religion and shamanic cosmovision is resolved by veneration of Fray Bartolomé as protector of the Indians, honored for his ingestion of *yagé.* However, native superiority is maintained, since he lacks the full shamanic power necessary to complete his journey to the sacred mine. Both cases show how the mechanism of mediation resolves the contradictions and domination from outsiders by means of magical power. Past events are raised to the mythic level and reinterpreted according to the native worldview.

We can also see that Catholic categories are similarly incorporated and reinterpreted into the shamanic system. Notions such as heaven and hell, not part of the native ideology, have been integrated and now exceed the limits they have in Christian doctrine. Evangelistic efforts are thus transformed into forces and representations that strengthen the shaman's power. As a result of the shamans' active trade participation, the shamanic system constitutes an open system, as Langdon has pointed out in shamanic treatment of disease (Langdon 1979b; 1991, 48). Rather than negating Western medicine or opposing its use, the shamans incorporate both pharmaceutical and medicinal herbs in their cures. In this way, both objects and liturgical symbols become part of the healing rituals and are used as instruments of shamanic power.

In the following, we offer additional examples of the incorporation of foreign elements into native categories. One Kamsá shaman tells us about his experience of ascending to the sky after ingesting *Cielohuasca,* "Heaven Yagé."

> I've flown up to heaven where there are benches, just like those we have here. There were a lot of remedies, as well as a man standing in the entrance, who might have been a saint. He came out while I was looking at him and asked, "Why have you come here?" I told him, "Well, I've just come here to visit, that's all." He replied, "It isn't time for you to come here. It seems to me that you know many remedies. There are many here and you can choose what you want. Come." He showed me the whole garden divided into big and small sections where there were all kinds of remedies. He collected some and gave them to me to bring and plant here on earth. In heaven our Lord sits as if enclosed in a cupboard surrounded by genuine crystal.

Yagé permits the shaman to travel wherever he wants, to meet and dominate those supernatural forces spoken of by the missionaries. On arrival, that heaven reflects the areas most significant for the expression of their social relations and magical power. The benches found in heaven and in shamans' houses are such an example. Through them circulate the oppositions of male/female, crystallizing in symbolic form the system of social organization. On the other hand, the shaman's garden with its medicinal and magical plants synthesizes the notion of the power of activity and movement. The Christian representations, such as the enclosed God, appear inactive and static.

Within the temporal category the conceptions of Catholicism and shamanism are mediated through the hallucinogenic ritual. For instance in the shaman's initiation ritual, he "travels to heaven." In this journey, the categories of Christianity are recognized, but only within the Sibundoy temporal category where it is possible to relive primordial time. Shamanic journeys with the aid of hallucinogens link the supernatural and ordinary world, contradicting Church dogma in which such a trip is reserved for those who have died. In the above vision, the man's comment that it is not time for the shaman to be in heaven is a reference that it is not his time to die; however, he gives the shaman further power and knowledge before his return to earth. The rupture of sacred and profane time disappears in the shamanic ritual where the shaman functions as mediator between the supernatural and real worlds. This mediation function is the foundation and support of shamanic activities.

The blending of the sacred and profane in shamanic journeys is evident in another shaman's description of the initiate's journey. He says the *Brugmansia* flowers take the initiated up to heaven, after first running through his body and irrigating it with his ancestors' blood, which is the quintessence of the sun's blood. This very first trip through the supernatural world must reveal its essential nature to the initiated, a nature that appears as a fluid world of images and rotating webs within webs in the same way one constellation enters another. This continuum of images is accompanied by choirs singing to the world's first dawn. Next the initiate begins an ascent to heaven. The shaman described this as an entrance to a great moving garden, whose image is seen in the distance. Farther off, floating churches lift off into flight; their bells are the flowers of heaven, and a cascade of polychromatic patterns, each one with its own sound, descends to earth.

In the same way that Heaven *Yagé* permits contact with the Christian religious domains, it is under *Intihuasca,* "Sun Yagé," that shamans relive their origin myth. The shaman establishes contact with the creators of color and sound, and with the Solar Men. The latter appear as midgets radiating a golden light and singing beautiful chants accompanied by flutes and drums as they descend with the *yagé* vine from heaven to earth. The ancestors tell about primeval times when the whole world was in darkness. It was already inhabited by all beings, including humans who lacked intelligence. The humans wandered throughout the earth in search of food when they stumbled onto the *yagé* vine. They cut it into portions; one was given to the women to try, and their menstruation began. The men tried another and became ecstatic when they saw how the remaining piece of *yagé* began to grow and to creep up to heaven. At the same time, shadows formed and their silhouettes glittered. In the depth of heaven, they saw *yagé* penetrate a huge flower that became the sun as it was fertilized. From there the Solar Men descended. Each one played a distinctive melody with his flute or drum, and each melody transformed into a different color. When they arrived on earth they dispersed, depositing light and color to each being there. When the world was illuminated, all this symphony of colors and music brought forth understanding to humankind, creating intelligence and language. *Yagé* has been used ever since by shamans to see the world as it really is, and to make everything clear and harmonious for the *curaca*'s spirit.

The hallucinogenic ritual fulfills two essential functions. First, it mediates a contact situation in favor of mythic categories and indigenous procedures. Second, it allows the reconstruction and reaffirmation of a worldview, much as Langdon (1979a, 85) has asserted for the Siona: "The Siona worldview derives much of its authority from the renewal and reaffirmation given to it by the ritual. Without the authoritative experience of the ritual, the system as an ordered whole will not persist in the face of increasing contact with Western culture."

The ethnic identity of the Sibundoy is a continuous affirmation intimately related to the blood's tenor, which renews itself in the *yagé* ritual. It is through this primeval myth, relived in the ritual, that a mediating model is generated to explain the separation of nature and culture, man and woman. The model establishes the dynamic of oppositions, and thus, those of the mediations that mark the dialectic. It is in primordial time that Man as a generic being finds *yagé* and experiences the mythic episode establishing sex differences. Women menstruate as they contact *yagé,* whereas the descent of the Solar Men colors the world and gives birth to intelligence and language. Thus, the opposites are established. Masculinity is linked to intelligence, to order, to culture, and to the spirit through the plant of highest importance. Femininity is linked to nature, to disorder, and to the body by means of the notion of animality.

This model is crystallized through the ritual manipulation of oppositions derived from the primary one of man/woman. Following these we have:

man	woman
culture	nature
right	left
even	odd
fermented corn	cooked corn
form	content
image	substance

The opposites are dynamic and become relativized depending on the real and immediate context. For example, when men meet to drink "chicha" (fermented corn beer), lower status males occupy the place of women; during pregnancy, women represent order because the fetus represents new life and perpetuation of social order. Female categories can be applied to a man, such as a sorcerer who represents disorder and death. His rituals involve the use of odd numbers and distribution on the left side. During the hallucinogenic ritual, the shaman is able to establish a transformative dialectic from that of masculinity and spirit to that of femininity and animality. Such occurs when he changes into the Jaguar Mother, establishing mediation and synthesis between such opposites.

In the same way, there are constant parameters that identify men and women in daily life. The Sibundoy display them on the forehead as a color spectrum whose intensity depends on two factors: age and the number of hallucinogenic trips realized. This, in its turn, defines gender and status within the group: nonpregnant and nonmenstruating women can be placed in the male category, and those men whose *pinta* (paint color) in the blood has been robbed by sorcery can be placed in the category of female.

THE SHAMANIC GARDEN

The Sibundoy world arises from the dominion over plants, and it invariably returns to them. The importance of plants is present in all social spheres. From birth to death, plants appear as revealers of the philosophic and supernatural background, used to determine or counteract destiny or to assist the passing of a diseased person's soul to the other world. With children, plants counter deadly influences and help them to enter the realm of culture through rites of passage. *Yagé* is the highest force over all plants and life contradictions. It initiates, activates, and allows the shaman to possess the power of the spirit.

Cultivation of magical and medicinal plants is a specialized knowledge and may be performed only by men. A garden should be fenced so that women cannot enter or touch the plants. This prohibition is related to the function and character of medicinal and magical plants. The forces that inhabit them are supernatural and consequently belong to the masculine sequence of life and spirit. The shaman has his plot of healing plants near the house where *yagé* is prepared. As one shaman explains, "Magical and medicinal plants are like human beings; they must live where they belong. They shouldn't mix with the cultivation of other plants, for they curtail one another. The spiritual force of remedies cannot be mixed with food. When we take remedies, we maintain a diet. The jungle's spirit and the earth's are like this. Each one has its head in its place, and likewise do all the parts of the body."

The garden of medicinal and magical plants is a microcosm containing the basic elements of the mythic world, as well as its animating forces. Gardens also have their guardians, which can be the forces of thunder and lightning or Catholic saints such as Saint Ciprianus. If one enters a garden without permission, one risks attack.

Plants are generally arranged by species. Foremost are the *Borracheros, Datura candida,* and *D. sanguinea,* of which Bristol has found ten and two varieties, respectively. They are used for treatment of illness: *Macan Borrachero* (*Iresine celocial*) is an anti-inflammatory, antirheumatic, menstrual regulator, and magical treatment; *Orejón Borrachero* (*Iresine rigens*) is used to remove evil and as a contraceptive. *Borracheros* potentiate and increase sensory capacities. The *Daturas* correspond to the classes of *yagé,* since the Sibundoy differentiate three genera of each. In both, the three genera represent animals, the sun, and thunder.

The *Cullaguillos* are in the second rank. These include *Cullaguillo Juá (Peperomia galioides)* and *Vinan* (*Pepermos* sp.), with its subvarieties of *Tausaivinan* and *Condorvian.* In general they have magical powers to prevent witchcraft, to seal the body, to attract people, and to impart wisdom.

The *Chondores* are in the third rank. *Cucochondor* withdraws evil spirits and prevents evil from penetrating. *Tigrechondor* and *Aichachondor* aid in animal reproduction, giving abundant offspring. *Frescochondor* is used for fever. *Guarmechondor* is for conquering women, and *Carechondor* for conquering men. *Cullanguillos* and *Chondores* are men and women and always go in pairs.

Medicinal plants used to resolve the illnesses or problems of whites are cultivated apart in order to separate them from the power of indigenous plants, and symbolically, to avoid confusion of ethnic identities. Native herbs "paint" the blood, whereas foreign plants, even though grown by Indians, do not have that quality. Their range of magical power is lower and purely functional, in the sense that they attract or expel spirits or the witchcraft of whites, generally considered inferior magical forces.

SHAMANISM AND POPULAR CULTURE

In general, both the highland and lowland Indian groups have undergone a progressive disintegration. They are increasingly isolated in miserable conditions in *resguardos* (reservations), or work as servants and laborers. Nevertheless, it is within the Sibundoy Valley, and specifically within the shamanic system, that we best observe a capacity for adaptation to the market-based class society.

Whereas the Sibundoy formerly depended on the lowland Amazonian groups for their acquisition of ritual knowledge and ceremonial careers, they have nearly liberated themselves from these teachers. Today, the Sibundoy Valley is a center of synthesis of native wisdom regarding the cosmos, nature, healing, and shamanic power. This is most evident in the shamanic gardens, laboratories of experiment and adaptation for plants from all over the country. In addition, their reputation as powerful shamans has increased as the lowland shamans have decreased in number. Many whites journey from other parts of Colombia for their magical cures, and Sibundoy shamans, particularly the Inga, make trips into the highlands and large cities as far as Venezuela.

Taussig (1980a) has argued that the reputation of the Sibundoy as great shamans has increased as the Amazonian groups have faced cultural deterioration and as the tensions between ethnic and class groups have increased. He attributes this to the economics of the sugarcane industry in the Cauca Valley. Thus, the Sibundoy have infiltrated as the mediators of interethnic conflicts. They continue to use hallucinogens in these healing rites, manipulating the visionary experience to allow the whites and others to interpret problems in terms of their own cosmogonic codes. In particular, one of the manners by which popular culture interprets illness and misfortune is through sorcery. Further, the effects of ethnic and class struggles have been interpreted within the causal framework of sorcery.

The increase in social conflicts is not limited to those regions affected by the sugarcane industry, but marks all areas of this developing country. With this, a wide network of healers throughout the country has established itself, creating a popular medical system that draws from prehispanic Indian knowledge, as well as from esoteric Afro-Caribbean cults, and European and North American witchcraft traditions (Pinzón and Suárez 1983). In Bogotá, where tensions have significantly increased in the last ten years, an exceptional variety of healers now flourishes. The variety of techniques and kinds of healers has been described by Press (1971). Although he found no Indian healers in Bogotá, the fame of Indian power and certain techniques, said to be learned from a shaman, were incorporated into the healing repertoires of several curers. Following Press, psychologists Rosa Suárez and Carlos Pinzón began a similar investigation of urban healers. During the first five years, they detected seventy types of different curers, although none had learned his duties from a shaman. In 1978, they finally discovered a Sibundoy shaman who was the son of one of the most famous Kamsá shamans in the valley. He was at that time training a curer from Boyacá, and he invited the investigators to begin the shamanic apprenticeship with him.

From the beginning of the apprenticeship, the shaman was emphatic in affirming that a non-Sibundoy could never become as knowledgeable as the Indians, for they learn about shamanism and how to "paint the blood" practically from birth. This particular shaman began at the age of five, when his maternal grandfather began to instruct him in *yagé,* the ritual chants, and plant lore. He claimed he had taught healers from different parts of the country, but that the rituals were different because it is the *Yagé* Spirit that determines, through visions, the point at which each individual can acquire supernatural wisdom. He said in addition, the novice must renounce any sorcery and divination techniques alien to the *yagé* tradition. According to him, no white healer had ever complied with this, and thus none had attained all that *yagé* had to offer. Two years after initiating his training, the Boyacán curer decided it was not necessary to take *yagé* so continually.

The psychologists investigated the differences in perception that the patients held toward the shaman and toward the healer, as well as the shaman's and healer's perceptions of each other. Eighty percent of the patients who consulted the Sibundoy shaman stated that his sorcery was more powerful than the others', since he made them "see," through *yagé* visions, how the harm was caused and who had caused it. In addition, they felt they could know about their futures, and that they had learned how to feel others' energy. They also affirmed that if they needed a healing again, they would do so with *yagé,* since in that way they would know what was happening to them or what might happen. This would prevent them from falling into charlatans' hands (who make up any kind of story just to steal their money). Twenty percent of the patients stated that they would not take *yagé* again since it caused very unpleasant sensations. They also said the Sibundoy shaman was an evil sorcerer, since they had seen demons and black witchcraft in the visions. The patients of the Boyacán healer stated that they understood better what he does and his manner of performing rituals. They felt him to be more accurate than Indians in solving marriage problems, because he knew whether they were actually resolvable. The Indians always promised to solve such problems and failed many times.

The shaman perceived the Boyacán healer as stubborn for insisting on the use of divination techniques, and he objected to the Boyacán's life-style. On the other hand, the Boyacán affirmed that the Sibundoy was efficient in curing magical spells but limited in dealing with other kinds of magic, illnesses, and domestic problems. He also perceived the shaman as very domineering.

After seven years of research with two thousand patients who have sought the Sibundoy's treatments, our conclusion is that each patient centers his beliefs and values within the experience of *yagé* visions. According to them, the shaman's power consists of "projecting us towards our supernatural world." It is because of this that we believe the Sibundoy shaman plays a "mirror-like" role among the popular classes (in the sense of Lacan), which permits reconstruction or affirmation of identity in reference to the total opposition of "the other."

This relation is made clearer by comparison of the learning process a Sibundoy receives from his shaman and that which a non-Indian receives from the shaman. In the first instance, they share similar beliefs in the world's origins, they experience all of the *pintas* (colors) in the rainbow, which are linked to the cosmos, to ecology, and to the animal allies and their power. This is in order to construct a "total image of the world" and to "imprint it in the blood." During the final test, when the novice is challenged to drink as much *yagé* as his master shaman, the color white, in the form of an animal, appears at the end of the session to confirm that the novice dominates "all levels of form as well as all visions of color." When the novice belongs to another ethnic group, the final test is never administered, for the shaman considers it obvious that the novice cannot reach the master's superiority. Also, the non-Indian is never obligated to learn the language, even though the use of chants and use of ceremonial garments are perceived as signs of power (Taussig 1980a).

The capacity to recognize the supernatural world in the *yagé* visions has awakened cultural forces that lie in the unconscious of the popular classes. In this sense, the Sibundoy have succeeded in returning the foundations of popular culture, and in inverting them as well.

> The structure of ideas and sentiments created by the Spanish conquest of the New World in the sixteenth century, pertaining to the ideology of cast and class relations lives on today as an active force. Folk healing sustains this structure of ideas. . . The evil and magic invested in the exploited people, essential to the colonial hegemony, become the means by which the colonizer seeks release from the civilization which assails him (Taussig 1980a, 251).

We are in agreement with Taussig as we continue with our research on popular culture and urban healers. Since meeting the first Sibundoy in Bogotá seven years ago, we have met several of his apprentices. We have also met several Inga shamans who are also teaching urban healers, and healers of various popular religions who include the ingestion of *yagé* as part of their ceremonial repertoires. Beyond the whole of Colombia, the ingestion of *yagé* has extended to Venezuela, Panama, and the United States. In Brazil, Peru, and Bolivia it has generated a religion of its own.

What is true is that a popular culture based on hallucinogens begins to unite threads that were loosened during the colonial period, spreading to all of Latin America and the Antilles. Because of this, we consider important the study of popular culture and its relationships with hallucinogens in the formation of a new Latin American identity.

Notes

1. This research was done during 1985 under the auspices of the Instituto Colombiano de Antropología—ICAN—(Colombian Institute of Anthropology). Fieldwork, secondary data, and interviews with Kamsá and Inga informants since 1977 have been our main sources.

2. Malpighiaceae family, genus *Banisteriopsis,* containing harmine, harmaline, and d-tetrahydroharmine as active ingredients (Schultes 1972, 38).

3. Shaman is the name (concept) that anthropologists designate for the native terms *Curaca* or *Taita;* these three denominations will be utilized at random to denote the expert who manages and controls supernatural, magical, or religious forces. He is also a botanical medicine man.

4. The shaman is a master shaman when he has complied with all rituals of initiation, the apprenticeship process, and the final decisive step; he also must have fifteen to twenty years of demonstrated experience in the community.

BIBLIOGRAPHY

ADAMS, PATRICIA

1962 Textos culina. *Folklore Americano* 10: 93–222.

1963 Some notes on the material culture of the Culina Indians. *Anthropológica* 12: 27–44.

1971 La cultura del grupo idiomático culina. Lima, Perú: Institute Lingüístico de Verano.

1976 Cerámica culina. *Cummunidades y Culturas Peruanas* 7. Lima, Perú: Instituto Lingüístico de Verano.

ALTSCHUL, SIRI VON REIS

1972 *The genus* Anadenanthera *in Amerindian cultures.* Cambridge: Botanical Museum of Harvard University.

AMÉRICA INDÍGENA

1986 Chamanismo e etnobotánica en la cuenca Amazónica. Edición especial 46 (1).

ANDRITZKY, WALTER

1989 Sociopsychotherapeutic functions of *ayahuasca* healing in Amazonia. *Journal of Psychoactive Drugs* 21 (1): 77–89.

D'ANGLURE, BERNARD SALADINO

1986 Du foetus au chamane: la construction d'un "troisième sex inuit." *Etudes Inuit/Studies* 10 (1–2): 25–113.

ARBMANN, ERNS

1931 Seele und Mana. *Archiv für Religionswissenschaft* 29: 293–394. Berlin.

ARDITTI, JOSEPH, AND ELOY RODRIGUEZ

1982 Dieffenbachia: Uses, abuses and toxic constituents: A review. *Journal of Ethnopharmacology* 5: 293–302.

ARENAS, P., AND J. BRAUNSTEIN

1981 Plantas y animales empleados en paquetes y otras formas de la magia amorosa entre los Toba *takšek. Parodiana* 1 (1): 149–69. Argentina.

ARÉVALO VALERA, GUILLERMO

1986 El *ayahuasca* y el curandero Shipibo-Conibo del Ucayali (Perú). *América Indígena* 46 (1): 147–61.

ARQUIVO DO AMAZONAS (AA)

1907 Revista destinada à vulgarisação de documentos geográficos e históricos do estado do Amazonas, vols. 1 and 2, nos. 2–7. Edited by Bento de Figueiredo Tenheiro Aranha.

ARQUIVO HISTÓRICO NACIONAL (AHN), Rio de Janeiro

1858 *Relatório do juiz municipal e delegado da polícia da capital do Amazonas (Marcos Antônio Rodrigues de Souza) apresentado ao Presidente da Província em 8 de setembro de 1858.* Ofícios do Ministério da Justiça. (unpublished).

AUSTIN, J.

1962 *How to do things with words.* Oxford: Clarendon.

AVÉ-LALLEMANT, ROBERT

1860 *Reise dürch Nordbrasilien im Jahre 1859.* Leipzig.

BAER, GERHARD

1982 Social aspects of the South American shaman. Paper presented at the 44th International Congress of Americanists, September, Manchester, England.

1984 *Die Religion der Matsigenka (Ost-Peru): Monographie zur Kultur und Religion eines Indianervolkes am Oberen Amazonas.* Basel: Wepf.

BAER, GERHARD, AND WAYNE W. SNELL

1974 An *ayahuasca* ceremony among the Matsigenka (eastern Peru). *Zeitschr. für Ethnologie* 99 (1/2): 64–80. Braunschweig.

BALL. J. VAN, AND W. E. A. VAN BEEK

1985 *Symbols for communcation.* Netherlands: van Gorcum.

BARTOLOMÉ, MIGUEL

1977 *Shamanismo y religión entre los Ava-katú-eté del Paraguay.* Mexico City: Instituto Indigenista Interamericano, Serie Antropología Social no. 17.

BASSO, ELLEN

1985 *A musical view of the universe: Kalapalo narratives and ritual performance.* Philadelphia: University of Pennsylvania Press.

BASTIDE, R.

1976 *El sueño, el trance y la locura.* Buenos Aires: Amorrortu.

BAUMAN, RICHARD

1977 *Verbal art as performance.* Rowley, Mass.: Newbury House.

BELLIER, IRÈNE

1986 Los cantos mai Huna del *yajé* (Amazonía Peruana). *América Indígena* 46 (1): 129–45.

BETTS, LAVERA

1967 Anthropological checklist. Report for the Summer Institute of Linguistics Technical Studies Department. Brasília: Instituto Lingüístico do Verão. Typescript.

BIDOU, PATRICE, AND MICHEL PERRIN (EDITORS)

1988 *Lenguaje y palabras chamánicas.* Quito, Ecuador: Ediciones ABYA-YALA.

BONILLA, VICTOR DANIEL

1972 *Servants of God or masters of men.* London: Penguin.

BOGORAZ, WALDEMAR G.

1904 *The Chukchee. Memoirs of the American Museum of Natural History,* vol. 16. New York: G. E. Stechert.

BOURDIEU, PIERRE

1977 *Outline of a theory of practice.* Translated by Richard Nice. New York: Cambridge University Press.

BRAUNSTEIN, J.

1981 Notas etnográficas de los Toba *takšek*: Introducción. *Entregas del Instituto Tilcara,* vol. 10. Buenos Aires: Universidad de Buenos Aires.

1983 Algunos rasgos de la organización social de los indígenas del Gran Chaco. *Trabajos de Etnología,* no. 2. Buenos Aires: Universidad de Buenos Aires, Facultad de Filosofía y Letras.

BRISTOL, MELVIN

1964 Philoglossa, a cultivar of the Sibundoy, Colombia. *Botanical Museum Leaflets* 21 (5). Cambridge: Harvard University.

1966a Notes on the species of tree Daturas. *Botanical Museum Leaflets* 21 (8). Cambridge: Harvard University.

1966b The psychotropic *Banisteriopsis* among the Sibundoy of Colombia. *Botanical Museum Leaflets* 21 (5). Cambridge: Harvard University.

1968 Sibundoy agriculture. *Actas y Memorias del XXXVII Congreso Internacional de Americanistas* 2: 575–602. Buenos Aires.

1969 Tree Datura drugs of the Colombian Sibundoy. *Botanical Museum Leaflets* 22 (5). Cambridge: Harvard University.

BROWN, MICHAEL

1984 The role of words in Aguaruna hunting magic. *American Ethnologist* 11 (3): 545–58.

1985 *Tsewa's gift: Magic and meaning in an Amazonian society.* Washington, D.C.: Smithsonian Institution Press.

BUCHILLET, DOMINIQUE

1983 Maladie et mémoire des origines chez les Desana du Uaupés brésilien. Thèse de doctorat de 3ème cycle, Université de Paris-X Nanterre.

BUCKWALTER, A.

1980 *Vocabulario Toba.* Buenos Aires: Talleres Gráficos Gracharoff.

BUENO, FRAY RAMON

[1800] 1965 *Tratado histórico y diario de Fray Ramon Bueno, misionero de Orinoco.* Fuentes para la Historia Colonial de Venezuela, no. 78. Caracas: Biblioteca de la Academia Nacional de Historia.

BUTT, AUDREY

1965–66 The shaman's legal role. *Revista do Museu Paulista, Nova Série,* 16: 151–86. São Paulo.

BUTT COLSON, AUDREY

1977 The Akawaio shaman. In *Carib-speaking Indians: Culture, society, and language,* edited by E. B. Basso, 43–65. Anthropological Papers of the University of Arizona, no. 28. Tucson: University of Arizona Press.

CAILLOIS, ROGER

1964 Problemas del sueño. In *Los sueños y las sociedades humanas.* Coloquio de Royaumont. Buenos Aires: Ediciones Sudamericana.

CALVO, CÉSAR

1981 *Las tres mitades de Ino Moxo y otros brujos de la Amazonía.* Iquitos, Peru: Proceso Editores.

CAMARA CASCUDO, LUIS DA

1983 *Geografia dos mitos Brasileiros.* São Paulo: Editorial Itatiaia.

CARNEIRO DA CUNHA, MANUELA

1973 Logique du mythe et de l'action: Le mouvement messianique Canela de 1963. *L'Homme* 13 (4): 5–37.

CASTANEDA, CARLOS

1968 *The teachings of Don Juan: A Yaqui way of knowledge.* Berkeley: University of California Press.

CHAUMEIL, JEAN-PIERRE

1982 Représentation du monde d'un chaman Yagua. *L'Ethnografie* 88 (87–88) (2–3): 49–84.

1983 *Voir, savoir, pouvoir: le chamanism chez les Yagua du nord-est Péruvien.* Paris: Editions de l'Ecole de Hautes Etudes en Sciences Sociales.

CHERNELA, JANET

1983 Hierarchy and economy of the Uanano (Kotiria) speaking peoples of the middle Uaupés basin. Ph.D. diss., Columbia University, New York.

CHEVALIER, JACQUES M.

1982 *Civilization and the stolen gift: Capital, kin and cult in eastern Peru.* Toronto: University of Toronto Press.

CHIAPPE, MARIO, MOISÉS LEMLIJ, AND LUIS MILLONES

1985 *Alucinógenos y shamanismo en el Perú contemporáneo.* Lima: Ediciones El Virrey.

CORDEU, E.

1969–70 Aproximación al horizonte mítico de los Toba. *Runa* 12 (1–2): 67–176. Buenos Aires: Universidad de Buenos Aires, Facultad de Filosofía y Letras, Instituto de Ciencias Antropológicas.

CORDEU, E., AND J. A. BRAUNSTEIN

1974 Los "aparatos" de un shamán chamacoco: Contribución al estudio de la parafernalia shamánica. *Scripta Ethnológica,* no. 2, pt. 2: 121–39. Buenos Aires.

CORDEU, E., AND A. SIFFREDI

1971 *De la algarroba al algodón: Movimientos milenaristas del Chaco Argentino.* Buenos Aires: Juarez Editor.

CORRY, STEPHEN

1984 Cycles in dispossession: Amazon Indians and government in Peru. In *Genocide in Bangladesh, Indians and government in Peru, Indians and the world bank and other articles* 43 (1983): 45–70. London: Survival International Review.

CRAPANZANO, VINCENT, AND VIVIAN GARRISON

1980 *Case studies in spirit possession.* New York: John Wiley and Sons.

CROCKER, JON CHRISTOPHER

1985 *Vital souls: Bororo cosmology, natural symbolism, and shamanism.* Tucson: University of Arizona Press.

CROCKER, WILLIAM

1967 The Canela messianic movement: An introduction. In *Atas do Simpósio sobre a Biota Amazônica,* vol. 2, Antropologia, 69–83. Rio de Janeiro: Conselho Nacional de Pesquisas.

DE BARANDIARÁN, DANIEL

1962 Shamanismo Yecuana o Makiritare. *Antropológica* 11: 61–90. Caracas.

DEGARROD, LYDIA

1989 Dream interpretation among the Mapuche Indians of Chile. Ph.D. diss., University of California, Los Angeles.

DEVEREUX, GEORGES

1958 Cultural thought models in primitive and modern psychiatric theories. *Psychiatry* 21: 359–74.

1970 Normal et anormal. In *Essais d'ethnopsychiatrie générale.* (Bibliothèque de Sciences Humaines.) Paris: Gallimard.

1972 *Ethnopsychiatrie complémentariste.* (Nouvelle Bibliothèque Scientifique). Paris: Flammarion.

DOBKIN DE RIOS, MARLENE

1972 *Visionary vine: Psychedelic healing in the Peruvian Amazonas.* San Francisco: Chandler.

1976 *The wilderness of mind: Sacred plants in cross-cultural perspective.* Sage Research Papers in the Social Sciences, vol. 5. Beverly Hills, Calif.: Sage.

DOLGIN, JANET, DAVID S. KEMNITZER, AND DAVID M. SCHNEIDER (EDITORS)

1977 *Symbolic anthropology: A reader in the study of symbols and meanings.* New York: Columbia University Press.

DONNER, FLORINDA

1984 *Shabono.* London: Granada.

DOORE, GARY (EDITOR)

1988 *Shaman's path: Healing, personal growth, and empowerment.* Boston: Shamabala.

DOUGHERTY, JANET, AND CHARLES KELLER

1985 Taskonomy: A practical approach to knowledge structures. In *Directions in cognitive anthropology,* edited by Janet Dougherty, 161–74. Urbana: University of Illinois Press.

DOUGLAS, MARY

1966 *Purity and danger.* London: Routledge and Kegan Paul.

1973 *Natural symbols: Explorations in cosmology.* New York: Pantheon.

DRUMMOND, LEE

1981 The serpent's children: Semiotics of cultural genesis in Arawak and Trobriand myth. *American Ethnologist* 8 (3): 633–60.

DUCCI, Z.

1904 *Los Toba de Tacaaglé, Missión San Francisco Solano.* Buenos Aires: Impr. y Lit. La Buenos Aires.

DURKHEIM, EMILE

[1912] 1965 *Elementary forms of religious life.* New York: Free Press.

EGGAN, D.

1949 The significance of dreams for anthropological research. *American Anthropologist* 51: 177–98.

1964 Los sueños en la perspectiva cultural. In *Los sueños y las sociedades humanas.* Coloquio de Royaumont. Buenos Aires: Editores Sudamericana.

EIDLER, Y. I., G. L. GENKINA, AND T. T. SHAKIROV

1975 Quantitative determination of furocoumarins in *Ficus carica* leaves. *Khimiya Prirodnykh Soedineii* 3: 349–51.

ELGAMAL, M. H. A., B. A. H. EL-TAWIL, AND M. B. E. FAYEZ

1975 The triterpenoid constituents of the leaves of *Ficus nitida. Naturwissenschaften* 62: 486.

ELIADE, MIRCEA

1961 *Mitos, sueños y misterios: Relaciones mágicas en el universo del espíritu.* Buenos Aires: Cía Gral Fabril Editora.

[1951] 1964 *Shamanism: Archaic techniques of ecstasy.* Translated by Willard R. Trask. Princeton, N.J.: Princeton University Press and the Bollingen Foundation.

ELICK, JOHN W.

1969 An ethography of the Pichis Valley Campa of eastern Peru. Ph.D. diss., University of California, Los Angeles.

ESTRADA, ALVARO

1977 *Vida de María Sabina, la sabia de los hongos.* Mexico City: Siglo XXI.

EVANS, F. J., AND C. J. SOPER

1978 The *Tigliane Daphnane* and *Ingenane Diterpenes*: Their chemistry, distribution, and biological activities: A review. *Lloydia* 4: 193–233.

FABIAN, JOHANNES

1981 *Time and the other: How anthropology makes its object.* New York: Columbia University Press.

FARON, DOUGLAS
1964 *Hawks of the sun: Mapuche morality and its ritual attributes.* Pittsburgh: University of Pittsburgh Press.

FAUST, NORMAN
1973 *Lecciones para el aprendizaje del idioma Shipibo-Conibo.* Lima, Perú: Instituto Lingüístico de Verano.

FEELY-HARNIK, GILLIAN
1984 The political economy of death: Communication and change in Malagasy colonial history. *American Ethnologist* 11: 1–18.

FISCHER, HANS
1965 *Studien über Seelenvorstellungen in Ozeanien.* Munich: Klaus Renner.

FONTANIER, P.
1968 *Les figures du discours.* Paris: Flammarion.

FRAZER, JAMES
[1890] 1980 *The golden bough: A study in magic and religion.* London: Macmillan.

FREUD, SIGMUND
1948 La interpretación de los sueños. In *Obras completas,* vol. 1. Madrid: Biblioteca Nueva.
1958 *The complete works of Sigmund Freud.* Vol. 16, Introductory lectures on psychoanalysis, 1916, edited by J. Strachey. London: Hogarth.

FRIEDBERG, CLAUDINE
1965 Des *banisteriopsis* utilisés comme drogue en Amérique du sud: Essai d'etude critique. *Journal d'Agriculture Tropicale et de Botanique Appliquée* 12 (9–12).

FRIEDEMANN, NINA S. DE, AND JAIME AROCHA
1982 *Herederos del jaguar y la anaconda.* Bogotá: Carlos Valencia Editores.

FRIEDRICH, PAUL
1986 *The language parallax: Linguistic relativism and poetic indeterminancy.* Austin: University of Texas Press.

GALVÃO, EDUARDO
1955 *Santo e visagens: Um estudo da vida religiosa de Itá, Amazonas.* São Paulo: Companhia Editora Nacional.
1959 Aculturação indígena no Rio Negro. *Boletim do Museu Paraense Emilio Goeldi, Antropologia* 7: 1–60.

GATES, BRONWEN

1982 *A monograph of* Banisteriopsis *and* Diplopterys Malpighiaceae. New York: New York Botanical Garden.

GEBHART-SAYER, ANGELIKA

1985 The geometric designs of the Shipibo-Conibo in ritual context. *Journal of Latin American Lore* 11 (2): 143–75.

1986 Una terapia estética: Los diseños visionarios de *ayahuasca* entre los Shipibo-Conibo. *América Indígena* 46 (1): 189–218.

1987 *Die Spitze des Bewusstseins: Untersuchungen zu Weltbild und Kunst der Shipibo-Conibo.* Hohenscäftlarn: Klaus Renner.

GEERTZ, CLIFFORD

1966 Religion as a cultural system. In *Anthropological approaches to the study of religion,* monograph no. 3: 1–45. London: Tavistock.

1973a Religion as a cultural system. In *The interpretation of culture.* New York: Basic Books.

1973b Ethos, world view, and the analysis of sacred symbols. In *The interpretation of culture.* New York: Basic Books.

1984 Distinguished lecture: Anti anti-relativism. *American Anthropologist* 86 (2): 263–78.

GENNEP, ARNOLD VAN

1903 De l'emploi du mot "chamanisme." *Revue de l'Histoire des Religions* 47 (1) (24e année): 51–57.

1909 *Les rites de passage.* Paris: Emile Nourry.

1960 *The rites of passage.* Chicago: University of Chicago Press.

GILLEN, JOHN

1948 Magical Fright. *Psychiatry* 11: 387–400.

GOLDMAN, IRVING

1963 *The Cubeo: Indians of the northwest Amazon.* Urbana: University of Illinois Press.

GONZÁLEZ HOLGUÍN, DIEGO

1989 *Vocabulario de la lengua general de todo el Perú llamada lengua Quichua o del Inca.* Lima: Universidad Nacional Mayor de San Marcos. Facsimile of the 1952 edition.

GONZÁLEZ VIAÑA, EDUARDO

1979 *Habla, Sampedro: Llama a los brujos!* Barcelona: Editorial Argos y Vergara.

GRAHAM, LAURIE

1986 Three modes of Shavante vocal expression: Wailing, collective singing, and political oratory. In *Native South American discourse,* edited by Joel Sherzer and Greg Urban, 83–118. Amsterdam: Mouton de Gruyter.

GREGOR, THOMAS

1977 *Mehinaku.* Chicago: University of Chicago Press.

GRENAND, P.

1980 *Introduction à l'étude de univers Wayapi: Ethno-écologie des Indiens de haut Oyapock.* Paris: SELAF.

GROF, STANISLAV

1985 *Beyond the brain: Birth, death and transcendence in psychotherapy.* New York: State University of New York at Albany.

GROOT, ANA MARÍA, LUZ PIEDAD CORREA, AND EVA HOOYKAS

1976 Estudio etnohistórico y arqueológico de la zona andina nariñense con el fin de establecer los límites de ubicación de los grupos indígenas y los alcances geográficos de las incursiones del Imperio Incaico. *Investigación para FINARCO.* Bogotá: FINARCO, unpublished research report.

GRUNEBAUM, G. E. VON

1964 Introducción al coloquio de Royaumont. In *Los sueños y las sociedades humanas.* Buenos Aires: Ediciones Sudamericana.

GUSS, D. M.

1980 Steering for dream: Dream concepts of the Makiritáre. *Journal of Latin American Lore* 6 (2): 287–312.

HALIFAX, JOAN

1979 *Shamanic voices: A survey of visionary narratives,* New York: E. P. Dutton.

HALLOWELL, I.

1964 El papel de los sueños en la cultura Ojibwa. In *Los sueños y las sociedades humanas.* Coloquio de Royaumont. Buenos Aires: Ediciones Sudamericana.

HANSSON, ANDERS, ET AL.

1986 Preclinical and clinical studies with latex from *Ficus glabrata* (*HBK*), a traditional intestinal anthelminthic in the Amazonian area. *Journal of Ethnopharmacology* 17: 105–38.

HARNER, MICHAEL

1972 *The Jivaro.* New York: Doubleday.

1973 The sound of rushing water. In *Hallucinogens and shamanism,* edited by Michael Harner. New York: Oxford University Press.

1982 *The way of the shaman.* New York: Bantam.

1988 What is a shaman. In *Shaman's path: Healing, personal growth, and empowerment,* edited by Gary Doore. Boston: Shamabala.

HEINZE, RUTH-INGE (EDITOR)

1987 *Proceedings of the third international conference on the study of shamanism and alternate modes of healing.* Madison, Wis.: A-R Editions.

1988 *Proceedings of the fourth international conference on the study of shamanism and alternate modes of healing.* Madison, Wis.: A-R Editions.

HEMMING, JOHN

1978 *Red gold: The conquest of the Brazilian Indians.* London: Macmillan.

HENMAN, ANTHONY RICHARD

1981 *Mama coca.* Bogotá: Editorial Oveja Negra.

1986 Uso del *ayahuasca* en un contexto autoritario: El Caso de la união do vegetal en Brasil. *América Indígena* 46 (1): 219–45.

HEREDIA, L.

1978 El fenómeno onírico entre los aborígenes Toba y Mataco del Gran Chaco. *Relaciones* 12 (Nueva Serie): 35–46. Buenos Aires: Sociedad Argentina de Antropología.

HIGHWATER, JAMAKE

1982 *The primal mind: Vision and reality in Indian America.* New York: Harper and Row.

HILL, JONATHAN

1983 Wakuénai society: A processual-structural analysis of indigenous cultural life in the upper Rio Negro basin, Venezuela. Ph.D. diss., Department of Anthropology, University of Indiana, Bloomington.

1984a Agnatic sibling relations and rank in northern Arawakan myth and social life. *Working Papers on South American Indians,* no. 7, edited by J. Shapiro and K. Kensinger, 25–33. Bennington, Vt.: Bennington College.

1984b Social equality and ritual hierarchy: The Arawakan Wakuénai of Venezuela. *American Ethnologist* 11: 528–44.

1984c Los misioneros y las fronteras. *América Indígena* 44 (1): 183–90.

1985 Myth, spirit-naming, and the art of microtonal rising: Childbirth rituals of the Arawakan Wakuénai. *Latin American Music Review* 6 (1): 1–30.

1987 Representaciones musicales como estructuras adaptativas. Translated by A. Pollak-Eltz and Y. Lecuna. *Montalbán* 17: 67–101.

1989 Review of *Icanchu's Drum: An Orientation to Meaning in South American Religions,* by Lawrence E. Sullivan. *American Anthropologist* 91 (4): 1073.

In press *Keepers of the sacred chants: The poetics of ritual power in an Amazonian society.* Tucson: University of Arizona Press.

HILL, JONATHAN (EDITOR)

1988 *Rethinking history and myth: Indigenous South American perspectives on the past.* Urbana: University of Illinois Press.

HOPPÁL, MIHÁLY

1987 Shamanism: An archaic and/or recent system of beliefs. In *Shamanism,* edited by Shirley Nicholson. Wheaton, Ill.: Theosophical Publishing House.

HUGH-JONES, CHRISTINE

1979 *From the Milk River.* New York: Cambridge University Press.

HUGH-JONES, STEPHEN

1979 *The palm and the Pleiades: Initiation and cosmology in northwest Amazonia.* New York: Cambridge University Press.

HUXLEY, ALDOUS

1954 *The doors of perception.* New York: Harper and Row.

IDOYAGA MOLINA, A.

1978–79 La bruja pilagá. *Scripta Ethnológica,* no. 2, pt. 2: 95–117. Buenos Aires.

ILLIUS, BRUNO

1987 *Aini Shinan: Schamanismus bei den Shipibo-Conibo.* Tübingen, Germany: S&F.

JACKSON, JEAN

1983 *The fish people: Linguistic exogamy and Tukanoan identity in northwest Amazonia.* New York: Cambridge University Press.

JAIN, RAVINDRA (EDITOR)

1977 *Text and context: The social anthropology of tradition.* Philadelphia: ISHI Press.

JANGOUX, JAQUES

1977 Preliminary observations on shamanism, curing rituals and propitiatory ceremonies among the Asurini Indians of the middle Xingu in Brazil. Typescript.

JILEK, WOLFGANG G.

1978 Native renaissance: The survival and revival of indigenous therapeutic ceremonials among North American Indians. *Transcultural Psychiatric Research Reviews* 15: 117–45.

JOCHELSON, WALDEMAR

1905 *Religion and myths of the Koryak. Memoirs of the American Museum of Natural History,* vol. 10 (2). New York: G. E. Stechert; Leiden, E. J. Brill.

JOURNET, NICOLAS

1981 Los curripaco del río Isana: Economía y sociedad. *Revista Colombiana de Antropología* 23: 127–83.

N.d. Sur les rites Chrétiens dans une société du Vaupés Colombien. Unpublished manuscript.

KAKAR, SUDHIR

1978 *The inner world: A psychoanalytic study of childhood and society in India.* Oxford: Oxford University Press.

KAMPPINEN, MATTI

1989 *Cognitive systems and cultural models of illness: A study of two mestizo peasant communities of the Peruvian Amazon.* Helsinki: Academia Scientiarum Fennica.

KAPLAN, JOANNA OVERING

1982 The paths of sacred words: Shamanism and the domestication of the asocial in Piaroa society. Paper presented at the 44th International Congress of Americanists, September, Manchester, England.

1984 Shamanism in lowland South American societies: A problem of definition. In *Past and present in the Americas: A compendium of recent studies,* edited by John Lynch, 167–72. Manchester: Manchester University Press.

KARSTEN, RAFAEL

1932 *Indian tribes of the Argentine and Bolivian Chaco.* Commentationes Humanarum Litteratum 4 (1). Ethnological Studies. Helsingfors: Societas Fennica.

1964 *Studies in the religion of the South American Indians east of the Andes.* Edited by Arne Runenberg and Michael Webster. Commentationes Humanarum Litterarum 29 (1). Helsinki: Societas Scientiarum Fennica.

KATZ, F., AND M. DOBKIN DE RIOS

1971 Hallucinogenic music: An analysis of the role of whistling in Peruvian *ayahuasca* healing sessions. *Journal of American Folklore* 84 (333): 320–27.

KAYE, J.

1965 Two conceptions of Desana phonology. Master's thesis, Columbia University, New York.

1970 The Desana verb: Problems in semantics, syntax, and phonology. Ph.D. diss., Columbia University, New York.

KENNEDY, JOHN

1973 Cultural psychiatry. In *Handbook of social and cultural anthropology,* edited by John J. Honigman. Chicago: Rand McNally.

KENSINGER, KENNETH

1973 *Banisteriopsis* usage among the Peruvian Cashinahua. In *Hallucinogens and shamanism,* edited by Michael Harner. New York: Oxford University Press.

KIEV, ARI

1962 The psychotherapeutic aspects of primitive medicine. *Human Organization* 21: 25–29.

1968 *Curanderismo: Mexican-American folk psychiatry.* New York: Free Press.

KIEV, ARI (EDITOR)

1964 *Magic, faith, and healing.* New York: Free Press.

KLEINMAN, ARTHUR

1980 *Patients and healers in the context of culture.* Berkeley: University of California Press.

KOCH-GRÜNBERG, THEODOR

1967 *Zwei Jahre unter den Indianern: Reisen in Nordwest Brasilien, 1903–5.* Australia: Akademische Druck, U. Verlagsanstalt.

KRACKE, WAUD

1979 Dreaming in Kagwahiv: Dream beliefs and their psychic uses. *Psychoanalytic Study of Society* 8: 119–71.

KUCZINSKI GODARD, MAXIME H.

1947 El pensamiento arcaicomítico del campesino peruano: Ensayo de interpretación. *Anales de la Sociedad Peruana de Historia de la Medicina,* vol. 9 (1–44).

KUMU, UMÚSIN PANLÕN, AND TOLAMÃN KENHÍRI

1980 *Antes o mundo não existia.* São Paulo: Livraria Editora Cultura.

LA BARRE, WESTON

1947 Primitive psychotherapy in native American cultures: Peyotism and confession. *The Journal of Abnormal and Social Psychology* 42: 294–309.

1969 *The Peyote Cult.* New York: Schocken Press.

LAMB, BRUCE F.

1985 *Río Tigre and beyond: The Amazon jungle medicine of Manuel Córdoba Ríos.* Berkeley: North Atlantic.

LANGDON, E. JEAN MATTESON

1979a The Siona hallucinogenic ritual: Its meaning and power. In *Understanding religion and culture: Anthropological and theological perspectives,* edited by John H. Morgan. Washington, D.C.: University Press of America.

1979b *Yagé* among the Siona: Cultural patterns in visions. In *Spirits, shamans, and stars,* edited by David L. Browman and Ronald A. Schwarz. The Hague: Mouton.

1981 Cultural bases for trading of visions and spiritual knowledge in the Colombian and Ecuadorian Montaña. In *Networks of the past: Regional interaction in archaeology.* Proceedings of the Twelfth Annual Conference, the Archaeological Association of the University of Calgary.

1983 *Dau:* Power of the shaman in Siona religion and medicine. Paper presented at the XI International Congress of Ethnological and Anthropological Sciences, Vancouver.

1985 Power and authority in Siona political process: The rise and demise of the shaman. In *Political anthropology of Ecuador,* edited by Jeffrey Ehrenreich. Albany, New York: Society for Latin American Anthropology and the Center for the Caribbean and Latin America.

1991 Interethnic processes affecting the survival of shamans: A comparative analysis. In *Otra America en construcción: Medicinas tradicionales, religiones populares,* edited by Carlos Ernesto Pinzón and Rosa Suárez P. Bogotá: Instituto Colombiano de Antropología/COLCULTURA.

In press A cultura Siona e a experiência alucinogênica. In *Iconografia e Grafismos Indígenas,* edited by Lux Vidal. São Paulo: Editor Nobel.

LANDGON, E. JEAN MATTESON, AND ROBERT MACLENNAN

1979 Western biomedical and Sibundoy diagnosis: An interdisciplinary comparison. *Social Science and Medicine* 13B: 211–19.

LANGDON, THOMAS

1975 Food restrictions in the medical system of the Barasana and Taiwano Indians of Colombian northwest Amazon. Ph.D. diss., Tulane University, Louisiana.

LAVONDES, H.

1963 Magie et langage: Note à propos de quelques faits malgaches. *L'Homme* 3: 109–17.

LEACH, EDMUND

1976 *Culture and communication.* New York: Cambridge University Press.

LÉVI-STRAUSS, CLAUDE

1958 L'efficacité symbolique. In *Anthropologie structurale* 1, 205–26. Paris: Plon.

1962 *La pensée sauvage.* Paris: Plon.

1963 The effectiveness of symbols. In *Structural anthropology,* vol. 1, 186–205. New York: Doubleday.

1966 *The savage mind.* Chicago: University of Chicago Press.

1969 *Mythologiques I: The raw and the cooked.* New York: Harper and Row.

LEWIN, LOUIS

[1927] 1980 *Phantastica: Die betäubenden und erregenden Genussmittel: Für Ärzte und Nichtärzte.* Linden: Volksverlag.

LEWIS, IOAN

1971 *Ecstatic religion.* Middlesex, England: Penguin.

LOEWEN, J., A. BUCKWALTER, AND J. KRATZ

1965 Shamanism, illness and power in Toba church life. *Practical Anthropology* 12: 250–80.

LUCE, GAY

1971 The importance of psychic medicine: Training Navaho medicine men. In *Mental Health Program Reports* 5, edited by Julius Segal. Washington, D.C.: National Institute of Mental Health.

LUNA, LUIS EDUARDO

1984a The healing practices of a Peruvian shaman. *Journal of Ethnopharmacology* 11: 123–33.

1984b The concept of plants as teachers among four Peruvian shamans of Iquitos, northeast Peru. *Journal of Ethnopharmacology* 11: 135–56.

1986 *Vegetalismo: Shamanism among the mestizo population of the Peruvian Amazon.* Stockholm, Sweden: Almquist and Wiksell International.

1989a Análisis iconográfico del mundo subacuático en la obra del pintor y ex-curandero amazónico peruano Pablo Amaringo. *Revindi* no. 1. Budapest.

1989b *The songs the plants taught us: An anthology of* icaros*—magical songs—recorded among* ayahuasqueros *in the Peruvian Amazon.* Berkeley: Lux Natura.

1991 Plant spirits in *ayahuasca* visions by Peruvian painter Pablo Amaringo: An analysis. *Integration: Zeitschrift für Psychoaktive Pflanzen und Kulture.* no. 1: 18–30. Knetzgau, West Germany.

LUNA, LUIS, AND PABLO AMARINGO

1991 Ayahuasca *visions: The religious imagery of Pablo Amaringo.* Berkeley: North Atlantic Books.

MABIT, JACQUES MICHEL

1988 L'hallucination par l'*ayahuasca* chez les Guérisseurs de la Haute-Amazonie Péruvienne (Tarapoto). *Bulletin Institut Français d'Études Andines.* Document de Travail 1/1988.

MCKENNA, DENNIS J., L. E. LUNA, AND G. H. N. TOWERS

1986 Ingredientes biodinámicos en las plantas que se mezclan al *ayahuasca:* Una farmacopea tradicional no investigada. *América Indígena* 46 (1): 73–100.

MALINOWSKI, B.

1974 *Les jardins de corail.* Paris: Maspero.

MALLOL DE RECASENS, MARÍA ROSA

1963 Cuatro representaciones de las imágenes alucinatorias originadas por la toma del *yagé. Revista Colombiana de Folclor* 3 (8): 59–79. Bogotá.

MALLOL DE RECASENS, M. R., AND JOSÉ DE RECASENS T.

1964–65 Contribución al conocimiento del cacique-curaca entre los Siona. *Revista Colombiana de Antropología* 13: 91–145. Bogotá.

MARRETT, ROBERT T.

1900 *The threshold of religion.* London: Methuen.

MASON, J. ALDEN

1926 Use of tobacco in Mexico and South America. *Anthropology Leafelt* 16. Chicago: Field Museum of Natural History.

MATOS ARVELO, MARTIN

1912 *Vida indiana.* Barcelona: Casa Editorial Maucci.

MATTHÄI, HILDEGARD

1977 *Die Rolle der Greifvögel, insbesondere der Harpey und des Königsgeiers, bei ausserandinen Indianern Südamerikas.* Müncherner Beiträge zur Amerikanistik, vol. 1. Munich: Klaus Renner.

MAUSS, MARCEL

[1902–3] Esboço de uma teoria geral de magia. In *Sociologia e antropologia,* vol.
1974 1: 37–172. São Paulo: E. P. U./E. D. U. S. P. [Original in French.]

MELATTI, JULIO C.

1972 *O Messianismo Kraho.* São Paulo: Editora Herder, Universidade de São Paulo.

MÉTRAUX, ALFRED

1937 Études d'ethnographie Toba-Pilag'a (Gran Chaco). *Anthropos* 32: 171–94, 378–402.

1941 Religion and shamanism. In *Handbook of South American Indians* 5, 559–99. Washington: Smithsonian Institution.

1944 Le shamanisme chez les indiens de l'Amerique de Sud tropicale. *Acta Americana* 2: 197–219, 320–41. Mexico.

1948 The Guarani. In *Handbook of South American Indians, vol. 3, The tropical forest Indians,* edited by Julian Steward, 69–94. Washington, D.C., Bureau of American Ethnology, Bulletin no. 143, vol. 3.

1967 Le chamane dans les civilisations indigènes des Guyanes et de l'Amazonie. In *Religions et magies indiennes d'Amérique de Sud.* Paris: Ed. Gallimard (Bibliothèque des Sciences Humaines).

MILLER, ELMER

1966 Toba kin terms. *Ethnology* 5 (2): 194–201.

1967 Pentecostalism among Argentine Toba. Ph.D. diss., University of Pittsburgh, Pennsylvania.

1970 The Christian missionary, agent of secularization. *Anthropological Quarterly* 43 (1): 14–22.

1977 Simbolismo, conceptos de poder y cambio cultural de los Tobas del Chaco Argentino. In *Procesos de articulación social,* edited by E. Hermitte and L. Bartolomé. Buenos Aires: Amorrortu.

1979 *Los Tobas argentinos: Armonía y disonancia en una sociedad.* México: Siglo XXI Editores.

MONTEIRO DA SILVA, CLODOMIR

1983 O palácio de Juramidan. Santo Daime: Um ritual de transcendência e despoluição. Master's thesis, Universidade Federal de Pernambuco. Recife, Pernambuco.

1985 La cuestión de la realidad en la Amazonía: Un análisis a partir del estudio de la doctrina del Santo Daime. *Amazonía Peruana* 6 (11): 87–106. Lima, Centro Amazónico de Antropología y Aplicación Práctica (CAAP).

MOORE, SALLY F.

1976 Epilogue. In *Symbol and politics in communal ideology,* edited by Barbara Myerhoff, 230–38. Ithaca: Cornell University Press.

MOORE, SALLY F., AND BARBARA MYERHOFF (EDITORS)

1977 *Secular ritual.* Assen: Van Gorcum.

MOTZKI, HARALD

1977 Shamanismus als Problem religionswissenschaftlicher Terminologie. In *Arbeitsmaterialien zur Religionsgeschichte,* 2. Köln.

MUNN, NANCY

1969 The effectiveness of symbols in Murngin rite and myth. In *Forms of symbolic action,* edited by R. F. Spencer, 178–206. Seattle: University of Washington Press.

1973 Symbolism in a ritual context: Aspects of symbolic action. In *Handbook of social and cultural anthropology,* edited by John J. Honigmann, 579–612. Chicago: Rand McNally.

MURPHY, JANE M.

1964 Psychotherapeutic aspects of shamanism on St. Lawrence Island, Alaska. In *Magic, faith, and healing,* edited by Ari Kiev. New York: Free Press.

MYERHOFF, BARBARA G.

1974 *Peyote hunt: The sacred journey of the Huichol Indians.* Ithaca: Cornell University Press.

1975 Peyote and Huichol worldview: The structure of a mystic vision. In *Cannabis and culture,* edited by Vera Rubin. The Hague: Mouton.

NADEL, S. F.

1946 Study of shamanism in the Nuba Mountains. *Journal of the Royal Anthropological Institute* 76: 25–37.

NIMEUNDAJÚ, CURT

1914 Die Sagen von der Erschaffung und Vernichtung der Welt als Grundlagen der Religion der Apapocuya-Guarani. *Zeitschrift für Ethnologie* 2/3: 284–403. Berlin.

1919–20 Bruchstücke aus Religion und Ueberlieferung der Sipáia-Indianer. *Anthropos* 14–15: 1002–39.

1921–22 Bruchstücke aus Religion und Ueberlieferung der Sipáia-Indianer. *Anthropos* 16–17: 367–406.

1952 *The Tukuna,* edited by Robert H. Lowie. Berkeley: Univ. of California, Publications in American Archaeology and Ethnology, vol. 45.

NOLL, RICHARD

1983 Shamanism and schizophrenia: A state-specific approach to the schizophrenia metaphor of shamanic states. *American Ethnologist* 10 (3): 443–59.

OHLMARKS, ÅKE

1939 *Studien zum Problem des Schamanismus.* Kopenhagen: Lund.

OLIVEIRA, ADELIA E., AND EDUARDO GALVÃO

1973 A situação atual dos Baniwa (Alto Rio Negro) 1971. In *O Museu Goeldi no Ano do Sesquicentenário.* Publicações Avulsas 20: 27–40. Belém, Pará, Brazil.

OLSEN, DALE A.
1975 Music-induced altered states of consciousness among Warao shamans. *Journal of Latin American Lore* 1 (1): 19–33.

ORTNER, SHERRY
1973 On key symbols. *American Anthropologist* 75: 1338–46.

OSSIO A., JUAN M.
1973 *Ideología mesiánica del mundo Andino.* Lima: Ignacio Prado.
1977 Myth and history: The seventeenth century chronicle of Guaman Poma de Ayala. In *Text and context: The social anthropology of tradition,* edited by Ravindra Jain, 51–94. Philadelphia: ISHI.

OTTO, R.
1925 *Lo santo.* Madrid: Revista de Occidente.

PAGÉS LARRAYA, F.
1982 *Lo irracional en la cultura.* Buenos Aires: FECIC, vol. 3.

PADILLA, ALFONSO
1984 The *icaros* of Don Emilio Andrade Gómez: Appendix to the concept of plants as teachers among four Peruvian shamans of Iquitos, northeast Peru. *Journal of Ethnopharmacology* 11 (2): 147–56.

PALAVECINO, ENRIQUE
1979 The magic world of the Mataco. Trans. and ed. by J. A. Vásquez. *Latin American Indian Literatures* 3 (2): 61–75. Pittsburgh.

PARK, MARINELLI, NANCY WEBER, AND VICTOR CENEPO SANGAMA
1976 *Diccionario quechua: San Martín.* Lima: Ministerio de Educación.

PEASE, HELEN
1968 Parintintin grammar. Report for the Summer Institute of Linguistics Technical Studies Department. Brasília: Instituto Lingüístico do Verão. Typescript.

PENTIKÄINEN, JUHA
1979 The symbolism of liminality. In *Religious symbols and their functions* 10, edited by Biezais Haralds, 154–66. Scripta Instituti Donneriani Aboensis. Uppsala.

PERE, M., D. PERE, AND P. ROUGE
1981 Isolation and studies of the psychochemical and biological properties of lectins from *Hura crepitans. Planta Medica* 41: 344–50.

PERRIN, MICHEL
1976 *Le chemin des Indiens morts.* (Bibliothèque Scientifique.) Paris: Payot 2d ed. 1983.

1979 Théories et pratiques médicales guajiro. *Actes du XLIIe Congès International des Américanistes* 6: 387–405.

1980 Un succès bien relatif: la médecine occidentale chez les Indiens Guajiro. *Social Science and Medicine* 14B: 279–87.

1982a *Antropólogos y médicos frente al arte Guajiro de curar.* Caracas/Maracaibo: Corpozulia/U. C. A. B.

1982b Pointe de vue anthropologique sur les drogues toxicomanogènes. In *Droque et civilisation: Refus social ou acceptation,* 127–38. Paris: Pergamon.

1985 Les fondements d'une catégorie étiologique (la notion de contamination chez les Guajiro). *L'Ethnographie* 81: 103–22.

1986a Une interprétation morphogénétique de l'initation chamanique. *L'Homme* 26/1–2: 107–23.

1986b *La pensée mythique en actes. Mythes et rêves, rituels et chamanisme: L'exemple des Indiens guajiro du Venezuela et de Colombie.* Thèse de Doctorat d'Etat, Université Paris V, Paris, 3 vols.

1986c *The way of the dead Indians,* Austin: University of Texas Press.

1987 Creaciones míticas y representación del mundo: El ganado en el pensamiento simbólico guajiro. *Antropológica* 67: 3–31. Caracas.

1988 Du mythe au quotidien, penser la nouveauté. *L'Homme* Numéro Spécial: "Le mythe et ses métamorphoses," 28 (106–7): 120–37.

1992 *Les praticiens du rêve: Un exemple de chamanisme.* Paris, PUF.

PETERS, LARRY G.

1982 Trance, initiation and psychotherapy in Tamang shamanism. *American Ethnologist* 9: 21–46.

PETERS, LARRY G. AND DOUGLASS PRICE-WILLIAMS

1980 Toward an experiential analysis of shamanism. *American Ethnologist* 7: 397–418.

PFISTER, OSKAR

1932 Instructive psychoanalysis among the Navajos. *Journal of Nervous and Mental Diseases* 76: 251.

PINKLEY, HOMER, AND J. LINDGREN

1972 Plant admixtures to *ayahuasca,* the South American hallucinogenic drink: Ethnobotanical and chemical investigations. *Economic Botany* 29: 101–29.

PINZÓN, CARLOS, AND ROSA SUAREZ

1979 Locos y embrujados. In *Actas del primer congreso mundial de medicina tradicional.* Lima: Universidad de San Marcos.

1983 La dialéctica de la medicina popular. In *Análisis del primer seminario de medicina tradicional,* vol. 1. Mexico City: Morelos.

POLARI DE ALVERGA, ALEX
1984 *O livro das mirações: Viagem ao Santo Daime.* Rio de Janeiro: Editora Rocco.

POLLOCK, DONALD
1985 Food and sexual identity among the Culina. *Food and Foodways* 1: 25–42.
1988 Indigenous health care among the Culina, western Brazil. *Cultural Survival Quarterly* 12 (1): 28–32.

PRESS, IRWIN
1969 Physicians, curers and dual use in Bogotá. *Journal of Health and Social Behavior* 10: 209–18.
1971 The urban curandero. *American Anthropologist* 73: 741–56.

PRICE, RICHARD
1983 *First-time: The historical vision of an Afro-American people.* Baltimore: Johns Hopkins University Press.

PRICE-WILLIAMS, DOUGLASS
1977 The waking dream in ethnographic perspective. In *Dreaming: Anthropological and psychological interpretations,* edited by Barbara Tedlock. New York: Cambridge University Press.

PRIMOV, GEORGE
N.d. A descriptive outline of the post-Columbian history of the territorio federal Amazonas until 1970. Unpublished manuscript.

PRINCE, RAYMOND (EDITOR)
1982 Issue on shamans and endorphins. *Ethos* 10 (4): 299–423.

RAMÍREZ DE JARA, MARÍA CLEMENCIA, AND CARLOS ERNESTO PINZÓN
1986 Los hijos del bejuco solar y la campana celeste. El *yagé* en la cultura popular urbana. *América Indígena* 46 (1): 163–88.

RAPPAPORT, JOANNE
1980 Mesianismo y las transformaciones de símbolos mesiánicos en Tierradentro. *Revista Colombiana de Antropología* 23: 367–413.
1985 History, myth, and the dynamics of territorial maintenance in Tierradientro, Colombia. *American Ethnologist* 12: 27–45.

RAPPAPORT, ROY
1979 *Ecology, meaning, and religion.* Richmond, Calif.: North Atlantic.

RASMUSSEN, KNUD

1929 *Intellectual culture of the Hudson Bay Eskimos.* Translated by W. E. Calvert. Report of the 5th Thule Expedition 1921–24. Vol. 7, no. 1. Copenhagen: Gyldendal.

REÁTEGUI, ULISES

1983 *Cushushca yushin: Bufeo colorado.* Chiclayo, Peru: Talleres de Editorial Offset "Kemoy" S. C. R. L.

REGAN, JAIME

1983 *Hacia la tierra sin mal. Estudio de la religión del pueblo en la Amazonía.* 2 vols. Iquitos, Perú: Ceta.

REICHEL-DOLMATOFF, GERARDO

1971 *Amazonian cosmos.* Chicago: University of Chicago Press.

1972 The cultural context of an aboriginal hallucinogen: *Banisteriopsis caapi.* In *Flesh of the Gods: The ritual use of hallucinogens,* edited by Peter Furst. New York: Praeger.

1975 *The shaman and the jaguar: A study of narcotic drugs among the Indians of Colombia.* Philadelphia: Temple University Press.

1976 Desana curing spells: An analysis of some shamanic metaphors. *Journal of Latin American Lore* 2 (2): 159–219.

1978 *Beyond the Milky Way: Hallucinatory imagery of the Tukano Indians.* Los Angeles: UCLA Latin American Center Publications.

REYBURN, W.

1954 *The Toba Indians of the Argentine Chaco: An interpretative report.* Elkhart, Ind.: Menonnite Board of Missions and Charities.

RIVIÈRE, PETER

1970 Factions and exclusions in two South American village systems. In *Witchcraft confessions and accusations,* edited by Mary Douglas. London: Tavistock.

RIVIER, LAURENT, AND JAN-ERIK LINDGREN

1972 *"Ayahuasca,"* The South American hallucinogenic drink: An ethnobotanical and chemical investigation. *Economic Botany* 26: 101–29.

RODRIGUES FERREIRA, ALEXANDRE

1885 Diário de viagem philosófica pela Capitania de São José do Rio Negro. *Revista do Instituto Histórico e Geográfico Brasileiro* 48 (1): 1–234.

ROE, PETER G.

1982 *The cosmic zygote. Cosmology in the Amazon basin.* New Brunswick, N.J.: Rutgers University Press.

ROMOLI DE AVERY, KATHLEEN

1978 Las tribus de la antigua jurisdicción de Pasto en el siglo XVI. *Revista Colombiana de Antropología* 21: 11–55.

ROSALDO, RENATO

1980 *Ilongot headhunting: 1883–1974: A study in society and history.* Stanford: Stanford University Press.

ROUGET, GILBERT

1980 *La musique et la transe: Esquisse d'une théorie générale des relations de la musique et de la possession.* Paris: Editions Gallimard.

RÜF, ISABELLE

1972 Le 'dutsee tui' chez les indiens Culina de Perou. *Bulletin de la Société Suisse de Americanistes* 36: 73–80.

SAHLINS, MARSHALL

1981 *Historical metaphors and mythical realities.* Ann Arbor: University of Michigan Press.

SAKATA, K., AND K. KAWASU

1971 Studies on a piscidal constituent of *Hura crepitans* D. Part 1, isolation and characterization of *Hura* toxin and its piscicidal activity. *Agricultural and Biological Chemistry* 35: 1084–91.

SAN ROMÁN, JESÚS

1975 *Perfiles históricos de la amazonía peruana.* Lima: Ediciones Paulinas.

SARGANT, WILLIAM

1973 *The mind possessed.* London: William Heinemann Ltd.

SCAZZOCCHIO, FRANÇOISE

1979 Ethnicity and boundary maintenance among Peruvian forest Quechua. Ph.D. diss., University of Cambridge.

SCHMIDT, FATHER WILHELM

1931 *The origin and growth of religion: Facts and theories.* New York: Lincoln, MacVeagh.

SCHULTES, RICHARD EVANS

1957 The identity of the Malpighiaceous narcotics of South America. *Harvard Botanical Museum Leaflets* 18: 1–56.

1972 An overview of hallucinogens in the western hemisphere. In *Flesh of the gods,* edited by Peter T. Furst. London: George Allen and Unwin.

1982 The beta-carboline hallucinogens of South America. *Journal of Psychoactive Drugs.* 14 (3): 205–20.

1986 El desarrollo histórico de la identificación de las malpigiáceas empleadas como alucinógenos. *América Indígena* 46 (1): 9–48.

SCHULTES, RICHARD EVANS, AND ALBERT HOFMANN

1980 *The botany and chemistry of hallucinogens.* Springfield, Ill.: Charles C. Thomas.

SCHUSTER, MEINHARD

1976 *Dekuana.* Munich: Klaus Reiner.

SCHWEDER, RICHARD A.

1979 Aspect of cognition in Zinacanteco shamans: Experimental results. In *Reader in comparative religion,* 4th ed., edited by William A. Lessa and Evon Z. Vogt. New York: Harper and Row.

SEEGER, ANTHONY

1986 Oratory is spoken, myth is told, and song is sung, but they are all music to my ears. In *Native South American Discourse,* edited by Joel Sherzer and Greg Urban, 59–82. Amsterdam: Mouton de Gruyter.

SEGUÍN, CARLOS ALBERTO

1979 *Psiquiatría folklórica: Shamanes y curanderos.* Lima: Ediciones Sermar.

SEIJAS, HAYDÉE

1969a Medical system of the Sibundoy Indians. Ph.D. diss., Tulane University, New Orleans, La.

1969b Algunos aspectos de la etnomedicina de los indios Sibundoy de Colombia. *Boletin Informativo* 6: 5–16. Caracas, Venezuela: Instituto Venezuelano de Investigaciones Científicas (IVIC).

1969c El susto como categoría etiológica. Paper presented at the 68th Annual Meeting of the American Anthropological Association, November, New Orleans, La.

1970 El crecimiento de población de los indios Sibundoy de Colombia. Paper presented at the XXXIX International Congress of Americanists, Lima, Peru.

SEITZ, GEORGE J.

1979 Epena, the intoxicating snuff powder of the Waika Indians and the Tucano medicine man, Agostino. In *Ethnopharmacologic search for psychoactive drugs,* edited by Daniel H. Efron, Bo Holsteadt, and Nathan S. Kline. New York: Raven.

SHARON, DOUGLAS

1978 *Wizard of the four winds: A shaman's story.* New York: Free Press.

SHERZER, JOEL

1983 *Kuna ways of speaking.* Austin: University of Texas Press.

SHERZER, JOEL, AND GREG URBAN (EDITORS)

1986 *Native South American discourse.* Amsterdam: Mouton de Gruyter.

SHIROKOGOROFF, SERGEI M.

1923 General theory of shamanism among the Tungus. *Journal of the Royal Asiatic Society, North China Branch* 62: 123–83. Shanghai.

[1935] 1980 *Psychomental complex of the Tungus.* London: Kegan Paul. (Reprinted, New York: AMS.)

SILVERMAN, J.

1967 Shamans and acute schizophrenia. *American Anthropologist* 69: 21–31.

SISKIND, JANET

1973a Visions and cures among the Sharanahua. In *Hallucinogens and shamanism,* edited by M. Harner. New York: Oxford University Press.

1973b *To hunt in the morning.* New York: Oxford University Press.

SKORUPSKY, J.

1976 *Symbol and theory: A philosophical study of theories of religion in social anthropology.* Cambridge: Cambridge University Press.

SOUKUP, J.

1970 *Vocabulario de los nombres vulgares de la flora peruana.* Lima: Colegio Salesiano.

SPENCER, B., AND F. J. GILLEN

1927 *The Arunta: A study of a stone age people.* London: Macmillan.

SPRUCE, RICHARD

1970 *Notes of a botanist on the Amazon and Andes.* Vol. 1. New York: Johnson Reprint Corporation.

STEINEN, KARL VON DEN

1904 *Diccionario Sipibo.* Berlin: Dietrich Reimer.

STEWARD, JULIAN, AND LOUIS C. FARON

1959 *Native peoples of South America.* New York: McGraw Hill.

STOCKS, ANTHONY

1979 Tendiendo un puente entre el cielo y la tierra en alas de la canción. *Amazonía Peruana* 2 (4): 71–100.

STOLLER, PAUL

1984 Sound in Songhay cultural experience. *American Ethnologist* 11 (3): 559–70.

SULLIVAN, LAWRENCE

1988 *Icanchu's drum: An orientation to meaning in South American religions.* New York: Macmillan.

SWANN, BRIAN (EDITOR)

1983 *Smoothing the ground: Essays on native American oral literature.* Berkeley, Calif.: University of California Press.

SWEET, DAVID

1974 A rich realm of nature destroyed: The middle Amazon Valley 1640–1750. Ph.D. diss., University of Wisconsin, Madison.

TAMBIAH, J.

1968 The magical power of words. *Man* 3: 175–208.

1973 Form and meaning of magical acts: A point of view. In *Modes of thought: Essays in thinking in Western and non-Western societies,* edited by R. Horton and R. Finnegan, 199–229. London: Faber and Faber.

TART, CHARLES T. (EDITOR)

1969 *Altered states of consciousness.* New York: Wiley.

1977 Putting the pieces together. In *Alternate states of consciousness,* edited by N. E. Zinberg. New York: Free Press.

TAUSSIG, MICHAEL

1980a Folk healing and the structure of conquest in southwest Colombia. *Journal of Latin American Lore* 6 (2): 217–78.

1980b *The devil and commodity fetishism in South America.* Chapel Hill: University of North Carolina Press.

1984 Culture of terror—space of death: Roger Casement's Putumayo report and the explanation of torture. *Comparative Studies in Society and History* 26 (3): 467–97.

1987 *Shamanism, colonialism, and the wild man: A study in terror and healing.* Chicago: University of Chicago Press.

TAVERA ACOSTA, B.

1927 *Rio Negro: Reseña etnográfica, histórica y geográfíca.* Maracay, Venezuela: Estado Araguá.

TEDLOCK, BARBARA

1981 Quiché Maya dream interpretation. *Ethos* 9 (4): 313–50.

1987 Dreaming and dream research. In *Dreaming: Anthropological and psychological interpretations,* 1–31. New York: Cambridge University Press.

TEDLOCK, BARBARA (EDITOR)

1987 *Dreaming: Anthropological and psychological interpretations.* New York: Cambridge University Press.

TESSMAN, GÜNTER

1930 *Die Indianer Nordost-Perus: Grundlegende Forschungen für eine Systematische Kulturkunde.* Hamburg: Friederichsen, de Gruyter.

TOMASINI, A.

1974 El concepto de *payák* entre los Toba de Occidente. *Scripta Ethnológica* 2 (1). Buenos Aires.

1976 *Dapitchí:* Un alto dios uránico de los Toba de Occidente. *Scripta Ethnológica* 4 (1): 69–87. Buenos Aires.

TOMASINA, A., AND J. BRAUNSTEIN

1975 Los Toba (familia linguística Guaycurú) de Misión Tacaagle. *Scripta Ethnológica* 3 (2). Buenos Aires.

TORREY, E. F.

1972 What Western psychotherapists can learn from witch doctors. *American Journal of Orthopsychiatry* 42 (1): 69–76.

TOVAR, ENRIQUE D.

1966 *Vocabulario del oriente peruano.* Lima: Universidad Nacional Mayor de San Marcos.

TOWNSEND, PATRICIA, AND P. ADAMS

1978 Estructura y conflicto en el matrimonio de los indios Culina de la amazonía peruana. Unpublished.

TURNER, TERENCE

1977 Transformation, hierarchy, and transcendence: A reformulation of van Gennep's model of the structure of rites de passage. In *Secular Ritual,* edited by Sally Moore and Barbara Myerhoff, 53–69. Assen: Van Gorcum.

1985 Animal symbolism, totemism, and the structure of myth. In *Animal myths and metaphors in South America,* edited by Gary Urton, 49–106. Salt Lake City: University of Utah Press.

TURNER, VICTOR

1966 *The ritual process.* Chicago: Aldine.

1967a A Ndembu doctor in practice. In *A forest of symbols.* Ithaca: Cornell University Press.

1967b *The forest of symbols.* Ithaca: Cornell University Press.

1974 *Dramas, fields, and metaphors.* Ithaca: Cornell University Press.

1977 Process, system, and symbol: A new anthropological synthesis. *Daedalus* 106: 61–79.

TYLOR, EDMUND
1871 *Primitive culture.* London: John Murray.

ULLMAN, M.
1960 The social roots of the dream. *American Journal of Psychoanalysis* 20 (2): 180–96.

ULMER, GREGORY
1983 The object of post-criticism. In *The anti-aesthetic: Essays on postmodern culture,* edited by Hal Foster, 83–110. Port Townsend, Washington: Bay Press.

URBAN, GREG
1985 Ergativity and accusativity in Shokleng. *International Journal of American Linguistics* 52 (2): 164–87.

USCATEGUI M. NÉSTOR
1959 The present distribution of narcotics and stimulants amongst the Indian tribes of Colombia. *Harvard Botanical Museum Leaflets,* 18: 273–304.

VAJDA, LASZLO
1959 Zur Phaseologischen Stellung des Schamanismus. *Ural-Altaische Jahrbücher, Gedenkband Julius V. Farkas* 31: 456–85.

VALDIZÁN, HERMILIO, AND ANGEL MALDONADO
1922 *La medicina popular peruana.* Vol. 1. Lima: Hospital Larco Herrera.

VENKATACHALAM, S. R., AND N. B. MULCHANDANI
1982 Isolation of phenanthroindolizidine alkaloid from *Ficus hispida. Naturwissenschaften* 69: 287–88.

VIERTLER, RENATE BRIGITTE
1981 Implicações de alguns conceitos ultilizados no estudo da religião e da magia de tribos Brasileiras. In *Contribuições à antropologia em homenagem ao professor Egon Schaden.* Coleção Museu Paulista, Série Ensaios, vol. 4, edited by Tekla Hartman e Vera Penteado Coelho. São Paulo: Universidade de São Paulo, Fundo de Pesquisas do Museu Paulista.

VIVEIROS DE CASTRO, EDUARDO
1978 *Relatório de trabalho de campo.* Brasília: Fundação Nacional do Indio.
1986 *Araweté: Os deuses canibais.* Rio de Janeiro: Jorge Zahar Editor/ANPOCS.

VUOTO, L.
1981 La fauna entre los Toba *Takšek. Entregas del Instituto Tilcara* 10: 77–138. Buenos Aires: Universidad de Buenos Aires.

VUOTO, P.

1981 Plantas útiles entre los Toba *Takšek*. *Entregas del Instituto Tilcara* 10: 1–76. Buenos Aires: Universidad de Buenos Aires.

WACHTEL, NATHAN

1977 *The vision of the vanquished*. Boston: Barnes and Noble.

WAGLEY, CHARLES

1943 Tapirapé shamanism. *Boletim do Museu Nacional Antropologia* no. 3. Rio de Janeiro: Museu Nacional.

1968 *Amazon town: A study of man in the tropics*. New York: Knopf.

1977 *Welcome of tears: The Tapirapé Indians of central Brazil*. New York: Oxford.

WAGNER, ROY

1972 *Habu: The innovation of meaning in Daribi religion*. Chicago: University of Chicago Press.

WALLACE, ALFRED R.

1890 *A narrative of travels on the Amazon and Rio Negro*. 3d ed. New York: Ward, Lock.

WALLACE, ANTHONY F. C.

1958 Dreams and wishes of the soul: A type of psychoanalytic theory among the seventeenth-century Iroquois. *American Anthropologist* 60: 252–58.

1966 *Religion: An anthropological view*. New York: Random House.

WASSEN, H., AND BO HOLMSTEDT

1963 The use of *paricá*, an ethnological and pharmacological review. *Ethnos* 1: 175–208. Lund, Sweden.

WASSON, R. G., F. COWAN, AND W. RHODES

1974 *María Sabina and her Mazatec mushroom velada*. New York: Harcourt Brace Jovanovich.

WEISS, GERALD

1973 Shamanism and priesthood in light of the Campa *ayahuasca* ceremony. In *Hallucinogens and shamanism*, edited by Michael Harner. New York: Oxford University Press.

1975 *Campa cosmology: The world of a forest tribe in South America*, 217–88. Anthropological papers of the American Museum of Natural History, vol. 52, pt. 5. New York.

WHITING, BEATRICE

1950 *Paiute sorcery*. New York: Viking Publications in Anthropology no. 15.

WHITTEN, NORMAN E., JR.

1978 Ecological imagery and cultural adaptability: The Canelos Quichua of eastern Ecuador. *American Anthrpologist* 80: 836–59.

1981 Amazonia today at the base of the Andes: An ethnic interface in ecological, social, and ideological perspectives. In *Cultural transformations and ethnicity in modern Ecuador,* edited by N. Whitten. Urbana: University of Illinois Press.

WILBERT, JOHANNES

1979 Magico-religious use of tobacco among South American Indians. In *Spirits, shamans, and stars: Perspectives from South America,* edited by David L. Browman and Ronald A. Schwartz. The Hague: Mouton.

1985 The house of the swallow-tailed kite: Warao myth and the art of thinking in images. In *Animal myths and metaphors in South America,* edited by Gary Urton. Salt Lake City: University of Utah Press.

1987 *Tobacco and shamanism in South America.* New Haven: Yale University Press.

WINKELMAN, MICHAEL

1986 Trance states: A theoretical model and cross-cultural analysis. *Ethos* 14 (2): 174–203.

WOLF, ERIC

1982 *Europe and the people without history.* Berkeley: University of California Press.

WRIGHT, PABLO

1981a Apuntes para la comprensión de la música en una comunidad Toba. Buenos Aires. Unpublished.

1981b Análisis hermenéutico de los sueños de una comunidad Toba *takšek* de la provincia de Formosa. Unpublished thesis for licenciatura. Buenos Aires, Universidad de Buenos Aires, Facultad de Filosofía y Letras.

1983a Presencia protestante entre aborígenes del Chaco Argentino. *Scripta Ethnología* 7: 73–84. Buenos Aires.

1983b Nombre aborigen e identificación étnica: una propuesta para su revalorización. Paper presented at the Congreso Argentino de Antropología Social, Posadas, Misiones.

1984a Análisis semántico preliminar de algunas ideas básicas en la morfología nominal y verbal Toba. Paper presented at the Tercero Congreso Argentino de Linguística, Morón, Buenos Aires.

1984b Quelques formes du chamanisme Toba. *Bulletin de la Société Suisse des Américanistes* 48: 29–35. Geneva.

1989 Collected Toba myths. In *Folk literature of the Toba Indians,* vol. 2, edited by J. Wilbert and Karin Simoneau. Los Angeles: University of Los Angeles Press.

WRIGHT, ROBIN

1981 The history and religion of the Baniwa peoples of the upper Rio Negro Valley. Ph.D. diss., Stanford University, California.

1983 Lucha y supervivencia en el noroeste de la Amazonia. *América Indígena* 43 (3): 537–54.

WRIGHT, ROBIN, AND JONATHAN HILL

1986 History, ritual, and myth: Nineteenth-century millenarian movements in the northwest Amazon. *Ethnohistory* 33 (1): 31–54.

WRIGHT, ROBIN, AND SALLY SWENSON (EDITORS)

1982 *The New Tribes mission in Amazonia.* ARC Bulletin 9. Boston: Anthropology Resource Center.

ZAMBRANO, MARTHA

1985 La población indígena de Colombia. Bogotá, Secretaría Ejecutiva Segunda Expedición Botánica.

ZOLLA, ELEMIRE

1983 A vindication of Carlos Castaneda. *Labrys* 8: 106. London.

C O N T R I B U T O R S

GERHARD BAER
Museum für Völkerkunde, Basel

DOMINIQUE BUCHILLET
ORSTOM, Institut Français de Recherche Scientifique pour le Dévelopement en Coopération

JONATHAN D. HILL
Southern Illinois University, Carbondale

BRUNO ILLIUS
Institut für Völkerkunde, Albert-Ludwigs-Universität, Freiburg

WAUD H. KRACKE
University of Illinois, Chicago Circle

E. JEAN MATTESON LANGDON
Universidade Federal de Santa Catarina, Florianópolis

LUIS EDUARDO LUNA
Swedish School of Economics, Helsinki

MICHEL PERRIN
Centre National de la Recherche Scientifique, Paris

DONALD POLLOCK
State University of New York, Buffalo

MARÍA CLEMENCIA RAMÍREZ DE JARA
CARLOS ERNESTO PINZÓN CASTAÑO
Instituto Colombiano de Antropología, Bogotá

PABLO G. WRIGHT
Consejo Nacional de Investigaciones Científicas y Técnicas, Centro Argentino de Etnología Americana, Buenos Aires

ROBIN M. WRIGHT
Universidade Estadual de São Paulo, Campinas

INDEX